MW00987115

Praise for *A Practical Guide to Fo*

"The interface of nursing, healthcare, and the law confronts nurses in all domains of practice. Angela Amar and Kathy Seukula's new book, A Practical Guide to Forensic Nursing, *represents a milestone to help guide nurses in their care of victims and their families. The authors have presented excerpts from actual situations of the many people involved in a crime, and the reader of these cases will quickly develop an understanding of the practice of forensic nursing. This is an important book that sheds light on difficult and stressful phenomenons of our times."*

–Ann Wolbert Burgess, DNSc, APRN, FAAN
Professor of Psychiatric Nursing, Connell School of Nursing, Boston College

"Amar and Sekula formalize the notion that all RNs practice forensic nursing. Then they lay a persuasive foundation of theories, forensic science concepts, existing evidence base, and practice exemplars of the common presentation when RN patient care intersects with legal systems. I highly recommend the book to academicians and RNs alike."

–Patricia M. Speck, DNSc, APRN, FNP-BC, DF-IAFN, FAAFS, FAAN
Professor and Program Director for Global Outreach
Department of Family, Community & Health Systems
The University of Alabama at Birmingham School of Nursing

"Amar and Sekula are to be praised for A Practical Guide to Forensic Nursing, *the latest forensic nursing textbook entrant. A must-have for students, practitioners, and associates, it is particularly strong in the areas of crime perpetration, victimization, and traumatization and how to approach the patient. A focus on principles keeps this book readable, and the tender care of the authoring nurses seeps through the pages. Case studies provide a basis for discussion in class."*

–Victor W. Weedn, MD, JD
Professor and Chair
George Washington University
Department of Forensic Sciences

A PRACTICAL GUIDE TO
FORENSIC NURSING

INCORPORATING FORENSIC PRINCIPLES INTO NURSING PRACTICE

Angela F. Amar, PhD, RN, FAAN | L. Kathleen Sekula, PhD, PMHCNS, FAAN

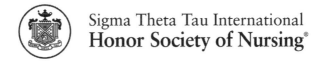
Sigma Theta Tau International
Honor Society of Nursing®

The Honor Society of Nursing, Sigma Theta Tau International (STTI) is a nonprofit organization whose mission is to support the learning, knowledge, and professional development of nurses committed to making a difference in health worldwide. Founded in 1922, STTI has more than 135,000 active members in 85 countries. Members include practicing nurses, instructors, researchers, policymakers, entrepreneurs, and others. STTI's 500 chapters are located at 699 institutions of higher learning throughout Armenia, Australia, Botswana, Brazil, Canada, Colombia, England, Ghana, Hong Kong, Japan, Kenya, Lebanon, Malawi, Mexico, the Netherlands, Pakistan, Portugal, Singapore, South Africa, South Korea, Swaziland, Sweden, Taiwan, Tanzania, Thailand, the United Kingdom, and the United States of America. More information about STTI can be found online at www.nursingsociety.org.

Sigma Theta Tau International
550 West North Street
Indianapolis, IN, USA 46202

To order additional books, buy in bulk, or order for corporate use, contact Nursing Knowledge International at 888. NKI.4YOU (888.654.4968/US and Canada) or +1.317.634.8171 (outside US and Canada).

To request a review copy for course adoption, email solutions@nursingknowledge.org or call 888.NKI.4YOU (888.654.4968/US and Canada) or +1.317.634.8171 (outside US and Canada).

To request author information, or for speaker or other media requests, contact Marketing, Honor Society of Nursing, Sigma Theta Tau International at 888.634.7575 (US and Canada) or +1.317.634.8171 (outside US and Canada).

ISBN: 9781940446349
EPUB ISBN: 9781940446356
PDF ISBN: 9781940446363
MOBI ISBN: 9781940446370

Library of Congress Cataloging-in-Publication data

A practical guide to forensic nursing : incorporating forensic principles into nursing practice / [edited by] Angela Amar, L. Kathleen Sekula.
    p. ; cm.
  Includes bibliographical references.
  ISBN 978-1-940446-34-9 (print : alk. paper) -- ISBN 978-1-940446-35-6 (epub) -- ISBN 978-1-940446-36-3 (pdf) -- ISBN 978-1-940446-37-0 (mobi)
  I. Amar, Angela, 1960- , editor. II. Sekula, L. Kathleen, 1943- , editor. III. Sigma Theta Tau International, issuing body.
  [DNLM: 1. Forensic Nursing. WY 170]
  RA1053
  614'.1--dc23
                           2015033597

First Printing, 2015

Publisher: Dustin Sullivan

Acquisitions Editor: Emily Hatch

Editorial Coordinator: Paula Jeffers

Cover Designer: Rebecca Batchelor

Interior Design/Page Layout: Rebecca Batchelor

Principal Book Editor: Carla Hall

Development and Project Editor: Rebecca Senninger

Copy Editor: Erin Geile

Proofreader: Todd Lothery

Indexer: Larry Sweazy

DEDICATION

We begin and end this journey with a tremendous amount of gratitude. What began as a vision shared through numerous discussions has now become a reality. We have long believed that *every nurse is a forensic nurse,* in that every nurse encounters patients with forensic issues at some and often multiple points in his or her practice. This book enables us to share our vision while providing information that can enhance and transform nursing practice. We dedicate this book to victims of violence throughout the world and hope that in some way this book will impact caregivers in such a way that care of victims across the continuum will improve as nurses become more and more knowledgeable about ways they can make a difference in victims' lives. We also acknowledge the complexity of issues related to perpetrators of violence, many of whom were also victims at a time in their lives. We look to a time when the healthcare system is fully prepared to provide optimal care for all forensic patients.

ACKNOWLEDGMENTS

I want to acknowledge my husband, Conway, for his continued support throughout my career. I also greatly appreciate my children, mother, sister and her family, and brothers and their families. I think that they built the wings that keep me afloat. I also thank my many coworkers and colleagues for the support offered while I worked on this book.

–Angela Amar

I thank my family for patience and understanding, especially my husband, Ray, as I took time away from "life" to work on this book, which I consider very important in improving care of the forensic patient. The encouragement I received from many in my life—family, friends, and close colleagues—was invaluable.

–Kathleen Sekula

We offer our sincere thanks to the authors with whom we worked for their wisdom and insight regarding forensic nursing practice. They shared their years of experience and knowledge at a level that all practicing nurses can understand and grasp. We hope that the readers of this book benefit and learn from reading it, as we did while working on it. We are also excited about the changes that will be seen in practice that can potentially affect the lives of myriad patients who are seeking healthcare and experiencing forensic issues.

Finally, we would be remiss if we didn't thank the editorial team that helped us through this process. Emily Hatch, our acquisitions editor, believed in us and provided encouragement and guidance throughout the process. Carla Hall, our principal book editor, and Rebecca Senninger, our project editor, were instrumental in crafting the final product. What they do to make each and every chapter special is a result of their vast expertise and editing abilities. Their patience and support was amazing. We learned so much from each of them as we worked through the creation of this book.

To each of you and to the entire behind-the-scenes folks at Sigma Theta Tau International, we extend heartfelt appreciation.

About the Authors

Angela F. Amar, PhD, RN, FAAN, is an associate professor and assistant dean for BSN education in the Nell Hodgson Woodruff School of Nursing at Emory University. She conducts research on dating violence, mental health responses to trauma, and strategies to increase help-seeking behavior. Her research consistently focuses on African-American women. She has conducted funded research, published more than 45 articles and book chapters on dating violence and sexual assault, and is active in university service related to violence and diversity. Amar is a fellow in the American Academy of Nursing, member of the Expert Panel on Psychiatric and Substance Abuse Care, and co-chair of its Expert Panel on Violence. Amar also serves on the Institute of Medicine Committee on the Biological and Psychosocial Effects of Peer Victimization: Lessons for Bullying Prevention. She is a distinguished fellow with the International Association of Forensic Nurses and received the 2015 Excellence in Practice and Policy award from the Nursing Network on Violence Against Women International. Amar is on the National Advisory Committee for the Robert Wood Johnson Future of Nursing Scholars program, a public voices fellow with the Op-Ed project, and an associate editor for the *Journal of Forensic Nursing*. Amar is certified as a clinical nurse specialist in advanced practice adult psychiatric and mental health and as an advanced forensic nurse. In her faculty role at Boston College, she developed a graduate program in forensic nursing and secured funding from the Health Resources and Services Administration for the program.

L. Kathleen Sekula, PhD, PMHCNS, FAAN, is a professor at Duquesne University School of Nursing in Pittsburgh, Pennsylvania. She has strengthened the role of forensic nursing regarding victims and perpetrators of violence through her leadership in evidence-based graduate programs and her continuing energy to expand forensic nursing science through her research and practice trajectory. Sekula created the graduate forensic programs (MSN, DNP, and PhD) at the School of Nursing with the support of two 3-year program grants from the Department of Health and Human Services. As an innovator in the area of forensic nursing practice, she provides guidance to forensic nurse professionals in the United States and other countries. She served as president of the International

Association of Forensic Nurses Certification Board and in that capacity worked to establish forensic nurse certification at the advanced practice level. She served on the editorial review board for the *International Journal of Forensic Nursing* for 6 years and continues as a reviewer for the journal. Sekula is a fellow in the American Academy of Nursing and serves on the Expert Panel on Violence. She is a recipient of the Virginia Lynch Pioneer in Nursing Award from the International Association of Forensic Nurses. She is an advanced practice adult psychiatric mental health clinical nurse specialist and maintains a faculty practice in the care of patients with depression and anxiety, many of whom are current and/or previous victims of violence. Sekula serves on the board of the Cyril H. Wecht Institute of Forensic Science and Law, as adjunct faculty in the School of Law, and as an advisor to the programs offered through the institute.

Contributing Authors

Paul Thomas Clements, PhD, APRN-BC, CGS, DF-IAFN, is an associate clinical professor and coordinator of the Forensic Trends in Healthcare Certificate program online at Drexel University in Philadelphia, Pennsylvania. His clinical experience includes previously serving as assistant director/bereavement therapist at the Homicide Bereavement Center at the Office of the Medical Examiner in Philadelphia, Pennsylvania. He is an experienced therapist, forensic consultant, and critical incident/trauma response specialist with many years of experience in management/administration and crisis intervention. Clements has provided counseling and crisis intervention to over 1,500 families of murder victims as well as to many surviving family members in the aftermath of suicide, industrial and occupational deaths, motor vehicle accidents, sudden infant death syndrome, and other types of sudden violent death, as well as to survivors of interpersonal violence such as sexual abuse, rape, and stalking. More recently, Clements traveled to Bolivia to work with agencies, including court judges and prosecutors, regarding the impact of childhood sexual abuse on women and children. Clements was inducted as a distinguished fellow in the International Association of Forensic Nurses in 2002.

Alison M. Colbert, PhD, PHCNS-BC, is an associate professor and the associate dean for academic affairs at the Duquesne University School of Nursing. She is a clinical nurse specialist in public/community health with 20 years of clinical experience. Named a Robert Wood Johnson Foundation Nurse Faculty Scholar in 2010, Colbert has centered her clinical practice and research on health promotion in vulnerable populations. Her current research focuses on the health and well-being of women recently released from incarceration. Colbert received her BA from the University of Arizona, her MSN from The University of Texas at Austin, and her PhD from the University of Pittsburgh. She teaches in the undergraduate and graduate programs, including in the graduate forensic nursing program. She is also active in the American Public Health Association/Public Health Nursing Section and the International Association of Forensic Nurses and is on the editorial board of the *Journal of Forensic Nursing.*

Stacy A. Drake, PhD, MPH, RN, AFN-BC, D-ABMDI, is an assistant professor at the University of Texas Health Science Center at Houston (UTHealth) School of Nursing. Drake received her PhD in nursing at Texas Woman's University, her MSN with a concentration in forensic nursing from the University of Colorado at Colorado Springs, her MPH from UTHealth School of Public Health, and her BSN from Bowling Green State University in Ohio. Drake has years of experience within various clinical and administrative positions including EMS/fire, trauma/burn/medical and surgical ICU, death investigation, and risk management. Drake teaches on a variety of topics and is involved with mentoring nurses in community-based clinical experiences. Her research interests include understanding deaths in the public sector for purposes of prevention and eliminating disparity, forensic nursing science education, and death investigation systems. Finally, she is practicing as a forensic nurse at the Harris County Institute of Forensic Sciences.

Di Fischer, MN, RN, PHN, received her bachelor of arts in linguistics, minor in GLBT studies, and master of nursing from the University of Minnesota. She has more than 5 years of experience working in progressive and comprehensive sexual healthcare services. Her interests lie in improving healthcare for marginalized and underserved communities. She currently performs home and school visits with pregnant and parenting adolescents.

Netanya Frohman, BSN, RN, received her BSN from Johns Hopkins University School of Nursing (SON), where she is currently a PhD student researching cardiovascular disease risk and outcomes related to exposure to violence, including family and partner violence and military service related PTSD. Prior to becoming a nurse, she received a BA from Dickinson College in Carlisle, Pennsylvania, where a diverse liberal arts education exposed her to the concept of spirituality as a mechanism of healing and communication. Through the mentorships of Jacquelyn Campbell, Phyllis Sharps, and others at the JHU SON, she has developed an interest in nursing's critical role in the prevention, intervention, and treatment of situations and outcomes related to human-on-human violence as well as the psychology of motivation and behavioral change. She envisions a career of making valuable contributions to the field of cardiovascular and violence research while playing an active role in educating incoming generations of nurse leaders, educators, and research scientists.

Lorie S. Goshin, PhD, RN, is an assistant professor at the Hunter-Bellevue School of Nursing. She received a master's degree in parent-child nursing from the University of Texas at Austin and a PhD and postdoctoral research scientist training at Columbia University. Goshin's research explores health inequities experienced by criminal justice–involved families. She began working with this population while providing clinical nursing care in a county juvenile jail. She was co-investigator on a National Institute of Nursing Research–funded study of long-term outcomes for women and children who lived together in a prison nursery. She is currently investigating alternatives to incarceration for women with children, as well as the needs of arrested veterans. She has received awards for this work from the American Public Health Association, National March of Dimes, and the Foundation for New York State Nurses. In August 2013, she was invited to the White House to speak about her research.

Stephen Goux, MSN, RN, AFN-BC, SANE-A, SANE-P, is a pediatric emergency nurse specializing in pediatric forensic nursing. He is certified as both a sexual assault nurse examiner-adult/adolescent (SANE-A) and sexual assault nurse examiner-pediatric (SANE-P) through the International Association of Forensic Nurses and is a board-certified advanced forensic nurse through the American Nurses Credentialing Center. Goux holds a baccalaureate degree in nursing and a master of science in forensic nursing. He is a doctoral student in the PhD program at Duquesne University, focusing on research related to the advancement of forensic nursing. He is a former law enforcement officer, having worked in many different areas including investigations, negotiations, and corrections. His teaching roles have included didactic nursing education, clinical faculty, and preceptor faculty for newly trained SANEs. His research interests include pediatric acute care clinical practice, forensic nursing practice, and the prevention of revictimization in male victims of sexual assault.

Anita G. Hufft, PhD, RN, is a professor and dean of the Texas Woman's University College of Nursing. Hufft is a veteran of the United States Army and is nationally recognized in the nursing profession as a consultant, a speaker at national conferences, and a frequent contributor to nursing publications in forensic nursing and nursing education leadership. She has served her profession as a member of various task forces, committees, and boards, such as the Georgia

Board of Nursing, the *Journal of Forensic Nursing* Editorial Board, the Southern Regional Education Board of the Council on Collegiate Education for Nursing, the International Association of Forensic Nursing, and the American Association of Colleges of Nursing.

Emily Ruth Johnson, MN, MA, RN, SANE-A, has been a sexual assault nurse examiner (SANE) since 2012. She works for two forensic nursing programs in the Minneapolis-St. Paul area. Her background is in emergency department, intensive care, telemetry, post anesthesia care, and post-partum nursing. In addition to being a registered nurse, she holds a bachelor of science degree in geological and environmental science and a master of arts in Russian and East European studies from Stanford University.

Brittany E. Kelly, BSN, is currently a graduating accelerated bachelor of nursing student at Johns Hopkins University School of Nursing (July 2015). She is a John I. and Marilyn S. Mandler Scholarship scholar and a Johns Hopkins Center For AIDS Research scholar. She is a native of Baltimore, Maryland, and is involved in community outreach and research in the Baltimore area, which includes linking patients to Hep C treatment at the Johns Hopkins Hospital emergency department and working for Johns Hopkins University Global Initiative Center and Community Department. She is currently involved in HIV prevention in the Greater Baltimore area. Her nursing interests include infectious disease prevention in at-risk adolescents and African-American women in the Baltimore and Washington, DC, metropolitan areas and internationally.

Adine Latimore, MSN, PPCNP-BC, SANE, has been a nurse for 31 years, and for the last 21 years, she has worked as a pediatric nurse practitioner. She has been working at the Children's Advocacy Center (CAC) of Suffolk County in Massachusetts as a forensic nurse for more than 9 years. In her role at the CAC, she examines children who have been victims of sexual abuse. She diagnoses and treats medical conditions that may be related to sexual abuse and documents any possible physical and forensic evidence. The purpose of these exams is to reassure the child that his or her body is OK, to collect evidence that may be present on the child's body, and to ensure the health and wellbeing of the child. "To have a child leave my office knowing that his or her body is fine is the best part of my job."

Annie Lewis-O'Connor, PhD, NP-BC, MPH, FAAN, is a board-certified nurse practitioner. She is the founder and director of the C.A.R.E Clinic (Coordinated Approach to Recovery & Empowerment) at Brigham and Women's Hospital in Boston. She is committed to addressing domestic and sexual violence from a research, policy, education, and clinical perspective. She holds faculty appointments at Harvard Medical School (instructor) and Boston College. Her current research focuses on the use of tablets and virtual appointments for patients affected by violence, exploring patient-centered outcomes research, and the evaluation of healthcare models in caring for patients affected by intentional violence. She serves on the executive board of Casa Myrna Vasquez Shelter and the board of EQUALHEALTH, a nonprofit that is developing health, medical, and nursing education in Haiti. She received a master of science in nursing from Simmons College in Boston, a master of science in public health from Boston University, and a PhD from Boston College.

Linda Mabey, DNP, APRN, PMHCNS, has taught undergraduate and graduate nurses the art and science of psychiatric nursing since 1995. She received her doctor of nursing practice from the University of Utah in 2009. She is an active member of the American Psychiatric Nurses Association (APNA) and serves as a board member of the Utah Chapter of APNA. Her clinical focus is on treatment of psychological trauma and PTSD, and she maintains an active clinical practice. Her special interest in treating patients with psychological trauma led her to pursue certification as an EMDR therapist, an evidenced-based practice for the treatment of post-traumatic stress disorder. She is a published author on trauma and has presented at international and national conferences on trauma and PTSD.

Leslie Miles, DNP, APRN, PMHNP, is an assistant professor of nursing at Brigham Young University and a psychiatric nurse practitioner in the community. She received her associate degree in nursing from Brigham Young University in 1983 and her bachelor of science in 1999. Miles graduated with her master of science in psychiatric-mental health nursing from the University of Utah in 2004. She continued her education at Rush University in Chicago to earn her doctorate of nursing practice in 2012. Miles has worked in a variety of psychiatric settings for more than 30 years and is active in the American Psychiatric Nurses Association; Sigma Theta Tau International, Iota-Iota Chapter; and is a designated examiner for civil commitments in the State of Utah.

Stacey A. Mitchell, DNP, MBA, RN, SANE-A, SANE-P, holds a doctorate in forensic nursing practice from the University of Tennessee Health Science Center; a master of science in nursing, focusing on trauma and forensic nursing, from the University of Virginia in Charlottesville; and a bachelor of science in nursing from the Medical College of Virginia. Her nursing career spans more than 25 years, with experience in critical care, emergency nursing, forensic nursing, and risk management. Mitchell began her forensic nursing career as coordinator of the forensic nurse examiners of St. Mary's Hospital in Richmond, Virginia. She served as director at-large for two terms, treasurer, president-elect, and president of the International Association of Forensic Nurses (IAFN). Mitchell held the position of deputy chief forensic nurse investigator at the Harris County Medical Examiner's Office in Houston, Texas, for 6 years. Currently, she is the administrative director of forensic nursing services and risk management and patient safety for the Harris Health System. The Texas Nurses Association District 9 honored Mitchell as one of the Top 20 Outstanding Nurses. She is the 2015 recipient of the Virginia Lynch Pioneer in Nursing Award from the IAFN.

Cindy Peternelj-Taylor, RN, MSc, DF-IAFN, focuses on professional role development for nurses and other healthcare professionals who work with vulnerable populations in forensic psychiatric and correctional settings, with particular emphasis on ethical issues that emerge from practice (e.g., boundary violations, whistleblowing, othering, and ethical decision-making). She is currently funded for two small-scale research projects by the Centre for Forensic Behavioral Science and Justice Studies: a mixed methods study exploring correctional nurses' roles, responsibilities, and learning needs; and a scoping review exploring palliative care in correctional settings. Previous research, a phenomenological study, explored the lived experience of nurse engagement with forensic patients in secure environments. She is currently the Chairperson of the Undergraduate Education

Committee, Editor-in-Chief, *Journal of Forensic Nursing*, and a Distinguished Fellow with the International Association of Forensic Nurses.

Carolyn M. Porta, PhD, MPH, RN, SANE-A, is a sexual assault nurse examiner-adult/adolescent (SANE-A) employed with the Region's SANE Program since 2007. She is an associate professor in the Population Health and Systems Cooperative in the School of Nursing at the University of Minnesota, and adjunct associate professor in the Division of Epidemiology and Community Health of the School of Public Health. Her clinical expertise includes adolescent health, public health nursing, and forensic nursing. Porta is a mixed-method researcher, with emphasis on development and testing of preventive interventions tailored to the needs and preferences of adolescents, young people, and their families. Use of innovative technologies characterizes her work. She teaches and conducts research that emphasizes physical and mental health promotion, particularly for underserved and under-resourced populations. Porta is currently involved in collaborative research across North America and Africa, addressing threats to health that range from lack of insurance and social stigmas to gender-based violence/interpersonal violence and zoonotic diseases.

Phyllis W. Sharps, PhD, RN, FAAN, is a professor and associate dean for Community and Global Programs at the Johns Hopkins University School of Nursing. Sharps leads the Center of Global Initiatives, directing and coordinating global nursing educational and capacity-building initiatives for faculty and students. She is also the director of three community health nurse–based centers. She has published numerous articles on improving reproductive health and reducing violence amongst African-American women, including the physical and mental health consequences of violence against pregnant and parenting women, infants, and very young children. She has been the principal investigator for two NIH-funded grants, including the Domestic Violence Enhanced Home Visitation Program (DOVE), a public health nurse intervention to reduce violence against pregnant women. She is a fellow of the American Academy of Nursing and a member of STTI's International Nurse Researcher Hall of Fame.

Mariah Eliza Smock, BA, BSN, received a classical high school education from the Highlands Latin School in Louisville, Kentucky. She received her bachelor of arts from Centre College in 2011. Smock received her associate in nursing from Midway College in 2014 and her bachelor of science in nursing in 2015, also from Midway College.

William S. Smock, MD, is the full-time police surgeon and directs the Clinical Forensic Medicine Program for the Louisville Metro Police Department. Smock joined the faculty at University of Louisville's Department of Emergency Medicine in 1994 and was promoted to the rank of full professor in 2005. He is currently a clinical professor of emergency medicine at the University of Louisville School of Medicine. He has edited three textbooks on clinical forensic medicine and published more than 30 chapters and articles on forensic and emergency medicine. He is an internationally recognized forensic expert and trains nurses, physicians, law enforcement officers, and attorneys in the investigation of officer-involved shootings, strangulation, gunshot wounds, injury mechanisms, and motor vehicle trauma. Smock is also the police surgeon for the Jeffersontown, Kentucky, and St. Matthews, Kentucky, Police Departments and serves as a tactical physician and detective for the Floyd County Sheriff's Department in Indiana.

Julie Valentine, MS, RN, CNE, SANE-A, is an assistant professor at Brigham Young University College of Nursing. Her clinical specialty and research focus areas are forensic nursing, violence against women, and sexual assault. Valentine is a certified sexual assault nurse examiner (SANE) with Salt Lake Sexual Assault Nurse Examiners and Primary Children's Medical Center, Salt Lake City, Utah. She is also a full-time student pursuing her PhD in nursing at Duquesne University, with completion expected in December 2015. She is principal investigator in a collaborative research project with the Utah state crime laboratory that is exploring the impact of new DNA testing methods, specifically Y-STR analysis, on evidence collection following sexual assault. In addition, she is the principal investigator in other studies exploring the impact of training law enforcement and prosecutors on the neurobiology of trauma, specifically in sexual assault cases.

Andrea M. Yevchak, PhD, RN, is an assistant professor at Duquesne University School of Nursing. She is a clinical nurse specialist in gerontological nursing with 10 years of clinical experience. In 2009–2011, she was named a John A. Hartford Building Academic Geriatric Nursing Capacity Scholar. Yevchak received her BSN, MSN, and PhD in nursing from the Pennsylvania State University College of Nursing. She has focused her teaching and scholarship on vulnerable older adults seen across settings of care.

TABLE OF CONTENTS

1 WHAT IS FORENSIC NURSING? 1

2 FORENSIC SCIENCE 101 19

3 NEUROBIOLOGY OF TRAUMA 37

FOREWORD

The field of forensic nursing has rapidly advanced throughout the past decades. Exciting new findings in forensic science such as the neurobiology of trauma have influenced our field, but as always, it is difficult for practitioners to find, consume, evaluate, and thoughtfully apply all of the new developments. It is sometimes tempting for clinicians to "throw the baby out with the bathwater" and rush to change their practice as a new development is trumpeted in the popular press—before the research has been evaluated and put within the context of prior findings and then with a consensus of experts applied into practice.

A Practical Guide to Forensic Nursing: Incorporating Forensic Principles Into Nursing Practice is a groundbreaking book because of its strong evidence base that is carefully evaluated and contextualized—and made understandable and actually usable by the leading practicing forensic nurses in the field. Many are researchers themselves, some currently conducting "cutting edge" forensic nursing research about which they write eloquently but in a totally understandable and applicable way. Others are more immersed in practice or forensic nursing education, but all have training in translational research and have clearly maintained an active research as well as practice interest—resulting in evidence that is current and practice guidelines that are appropriate for today's and tomorrow's practitioners.

The chapters are short, with definitions provided, and combine a strong blend of science and legal implications. In addition to research evidence, theoretical concepts are presented in usable, practical fashion. Part of the forensic nurse's job in any setting is explaining evidence to nonscientists, and this book is incredibly helpful in its clarity in presenting the scientific basis of evidence.

Angela Amar and Kathleen Sekula, two of the most outstanding leaders in forensic nursing, have provided an incredible resource to forensic nursing educators teaching at all levels as well as to current practitioners. Publication of this book advances the exciting potential of forensic nursing in the future for helping victims obtain justice and gain understanding of and appropriate treatment for the holistic nature of their responses to trauma. It also advances the ability of forensic nurses to be an integral and highly respected part of the interdisciplinary community of scholars and clinicians working toward the prevention of violence.

–Jacquelyn Campbell, PhD, RN, FAAN
Anna D. Wolf Endowed Chair and Professor
Johns Hopkins University School of Nursing

INTRODUCTION

An 8-year-old boy is brought to the school nurse for sleeping in class. His teacher is concerned because every Monday, he is belligerent, distracted, and sleepy. The school nurse learns that he spends weekends with his father. His mother is concerned that the father is sexually abusing her son.

The visiting nurse is concerned about Margaret, an 82-year-old woman who lives with her granddaughter. On her most recent visit, the electricity was not working, and Margaret said she hadn't eaten in a few days. Margaret asked the visiting nurse not to "make a fuss" because she didn't want to upset her granddaughter.

> **CAUTION:** As healthcare clinicians, we must all be aware of our own behavior when working with victims so that we do not cause secondary victimization through victim blaming. We must be able to set aside our own biases when working with patients.

A 19-year-old college student is brought to the campus clinic. The student says her friends made her come. She tells the nurse that two nights ago she woke up in the lobby of her building. Her clothes were on backwards and she wasn't wearing underwear. The last thing she remembers is drinking and dancing at a party in another residence hall.

All of the patients above have markers that have criminal or civil forensic medical implications and potential court involvement. Violence and crime unite two of the most powerful systems in the world: criminal justice and healthcare. These two systems work together to ensure that justice, health, and public safety are restored and maintained. Forensic nursing, a fast-growing specialty, sits at the intersection of violence and health. *Forensic nursing* is the application of nursing science to public or legal proceedings. The practice of forensic nursing facilitates connections among the healthcare, social services, and criminal justice systems to assist victims, perpetrators, and their families to receive assistance, services, and resources. While all nurses are familiar with the healthcare system, fewer nurses are familiar and comfortable with legal proceedings. Unfortunately, education and training in most nursing schools does not prepare nurses entering the general workforce to provide care to patients who are victims of violence, nor perpetrators of violence who require healthcare services.

Violence is a major factor in healthcare today. Regardless of where a nurse works within the healthcare system, he or she will care for many victims and perpetrators of violence throughout his or her career. Exploring how to care for these patients, and the theoretical underpinnings of violence, are among the goals for this book. The psychological trauma experienced by victims of violence places them at risk for long-term mental health issues, including post-traumatic stress disorder (PTSD) and other comorbidities (Bonanno, 2004). Nurses in the generalist settings are most often the first to interact with a victim. For this reason, all nurses should have a basic understanding of forensic issues that affect their practice and ultimately their patients.

The purpose of this book is to provide nurses with essential information that can be incorporated into practice. The goal is to provide nurses with a practical, evidence-based guide to understanding and applying forensic nursing science in their practices. This book will introduce nurses to theoretical perspectives on violence, concepts essential to understanding forensic science and applying it in practice, and violence-prevention strategies. The book will highlight sociocultural diversity and relevant legal, ethical, societal, and policy issues. The information in the chapters will also include challenges in the practice area and potential solutions.

In 2013, an estimated 6.1 million United States adolescents and adults experienced a violent victimization (Truman & Langton, 2014). Violent crime, which includes rape or sexual assault, robbery, and aggravated and simple assault, often results in injury, pain, and physical and emotional trauma. Burglary is more often reported to the police; rape is least reported to the police (Hart & Rennison, 2003; Rennison, 2002). In crimes that are reported to the police, the victim is also more likely to receive healthcare (Tjaden & Thoennes, 2000). An estimated $105 billion per year is spent on medical care, mental health services, victim services, property loss or damage, and reductions in work productivity due to crime (Wright & Vicneire, 2010).

Crimes are offenses or omissions that are punishable by law. Crimes typically involve victims and offenders. *Victims* may be harmed, injured, or killed by crime and violence, an accident, or action. Some crimes are considered victimless:

actions that are against the law but involve consenting adults. *Offenders* (perpetrators) are persons who commit a criminal act.

Crimes can be prosecuted in civil and/or criminal courts. Civil courts handle non-criminal actions, such as disputes between two persons that they cannot resolve, like property disputes. On the other hand, criminal courts have the authority to punish offenders when found guilty of the crime. The founders of the United States specifically conceived of a criminal justice system to ensure that every person is innocent until proven guilty. The criminal justice system provides safeguards that are designed to protect the rights of the accused. In order to be found guilty in a criminal court, the burden of proof is "beyond a reasonable doubt." In the civil court, the burden of proof is "more likely than not." As an example, the 1994–95 criminal trial prosecuting O. J. Simpson for the murders of Nicole Brown Simpson and Ronald Lyle Goldman did not prove guilt beyond a reasonable doubt, and so Mr. Simpson was acquitted. In the civil case against him, however, he was found guilty because the burden of proof was that a reasonable person would agree that it was more likely than not that he committed the crime.

It's important to consider the effects of the criminal justice system on victims. For a criminal complaint, the victim does not decide whether a case will go to court or not. The *state* makes that decision, and in most cases it is the district attorney or a grand jury that serves as the state in making that decision—it is the *state* vs. the offender. The victim usually testifies in the criminal case. A civil case is brought before the court by the victim (grievant), usually with the assistance of a lawyer.

Victims have established rights in criminal proceedings, including the right to attend the criminal justice proceedings and the right to be heard. Victims have the right to be notified when offenders are released or escape from incarceration. Provisions are made through the Office of Victims of Crime for *victim compensation*, which is a government program that provides reimbursement of expenses related to the crime to victims of violent crime. Compensation even extends to surviving or affected family members. Law enforcement or the district attorney usually notifies victims that they are eligible to apply for funds. Compensation can be paid even when no one is arrested or convicted of the crime.

The term *secondary victimization* is characterized by victim-blaming attitudes, behaviors, and practices, which result in additional trauma to the victim (Campbell & Raja, 1999). The victim may not feel supported by family, friends, and professionals/clinicians, which leads to additional emotional harm. Victims may feel secondary revictimization in a criminal justice system that makes them recount their stories multiple times to various individuals involved in the case. A common example of secondary victimization occurs when the victim of sexual assault is blamed for the clothes she was wearing, or the alcohol she drank, or for her life choices. And when she is made to repeat her story many times, defense lawyers will focus on any discrepancies among the various reports that are made when the victim repeats her story.

Using victim advocates can be a helpful provision when assisting a patient. Advocates are professionals who are trained to provide support and resources to victims of crime. Advocates assist the victims while in the healthcare system and throughout their legal case. Nurses should be aware of this resource within their community and know how and when to refer victims.

As the largest sector of healthcare employees, nurses are in hospitals, clinics, correctional facilities, schools, and other healthcare settings. Forensic nursing entails skills in assessing and treating victims of violence, evidence collection and preservation, documentation, and understanding the legal system (Burgess, Berger, & Boersma, 2004). The medicolegal aspects of providing care to victims necessitate having background knowledge of violence and crime, which prepares the nurse to provide more comprehensive care. Because so few healthcare education programs, including nursing, provide forensic education and training, few healthcare clinicians are prepared to meet the responsibilities involved with caring for victims and perpetrators (Henderson, Harada, & Amar, 2012). While criminal investigations are within the purview of law enforcement, it is incumbent upon providers to understand forensic issues in their evaluation and plan of care for patients. The International Association of Forensic Nursing and its publication, the *Journal of*

Forensic Nursing, are resources for nurses wishing to learn more about forensic nursing.

The chapters in this book are designed to provide a basic understanding of forensic nursing and the many roles forensic nurses perform. The early chapters focus on forensic science and assessment of wounds and injuries. Theoretical perspectives on violence, victimization, and perpetration are provided to increase the nurse's understanding of victims and offenders. Neurobiological, psychological, social, physical, and behavioral responses to trauma are presented so that nurses can recognize the immediate and long-term effects of violence on health. The middle section of the book provides information on various crimes. Each chapter contains background information, relevant laws and statutes, assessment, and treatment. Case studies are provided to illuminate the content. The final section contains information on community strategies for violence prevention and intervention. Strategies to institute trauma-informed care in healthcare settings are provided. These chapters are not meant to explain all aspects of forensic care. Rather, they provide a starting point for the non-forensic nurse to begin to transform practice.

References

Bonanno, G. A. (2004). Loss, trauma, and human resilience: Have we underestimated the human capacity to thrive after extremely aversive events? *American Psychologist, 59*(1), 20–28. doi: 10.1037/0003-066X.59.1.20

Burgess, A. W., Berger, A. D., & Boersma, R. R. (2004). Forensic nursing: Investigating the career potential in this emerging graduate specialty. *AJN: The American Journal of Nursing, 104*(3), 58–64.

Campbell, R., & Raja, S. (1999). The secondary victimization of rape victims: Insights from mental health professionals who treat survivors of violence. *Violence and Victims, 14,* 261–275.

Hart, T. C., & Rennison, C. M. (2003). *Reporting crime to the police, 1992–2000.* U.S. Department of Justice, Office of Justice Programs.

Henderson, E., Harada, N., & Amar, A. (2012). Caring for the forensic population: Recognizing the educational needs of emergency department nurses and physicians. *Journal of Forensic Nursing, 8*(4), 170–177.

Rennison, C. M. (2002). *Rape and sexual assault: Reporting to police and seeking medical attention, 1992–2000*. Washington, DC: Bureau of Justice Statistics.

Tjaden, P., & Thoennes, N. (2000). *Extent, nature, and consequences of intimate partner violence*. Washington, DC: National Institute of Justice and the Centers for Disease Control.

Truman, J. L., & Langton, L. (2014). *Criminal victimization, 2013*. Washington, DC: Bureau of Justice Statistics.

Wright, E., & Vicneire, M. (2010). Economic costs of victimization. In B. S. Fisher & S. P. Lab (Eds.), *Encylopedia of victimology and crime prevention* (pp. 344–348). Thousand Oaks, CA: SAGE.

What Is Forensic Nursing?

L. Kathleen Sekula, PhD, PMHCNS, FAAN

Key Points in This Chapter

- All nurses are forensic nurses.

- The nurse generalist should become familiar with forensic procedures that can help provide the best care for patient cases that have legal implications.

- There are many roles that a forensic nurse can perform.

- Collaboration among professionals in a forensic case is key to good care.

- Every nurse should consider lifelong learning as a part of practice.

Forensic nursing is an evolving nursing specialty that focuses on healthcare when legal issues are involved. Forensic practice in nursing is now recognized as its own practice area, whereas in the past it had only been practiced informally, because there were no standards of education relating to forensic science for nurses.

The role of the forensic nurse evolved out of the practice of *clinical forensic medicine,* a subspecialty of forensic medicine defined as the application of forensic medical knowledge and techniques to living patients. This role has been evident in the United Kingdom and many other countries for over two centuries. However, as the role emerged in healthcare in the United States as a medical specialty, forensic medicine was considered to be the domain of physicians alone. It was not until the 1980s that the need for expansion of the role was identified. In a 1983 article, Smialek highlighted the need for knowledgeable clinicians in the emergency departments regarding forensic cases, because evidence was being lost by commission or omission during trauma treatment. For this reason, it became apparent that all nurses working throughout the healthcare system, and specifically in settings where trauma patients present, must have some baseline knowledge of how to assess patients, preserve evidence, and interface with the legal system in order to mitigate negative consequences for both the patient and the system.

While practicing as a death investigator and as one of the first nurses to become a member of the American Academy of Forensic Sciences, Lynch advocated for the value of forensic education in nursing schools and for the role of nurses in forensic practice. She proposed the development of forensic nursing as a specialty in 1986 (Lynch, 2013). And although her early vision of forensic nursing focused on the role of the death investigator, she quickly saw the need for an expanded role that encompassed a broader clinical forensic nursing practice.

The earliest example of forensic nursing practice involved sexual assault nurse examiners (SANEs). In the early 1990s, a group of nurses recognized the lack of appropriate care for victims of sexual assault and developed training for nurses to prepare them to properly assess patients, collect evidence, document findings, and interface with the legal system in caring for victims of sexual assault. This same group of nurse clinicians established the International Association of Forensic Nurses (IAFN) in 1995 (Sekula & Burgess, 2006). Over the years, the practice of forensic nursing has expanded to include the care of patients throughout the healthcare system who require consideration of the legal implications related to their care.

The specialty of forensic nursing was formally recognized by the American Academy of Forensic Sciences (AAFS) in 1991 (American Academy of Forensic Sciences, 2010) and by the American Nurses Association (ANA) in 1995 (American Nurses Association, 2009). In 1997, the *Scope and Standards of Forensic Nursing Practice* was developed and published through the joint effort of the IAFN and the ANA. Forensic nurses now practice as advanced practice nurses in hospitals and community settings where they support fellow professionals in applying medicolegal principles while caring for both victims and perpetrators of violence.

According to the World Health Organization (WHO), each year over 1.6 million people receive medical treatment for an injury that is violence-related ("The global burden of disease: 2004 update," 2008). Approximately 5.8 million people die each year as a result of injuries, accidental or intentional (World Health Organization, 2002). The first contact in the healthcare system is often the nurse who responds in various settings. For this reason, all nurses must be prepared to meet the needs of such patients.

While not all nurses receive education in the principles of forensic practice, the purpose of this book is to acquaint all nurses with basic forensic knowledge that can, and should, be applied in situations where legal implications may arise. We no longer can ignore the importance of assessing for how the injuries occurred in relationship to criminal or negligent behavior. Nurses must be prepared to serve a broader role in forensic practice.

Forensic nurses now serve in roles as advanced practice clinical nurse specialists, forensic nurse examiners, sexual assault forensic examiners, risk managers, death investigators, forensic psychiatric nurses, nurse coroners, nurse attorneys, legal nurse consultants, and forensic corrections nurses, among others.

FORENSIC NURSING THEORY

Nursing theory provides a conceptual framework by which nurses frame their practice. A framework addresses the concepts important to increasing the understanding of the human experience within a particular area of practice. In order to advance the practice of forensic nursing, nurses must define a body of knowledge that is unique to this application of nursing in the various clinical and community settings. Figure 1.1 shows the integrated practice model for forensic nursing science.

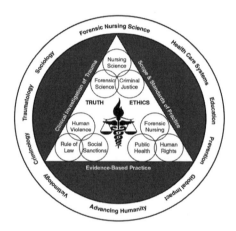

FIGURE 1.1 INTEGRATED PRACTICE MODEL FOR FORENSIC NURSING SCIENCE.

© COPYRIGHT VIRGINIA A. LYNCH, 1990. USED WITH PERMISSION.

DEFINITIONS REGARDING THE FORENSIC FIELD

The field of forensic nursing is new and can be complex and at times confusing. You will come across various terms and definitions in the course of your practice that may challenge you with relationship to practice. For the purpose of this book, these are the terms and definitions you should be familiar with:

- **Forensic nursing:** The application of the nursing process to public or legal proceedings, and the application of forensic healthcare in the scientific investigation of trauma- and/or death-related abuse, violence, criminal activity, liability, and accidents (Lynch & Duval, 2011).

■ **Forensic science:** The forensic sciences are used around the world to resolve civil disputes, to justly enforce criminal laws and government regulations, and to protect public health. Forensic scientists may be involved anytime when an objective, scientific analysis is needed to find the truth and to seek justice in a legal proceeding (American Academy of Forensic Sciences, 2010).

■ **Clinical forensic practice:** The application of medical and nursing sciences to the care of living victims of crime or liability-related accidents (Lynch, 2013).

The Role of the Emergency Department Nurse

Lynch (1990) studied the role behaviors and role expectations of emergency department (ED) nurses; her study identified the need for a multidisciplinary team approach to identifying forensic trauma, care and collection of evidence, and the preservation of evidence. More recently, Foresman-Capuzzi (2014) stressed the importance of evidence collection in the ED and introduced the reader to the basics of evidence collection and preservation of the chain of custody of that evidence. Based on the Emergency Nurses Association (ENA) position statement regarding forensic evidence collection, three statements define the emergency nurse position (Emergency Nurses Association, 2010). The emergency nurse:

■ Provides physical and emotional care to patients, and also helps preserve the evidentiary material collected in the emergency department

■ Collaborates with emergency physicians, social service, and law enforcement personnel to develop guidelines for forensic evidence collection, preservation, and documentation in the emergency care setting

■ Is familiar with the concepts and skills of evidence collection, written and photographic documentation, as well as testifying in legal proceedings

INSTITUTE OF MEDICINE REPORT ON FORENSIC NURSING

In 2010, the Robert Wood Johnson Foundation and the Institute of Medicine joined forces to make recommendations that would guide the transformation of nursing in order to meet the current and future challenges in healthcare (Sekula, Colbert, Zoucha, Amar, & Williams, 2012). This report, referred to as the *IOM Report on the Future of Nursing,* affects all areas of nursing as well as each entry level to nursing practice. Nurses in all clinical areas should be aware of the implications of practicing in the new healthcare system. The committee developed four key messages:

- Nurses should practice to the full extent of their education and training.

- Nurses should achieve higher levels of education and training through an improved education system that promotes seamless academic progression.

- Nurses should be full partners with physicians and other health professionals in redesigning healthcare in the United States.

- Effective workforce planning and policy-making require better data collection and an improved information structure.

These recommendations support nurses in gaining parity in the workforce by advancing their education and training and by assuring nurses have input in redesigning the healthcare system. Forensic nurses are taking that mandate seriously as they advance their practice, establish educational standards, and engage in forensic research. Each nurse in practice must advance his or her understanding of forensic issues in communities and in the healthcare system given the increase of violence in society.

By their very scope of practice, all nurses are *forensic* nurses. With the increase in violence in society, the acuity in patient care, and the need for closer attention to the legal implications when certain patients present in the healthcare system, all nurses can and should be prepared at some level to recognize and respond to those needs; having a basic understanding of what those needs might be is an important first step in advancing practice. Collaborating with advanced practice forensic nurses, reading pertinent literature in the area of forensics, participating in continuing education in the area of forensic nursing practice, and learning to address the impact of proper nursing care on the outcomes for patients with forensic issues are important first steps in advancing any nurse's practice in this important area.

FORENSIC NURSING IN THE UNITED STATES

When forensic nursing first became recognized in the United States, the focus was on the care of the victim. In Canada and the United Kingdom, where forensic nursing was recognized well before being recognized in the U.S., the term *forensic nursing* was most commonly associated with care of the psychiatric patient in secure settings, and therefore more focused on care within the corrections systems (Hammer, Moynihan, & Pagliaro, 2013). In the United States, the term was most commonly associated with practice within the forensic medical systems, and as such focused more on the victim of violence. However, in recent years the focus of forensic nursing in all countries has broadened to include both victims and perpetrators, as well as their families.

INTERFACING WITH FORENSIC NURSES

Emergency department (ED) nurses as well as trauma team nurses are often the first to encounter a patient with forensic issues. Patients who have been assaulted or who are victims of any type of violence or negligence, and perpetrators with various types of injuries or psychological problems present with unique needs. Nurses can no longer focus on treatment of physical injuries alone. Essential evidence that is highly perishable and fragile such as DNA evidence is often the most essential evidence linking the perpetrator to the crime (Lynch, 2013). Nurses must know when and how to collect evidence and how to preserve the chain of custody of that evidence. Assessing the patient for the possibility of being a victim, collecting the proper evidence as indicated, taking photographs, and properly informing the patient are all elements of proper care. These tasks are not difficult, but nurses need training in order to complete them properly. In addition, the nurse has an ethical responsibility to advocate for all patients, both victims and offenders. It is not the nurse's role to determine guilt or innocence. The nurse must provide holistic nursing care for each patient while being unbiased and an advocate for truth and justice (Lynch, 2013).

The purpose of this book is to offer an in-depth view of forensic nursing for nurses in the generalist settings. All nurses should have an understanding of the major practice areas that make up forensic nursing. Nurses must understand the implications when a patient presents in any setting with forensic issues. The nurse-patient relationship occurs in forensic nursing when the possibility arises that the patient is a victim of a crime or maybe committed a crime (Sekula & Colbert, 2013).

The following sections discuss the different aspects of forensic nursing practice. Regardless of the specific role, the nurse brings the holistic view of the patient and family. This holistic view is the unique contribution of nursing, and when forensic expertise is added, everyone benefits.

FORENSIC CLINICAL NURSE SPECIALIST

The clinical forensic nurse can function in various settings throughout the hospital, clinic, or community. Forensic clinical nurse specialists are prepared to provide expert forensic patient care while also serving colleagues as consultants, educators, and researchers (Sekula, 2005). Thus, they provide expert consultation related to identifying, assessing, collecting evidence, documenting, and testifying when forensic issues arise. In this role, the nurse is prepared with advanced education and training and recognizes the importance of a team approach to caring for both victims and perpetrators. The nurse serves as an unbiased expert who is focused on the facts and fairness of treatment. It is not the role of the clinical forensic expert to decide who is guilty or innocent but to collect evidence in an objective manner and to deliver care objectively.

FORENSIC NURSE EXAMINER/SEXUAL ASSAULT NURSE EXAMINER

The forensic nurse examiner (FNE), or sexual assault nurse examiner (SANE), was the first specialized forensic role for nurses and represents the largest subspecialty in forensic nursing. Nurses can take specialty training in both care of the adult and adolescent, and the child victim of sexual assault. The IAFN has established clear guidelines for the preparation and training of SANEs and provides certification at the national level for SANE practice. National guidelines are established by the Centers for Disease Control and Prevention (CDC) for the care of the sexual assault victim regarding HIV, STDs, and other communicable diseases (Centers for Disease Control and Prevention, 2010). Clear treatment guidelines are established, and all forensic nurse examiners are expected to follow the guidelines. Research supports that when a forensic nurse examiner is involved in the care of a sexual assault patient, successful prosecution rates increase and improved healthcare is achieved (Campbell, Townsend, Shaw, Karim, & Markowitz, 2014).

NURSE DEATH INVESTIGATOR

As one of the first areas of practice for forensic nurses, nurse death investigators offer a holistic assessment of the death scene. Nurses understand the importance of considering the impact of all aspects of the person's life in relationship to his or her death. The forensic nurse is often most prepared to deal with grieving relatives, the physiology and pharmacology implications in death cases, and the holistic view of the patient's life and intervening variables that may affect the overall outcome of the investigation. Some forensic nurse investigators serve as coroners in districts where the coroner system is in place. Others serve as investigators in both coroner jurisdictions, as well as medical examiner jurisdictions in which a forensic pathologist who is a physician leads the team.

Nurse Coroner

Because of the role of the death investigator in exploring all aspects of a death, the nurse coroner brings to the position a broader view of the life of one who has died. As previously described in the role of the forensic nurse in death investigation, the nurse coroner is a nurse who has experience as a death investigator and brings to the role a broad perspective when investigating circumstances that lead to death.

Forensic Correctional Nurse

In an enlightening statement, Hufft (2013) says that in order to understand society, one only needs to look within the prison system to see people affected by racism, poverty, and illiteracy. It is clear that the majority of prisoners are people of color and underrepresented minorities. As nurses we are geared to view each person as an individual and to treat that person in a way that is most humane. Advanced practice forensic nurses who work in corrections provide direct care to incarcerated persons. Some nurses working in corrections have advanced practice educations; others do not. Nurses must understand that there must be a balance between caring and custody (Holmes & Jacob, 2012; Holmes & Murray, 2011). The impact of restrictions in movement, interactions with caretakers, and other physical barriers create challenges to the care of this population. All nurses who practice in correctional settings need to advance their practice by coming to an understanding of the variables in play that contribute to the vulnerability of incarcerated individuals.

Forensic Psychiatric Nurse

A forensic psychiatric nurse is prepared as a generalist or at the advanced practice level to function as a direct care provider and patient advocate in caring for a most vulnerable population—those patients who suffer with mental illness and are also engaged in the legal system (Sekula & Colbert, 2013). Forensic nurses who are also prepared as psychiatric nurses address issues related to competency within the legal system. Advanced education is required for this role. However, generalist nurses are most often the ones who document the mental capacity of the patient on a day-to-day basis.

Legal Nurse Consultant and Nurse Attorney

Attorneys have utilized the expertise of nurses since the 1970s. Nurses were first seen in the legal arena as expert witnesses in nursing malpractice cases. As their expertise became more and more recognized, and as the courts recognized that nurses, rather than physicians, should define and evaluate the standards of nursing practice, nurses were sought out to review cases and offer opinion testimony about nursing care (Magnusson, Joos, Pike, Janes, & Beerman, 2003). During the 1980s, the role expanded further as it became clear that nurses are uniquely qualified to assist attorneys in their medical-legal practices. Most litigation practices now employ legal nurse consultants as full-time employees and as active members of the legal team.

The nurse attorney is qualified as an RN along with having the juris doctor degree. The combination of degrees prepares nurse attorneys to practice law, generally specializing in civil and criminal cases involving healthcare-related issues (Lynch, 2013).

Risk Manager

With a strong background in forensic science, nurses with advanced degrees in forensics are well prepared to serve as forensic investigators and as experts in risk management. When nurses master forensic content and incorporate that knowledge into clinical practice, forensic sciences can then serve as a framework for intuition by increasing the suspiciousness factor (Winfrey & Smith, 1999). It is often going beyond what is *seen* that compels a nurse to look further, and that hunch then leads to acting on a suspicion. Much information can be lost when one does not see beyond the obvious.

Many areas within the hospital system—including patient and family concerns about care, criminal behaviors among staff, suspicious or unexpected patient death, use of restraints, the occurrence of pressure ulcers, and drug diversion by staff—are addressed by risk managers. A risk manager with a forensic background can serve well in this capacity.

> ## JOINT COMMISSION STANDARD
>
> Joint Commission Standard PC.01.02.09 clearly outlines the responsibility of each hospital to establish objective criteria for identifying and assessing patients who are victims of physical assault, sexual assault, and other types of abuse and neglect. All providers are to be trained in the use of the established criteria (Joint Commission, 2014). In 2004, the Joint Commission instituted new standards for hospitals on how to respond to domestic abuse, neglect, and exploitation, and revised the standards in 2009. To assist hospitals in complying with the requirements, Futures Without Violence summarized the standards and provided recommendations for each with links to online resources and tools. The primary resource is the *National Consensus Guidelines: On Identifying and Responding to Domestic Violence Victimization in Health Care Settings* (Family Violence Prevention Fund, 2004). All nurses should be aware of these standards and how to meet the requirements in their practice.

EDUCATION OF THE FORENSIC NURSE

As of 2015, few associate degree or baccalaureate programs include forensic content in their programs. However, as stated previously, all nurses should have a working knowledge of issues related to care of patients when legal implications are involved; these issues demand the attention of the nurse when first interacting with the patient. Many RN programs (AD, diploma, and baccalaureate) have begun to add forensic content by threading it throughout courses, making students aware of where and when they might interface with forensic issues and how then to address forensic issues.

This book is intended to give nurses that basic understanding of forensic practice and some tools to ensure that all nurses practice to the fullest extent of their education when caring for victims and perpetrators of violence, or any patient who has experienced trauma.

Nurses practicing in any healthcare setting are well served to determine if a forensic clinician practices in their setting. If so, collaborate with that person and learn from the person. Take advantage of continuing education opportunities to increase knowledge related to forensic practice. There are many websites that offer free webinars in specific areas of forensics, such as End Violence Against Women International (EVAWI, www.evawintl.org); the International Association of Forensic Nurses (IAFN, www.forensicnurses.org); the Office on Violence Against Women (www.justice.gov/ovw); the Department of Justice (www.justice.gov); and Research Triangle International (RTI, www.rti.org). Most of these sites are available to register for free webinars, often for continuing education credits. Participants need to simply establish a login account and then choose webinars of interest.

Lastly, more and more nurses are advancing their education in forensic studies at the baccalaureate level. Associate degree and diploma prepared nurses are entering RN-BSN programs, some of which have a focus area in forensics. The key recommendation of the IOM report that encourages all nurses to engage in life-long learning is now being heeded. And it is the responsibility of nurses who are educated at higher levels and who are in positions of leadership to encourage nurses who work within their settings to advance their education. These same nurses can and should serve as mentors for nurses trying to achieve advanced education by encouraging them, helping them to find scholarships and financial aid, and otherwise being their advocates.

CASE STUDY: THE ROLE OF THE EMERGENCY NURSE

Nurses working throughout the healthcare system should be aware of potential forensic issues with all patients. With respect to what you have learned in this chapter, consider the following scenario and think about how you would address the issues that this nurse is faced with.

You are a nurse in a surgical unit in a large rural community hospital. You are on weekend call and are called in for an emergency surgical case late on a Saturday evening. Upon arrival, staff from the emergency department report that the patient, Karen, was brought in by ambulance after her boyfriend, James, called 911. He states that "Karen has not been feeling well for the past few weeks, must have gotten dizzy and fell down the steps" in their home. Among the surgical team are the surgeon, two nurses, a surgical technician, and others.

The team determines that Karen's injuries are life-threatening and therefore follow their emergency procedure for preparing the surgical suite for an urgent patient. The nurse questions whether the injuries are in fact a result of a fall down stairs. She sees discrepancies between James's description of events and the injuries. She asks the surgical team not to discard the patient's clothing and to allow her to quickly take photos of the injuries (there is a digital camera in the surgical suite). Her intuition is that Karen is a victim of violence, not of having fallen down the stairs. The surgeon in charge states that there is no time and that it is not "our job" to determine how Karen's injuries occurred. The team continues to prepare the patient and does not attend to the nurse's concerns. The patient goes into surgery, clothing is discarded, no photos are taken, and the only documentation of the nurse's concerns is noted in the patient's chart.

The nurse is frustrated and wonders what she can do in the future to help patients like this, if in fact Karen is a victim of violence rather than an accidental fall victim.

Some questions to consider as a nurse in this situation:

- What might you do as the nurse at this point to assure better forensic care in the future?

- How can you make a policy change within your hospital to establish precedent for taking forensic issues into consideration for all patients?

- How would you use current policies to support your concerns?

Think about what you have read in this chapter and how you might utilize what you know to establish better practice guidelines for all clinicians in your hospital regarding forensic patients. Who might you contact to voice your concerns? What information might you access in order to make your case for better forensic care? How would you use Joint Commission Standards to support your goals? How might you establish policies and procedures and then educate the staff regarding these policy changes? How would you interface with management to accomplish your goals?

Summary

What is most important for all nurses to know is that we must work together to provide the best care possible for all patients who have legal issues related to their care, whether they are sexual assault patients, child abuse victims, inmates, victims of fraud, victims of suspicious death, victims of healthcare malpractice, or victims of false accusations of healthcare malpractice.

Most importantly, all nurses must understand their role in forensic cases and that each of us can make a difference. The purpose of this book is to provide guidance for nurses in practice who have the ability to discern cases where the legal system may be involved in future litigation. Being an objective observer is paramount to good practice. The following chapters expand on this chapter by exploring specific issues in forensic nursing practice and by providing the generalist with techniques for forensic practice and practice guidelines in various areas of forensics.

Additional Resources

End Violence Against Women International (EVAWI): http://www.evawintl.org/

International Association of Forensic Nurses (IAFN): http://www.forensicnurses.org/

Office on Violence Against Women (OVW): http://www.justice.gov/ovw

References

American Academy of Forensic Sciences. (2010). Retrieved January 2015, from http://www.aafs.org

American Nurses Association. (2009). *Scope and standards of clinical nursing practice*. Silver Spring, MD: American Nurses Publishing.

Campbell, R., Townsend, S. M., Shaw, J., Karim, N., & Markowitz, J. (2014). Evaluating the legal impact of Sexual Assault Nurse Examiner programs: An empirically validated toolkit for practitioners. *J Forensic Nurs, 10*(4), 208–216. doi: 10.1097/JFN.0000000000000049

Centers for Disease Control and Prevention. (2010). Sexually transmitted diseases: Treatment guidelines Sexual Assault and STDs (pp. 1–80). *Morbidity and Mortality Weekly Report.*

Emergency Nurses Association. (2010). Position statement on forensic evidence collection.

Foresman-Capuzzi, J. (2014). CSI & U: Collection and preservation of evidence in the emergency department. *J Emerg Nurs, 40*(3), 229–236; quiz 294. doi: 10.1016/j.jen.2013.04.005

The global burden of disease: 2004 update. (2008). Geneva, Switzerland: World Health Organization.

Hammer, R. M., Moynihan, B., & Pagliaro, E. M. (Eds.). (2013). *Forensic nursing: A handbook for practice* (Vol. 1). Burlington, MA: Jones & Bartlett.

Holmes, D., & Jacob, J. D. (2012). Between care and punishment: The difficult coexistence of nursing care and prison culture. *Rech Soins Infirm* (111), 57–66.

Holmes, D., & Murray, S. J. (2011). Civilizing the 'Barbarian': A critical analysis of behaviour modification programmes in forensic psychiatry settings. *J Nurs Manag, 19*(3), 293–301. doi: 10.1111/j.1365-2834.2011.01207.x

Hufft, A. G. (2013). Correctional nursing. In R. M. Hammer, B. Moynihan, & E. M. Pagliaro (Eds.), *Forensic nursing: A handbook for practice* (Vol. 1, pp. 375–399). Burlington, MA: Jones & Bartlett.

Institute of Medicine. (2010). *The Future of Nursing: Leading Change, Advancing Health.* Washington, DC: The National Academies Press.

The Joint Commission. (2014). Revisions to deemed program requirements for hospitals Joint Commission Standard PC.01.02.09 on victims of abuse. Washington, DC: Futures Without Violence.

Lynch, V. A. (1990). Clinical forensic nursing: A descriptive study in role development. Master's thesis. University of Texas Health Science Center.

Lynch, V. A. (2013). Forensic nursing science. In R. M. Hammer, B. Moynihan, & E. M. Pagliaro (Eds.), *Forensic nursing: A handbook for practice* (Vol. 1, p. 518). Burlington, MA: Jones & Bartlett.

Lynch, V. A., & Duval, J. B. (2011). *Forensic nursing science* (2nd ed.). St. Louis, MO: Elsevier.

Magnusson, J. K., Joos, B., Pike, J. B., Janes, R., & Beerman, J. (2003). The history and evolution of legal nurse consulting. In P. W. Iyer (Ed.), *Legal nurse consulting: Principles and practice* (2nd ed., Vol. 1, pp. 145–164). New York, NY: CRC Press.

National Consensus Guidelines: On identifying and responding to domestic violence victimization in health care settings. (2004). San Francisco, CA: Family Violence Prevention Fund.

Sekula, L. K. (2005). The advance practice forensic nurse in the emergency department. *Topics in Emergency Medicine,* January/March, 27(1), 5–14.

Sekula, L. K., & Burgess, A. W. (Eds.). (2006). *Forensic and legal nursing* (Vol. 1). Boca Raton, FL: CRC Press.

Sekula, L. K., & Colbert, A. M. (2013). Forensic psychiatric nursing. In E. Varcarolis & M. B. Halter (Eds.), *Foundations of psychiatric mental health nursing* (7th ed., pp. 598–610). St. Louis, MO: Elsevier.

Sekula, L. K., Colbert, A. M., Zoucha, R., Amar, A. F., & Williams, J. (2012). Strengthening the science of forensic nursing through education and research. *Journal of Forensic Nursing, 8*(1), 1–2. doi: 10.1111/j.1939-3938.2012.01136.x; 10.1111/j.1939-3938.2012.01136.x

Winfrey, M. E., & Smith, A. R. (1999). The suspiciousness factor: Critical care nursing and forensics. *Critical Care Nursing Quarterly, 22*(1), 1–7.

World Health Organization (WHO). (2002). World report on violence and health: summary. Geneva, Switzerland: Author.

World Health Organization (WHO). (2008). The global burden of disease: 2004 update. Geneva, Switzerland: Author.

FORENSIC SCIENCE 101

Stephen Goux, MSN, RN, AFN-BC, SANE-A, SANE-P

KEY POINTS IN THIS CHAPTER

▪ When a nurse encounters a person who was involved in violence and crime, the nurse may also unknowingly encounter evidence that can be used by law enforcement to investigate the crime.

▪ An understanding of the processes regarding collection and analysis of evidence can be incorporated into the nurses' assessment practices and help to avoid contamination and degradation of samples.

▪ Care provided to individuals who experienced violence is enhanced by knowledge of the legal and ethical requirements of handling evidence.

The term *forensic science* can mean many different things to different people. With the influence of such TV programs as *CSI, Forensic Files,* and *Law and Order,* the public's perception of what forensic science is can be debated. Those who work in the field spend much of their time educating others on what the field actually entails and just how far this specialty has come since its development many years ago. The field of forensic science has advanced almost two-fold since its inception and continues to evolve. Without forensic science technology, the criminal justice system would be at a loss in how the legal process is conducted and carried out (Shipley & Arrigo, 2012).

The word *forensic* comes from the Latin word *forensis.* A relevant, contemporary definition of forensic is: relating to or dealing with the application of scientific knowledge to legal problems (forensic, n.d.). Any science used for the purposes of the law is considered a forensic science. Forensic science, sometimes referred to as *criminalistics,* applies the knowledge of science to the definition and enforcement of laws. Criminalistics is a branch of forensic science that is involved in the collection, analysis, and interpretation of physical evidence produced by criminal activity.

Forensic science embraces all branches of science and applies scientific techniques to the purpose of law. Originally all the techniques were borrowed from various scientific disciplines such as chemistry, medicine, biology, and photography. However, over the past several years, it has developed its own branches, which are more or less exclusive domains of forensic science. More recently, significant advances have been made in serology, voice analysis, odor analysis, and in studies relating to nose prints and ear patterns (Saferstein, 2013). Many different disciplines fall under the umbrella of forensic science.

The traditional forensic science disciplines are:

- Toxicology: The study of alcohol and drugs.

- Serology: Study of blood and other biological fluids.

- Questioned document examination: Examination of documents, handwriting comparison, study of inks, typewriter imprints, counterfeiting, etc.

- Forensic chemistry: The application of facts related to findings in chemistry to issues of civil and criminal law.

- Firearms identification and ballistics: Study of marks and striations on bullets.

- Hair and fiber analysis: Types of trace evidence that can be analyzed for classification as to origin of the hair or the fiber, or for contents such as use of drugs in hair analysis (Woods, 2006).

- Forensic pathology: That branch of natural science concerned with the causes and nature of disease processes, together with the anatomic and functional changes that occur in conjunction with them, and their application to medical-legal matters.

- Odontology: Study of bite marks and teeth structure.

The forensic science disciplines that are still emerging are:

- Disaster identification: Identifying bodies, cause of death, etc.

- Cheiloscopy: Analysis of lip prints.

- Forensic engineering: Investigation of materials, products, structures or components that fail or don't operate or function as intended and cause personal injury or damage to property, as well as accident reconstruction.

- Meteorology: Study of the impact of weather on a case.

- Blood spatter identification: The study of the patterns of blood stains that help identify the point of origin, relative positions of the victim and perpetrator at the time of bloodshed, mechanism that generated the bloodstain, etc. (Meyers, 2006).

- Voice print analysis: A graphic representation of a person's voice, showing the component frequencies as analyzed by a sound spectrograph (voiceprint; n.d.).

- Retinal scanning: Biometric technique that uses the unique patterns on a person's retina blood vessels for identification (e.g., for identification purposes).

▪ Forensic entomology: The study of insects related to cases where dead humans are found.

▪ Forensic anthropology: Concerned with the identification of human remains in a legal context.

History of Forensic Science

The idea of forensic science as a discipline and a career is barely 100 years old; however, the use of science in criminal investigations has been around since before the Roman Empire (Saferstein, 2011). It has only been within the last century that law enforcement agencies and the criminal justice system have come to rely so heavily on the use of scientific practices in criminal investigations. Until the mid-19th century, the use of science in investigations was discussed, but the appropriate application of scientific principles had not yet been fully implemented.

Throughout history, several examples of various pieces of evidence (which we would now call forensics) led to convictions or acquittals. During the 1800s, the application of scientific principles to criminal investigations accelerated. Clothing and vegetable grains could be used to place suspects at the scenes of crimes. The invention of the camera led to the use of photography to document and preserve crime scenes. Hydrogen peroxide was discovered to foam as it oxidized when it contacted hemoglobin. This demonstrated the ability to test for the presence of blood and was considered seminal in the study of serology.

These examples were all significant steps toward the development of forensic science as a discipline and included many forensic science pioneers. The independent works of Englishmen Henry Faulds and William Herschel, as well as American scientist Thomas Taylor, detailed the uniqueness of human fingerprints and their potential use in identifying people that led to the codification and standardization of accepted practices within forensic science. Dr. Edmond Locard, a French scientist and criminologist who had studied law and medicine, proposed the notion that "everything leaves a trace," a principle that prevails today in crime scene investigation. Locard's exchange principle put forth the idea that everything and everyone that enters a crime scene leaves some piece of evidence behind. Equally, everyone and everything takes some piece of the crime scene with them when they leave. Pursuant to Locard's initial work, the police department in Lyon, France, allowed him to work in its precinct, and thus, the world's first crime laboratory was built. The department provided him with a staff of two assistants to analyze evidence obtained from local crime scenes (Riley, 2005). The advancements of the 20th century were built largely upon the groundwork laid in the 19th century, refining techniques in the collection of and preservation of evidence and DNA analysis.

TYPES OF EVIDENCE

In forensic science, many different types of evidence can be collected and analyzed. Forensic evidence is collected at a crime scene, analyzed in a laboratory, and often presented in court. Each crime scene is unique, and each case presents its own challenges. Table 2.1 lists different types of forensic evidence.

TABLE 2.1 TYPES OF FORENSIC EVIDENCE

Type of Forensic Evidence	Example
DNA	Blood, saliva, semen, skin cells, tissue
Trace	Fibers, hairs
Toxicology	Blood, urine, tissue
Pathology	Bone, tissue, blood
Digital	Photographs, digital images, Internet sources
Impression and Pattern	Footprints, firearms, fingerprints
Controlled Substance	Narcotics, opioids
Anthropology and Dental	Bite marks, skeletal remains

Anytime forensic evidence is collected, the chain of custody must be followed (National Institute of Justice [NIJ], 2012c). The *chain of custody of evidence* is a record of every individual who has had physical possession of the evidence. Every time the evidence is opened from its collection container and the evidence seal is broken, or moved, there must be a log of that activity. Documentation is essential to maintaining the integrity of the chain of custody. Maintaining the chain of custody is necessary for any and all types of evidence. If laboratory analysis reveals that evidence was contaminated, or that there was a possibility of contamination at some point in the transfer of evidence, it may be necessary to identify all those who have handled that evidence. In collecting and processing evidence, the fewer people who handle that evidence, the better. There is less chance of contamination and a shorter chain of custody for court admissibility (NIJ, 2012c).

DNA EVIDENCE

One-tenth of a single percent of DNA (about 3 million bases) differs from one person to the next (NIJ, 2012a). Forensic scientists can use almost all of these variable regions to generate a DNA profile of an individual, utilizing samples from blood, hair, bone, and body tissues. Typically, in criminal cases, samples are gathered from crime-scene evidence and a suspect (Bevel & Gardner, 2012). DNA is then extracted and analyzed for the presence of a set of specific DNA markers. Simply put, if the sample profiles do not match, the suspect did not contribute the DNA at the crime scene. Physical evidence is any tangible object that can connect an offender to a crime scene. Biological evidence, which contains DNA, is a type of physical evidence. However, biological evidence is not always visible to the naked eye. DNA testing has expanded the types of useful biological evidence. Any and all biological evidence found at crime scenes can be subjected to DNA testing (NIJ, 2012a). Table 2.2 highlights types of evidence and the possible location where DNA can be found on the object (NIJ, n.d.).

TABLE 2.2 DNA EVIDENCE AND ITS SOURCES

Evidence Type	Possible Location of DNA	Source of DNA
Baseball bat or metal pipe	Handle, end	Sweat, skin, blood, tissue
Hat or mask	Inside brim area, inside mask	Sweat, hair, dandruff, skin cells
Eyeglasses	Nose piece, lens	Sweat, skin cells
Facial tissue, cotton swab	Surface area	Mucus, blood, sweat, semen, ear wax, skin cells
Clothing	Surface area	Blood, sweat, skin cells, semen, hair
Used cigarette	Cigarette butt	Saliva
Stamp or envelope	Licked area	Saliva
Tape or ligature	Inside/outside surface	Skin cells, sweat
Bottle, can, or glass	Sides, mouthpiece	Saliva, sweat, skin cells
Used condom	Inside/outside surface	Semen, vaginal and/or rectal fluid
Bite mark	Skin or clothing	Saliva
Fingernail	Scrapings	Blood, sweat, skin cells, tissue, semen

Several basic steps are performed during DNA testing regardless of the type of test being performed (NIJ, 2012b).

1. Isolate the DNA from an evidence sample that contains DNA of unknown origin. Isolate DNA from a sample (e.g., blood) from a known individual.

2. Process the DNA and obtain test results.

3. Determine the DNA test results (or types) from specific regions of the DNA.

4. Compare and interpret the test results from the unknown and known samples to determine whether the known individual is the source of the DNA or is included as a possible source of the DNA.

Each additional test at a previously untested locus (location or site) in the DNA provides an additional opportunity for the result of "exclusion" if the known individual being used for comparison is not the source of the DNA from an evidence sample of unknown origin. When a sufficient number of tests have been performed in which an individual cannot be excluded as the source of the DNA by any of the tests, the point is reached at which the tests have excluded virtually all of the world's population, and the unique identification of that individual as the source of the DNA has been accomplished (NIJ, 2012b).

Polymerase Chain Reaction
The evolution of DNA testing advanced significantly when Dr. Kary Mullis discovered that DNA could be copied in a laboratory setting (NIJ, 2012b). The copying process, known as *polymerase chain reaction* (PCR), uses an enzyme (polymerase) to replicate DNA regions. By repeating the copying process, a small number of DNA molecules can be reliably increased up to billions within a certain time frame. PCR analysis requires only a microscopic quantity of DNA, which allows the laboratory to analyze highly degraded evidence for DNA. Due to the sensitive PCR technique, in which the process replicates any and all of the DNA contained in an evidence sample, greater attention to contamination issues are necessary when identifying, collecting, and preserving DNA evidence. All of these factors are important when evaluating unsolved cases in which evidence might have been improperly collected or stored over time (Butler, 2012).

Short Tandem Repeat Technology and CODIS
Short tandem repeat (STR) technology is a forensic analysis technique that evaluates specific loci found on nuclear DNA. The variable nature of the STR regions that are analyzed for forensic testing increases the discrimination between one DNA profile and another (NIJ, 2012b). The Federal Bureau of Investigation (FBI) has chosen 13 specific STR loci to serve as the standard for the Combined DNA Index System (CODIS). CODIS is a software platform that blends forensic science

and computer technology. The FBI uses it to "develop, provide, and support the CODIS Program to federal, state, and local crime laboratories in the United States and selected international law enforcement crime laboratories to foster the exchange and comparison of forensic DNA evidence from violent crime investigations" (FBI, 2010). The purpose of establishing a core set of STR loci is to ensure that all forensic laboratories can establish uniform DNA databases and, most importantly, share valuable forensic information. In order to utilize the CODIS index, DNA profiles must be generated using STR technology and the specific 13 core STR loci selected by the FBI (NIJ, 2012b).

Genetic Markers

Scientists have identified several genetic markers on the Y-chromosome that can be used in forensic science applications. Y-chromosome markers target only the male fraction of a biological sample. Using this technique can therefore be very valuable if the laboratory detects complex combinations (multiple male contributors) within a biological evidence sample (NIJ, 2012b). Because the Y-chromosome is transmitted directly from a father to all of his male offspring, it can also be used to trace family relationships among male family members. Advancements in Y-chromosome testing could eventually eliminate the need for laboratories to extract and separate semen and vaginal cells (from a vaginal swab of a sexual assault kit) prior to analysis. This would lead to an increase in sexual assault kit analysis and a decrease in the backlog of kit testing that many cities currently face around the country. By testing sexual assault kits with a "male specific verification" analysis technique (SRY Gene Screening Kit), a laboratory can more rapidly process rape kits. Instead of taking several hours to manually examine slides, attempting to identify sperm, many cases can be analyzed simultaneously, using a gene sequencer to identify only Y-chromosome data (Johnson, Peterson, Sommers, & Baskin, 2012).

Mitochondrial DNA

Mitochondrial DNA (mtDNA) analysis allows forensic laboratories to develop DNA profiles from evidence that may not be suitable for PCR or STR analysis. Whereas those techniques analyze DNA extracted from the nucleus of a cell, mtDNA technology analyzes DNA found in a different part of the cell, the mitochondrion (NIJ, 2012b). Remains and evidence lacking nucleated cells (e.g., hair shafts, bones, and teeth) that are unusable for PCR and STR testing may yield results when mtDNA analysis is performed. Mitochondrial DNA testing can be useful in the investigation of an unsolved case or one where new DNA has been recovered but that DNA was improperly stored for a long period of time. It is important to note that all maternal relatives (e.g., a person's mother or maternal grandmother) have identical mtDNA. Therefore, forensic scientists can analyze and compare unidentified remains to the mtDNA profile of any maternal relative for the purpose of assisting missing persons or unidentified remains investigations.

Trace Evidence

Fibers, hair, soil, wood, gunshot residue, and pollen are several examples of trace evidence that may be transferred among people, objects, or the environment during a crime. When Locard developed his exchange principle, it was primarily trace evidence that he had in mind. Investigators can potentially link a suspect and a victim to a mutual location through trace evidence. For example, a fiber sample obtained from a deceased victim can be identified through trace-evidence analysis as originating from the vehicle carpet of the suspected perpetrator. The analysis of the fiber evidence can help establish if the victim and suspect were in the same area (Blackledge, 2007).

Toxicology Evidence

Forensic toxicology is the analysis of biological samples for the presence of toxins, including drugs and alcohol. The toxicology report can provide key information as to the type of substances present in an individual and if the amount of those substances is consistent with a therapeutic dosage or is above an unsafe level. These results can be used to make determinations when establishing whether a substance had a potential effect on an individual's death, illness, or mental or physical impairment. Forensic toxicology is a continually advancing discipline.

New drugs are always being developed, which creates a constant need to design novel approaches for their detection. Toxicology analysis is most commonly used when determining if a driver was impaired during an automobile accident (James, Nordby, & Bell, 2009).

PATHOLOGY EVIDENCE

Human remains are treated as a separate and unique type of forensic evidence and analysis. When an autopsy of the remains is completed, the cause and manner of any death that was possibly violent, unusual, or untimely can be determined. A forensic pathologist will conduct a post-mortem examination of the remains and consider death scene findings. The pathologist will also review the individual's medical history to help determine if the death was natural, accidental, or criminal. During the exam, the pathologist may recover critical evidence such as a bullet, which may help to determine the cause and manner of death. If a wound pattern is identified, it can possibly be matched to a specific weapon in deaths involving firearms and other projectiles (Maio & Maio, 2001).

DIGITAL EVIDENCE

Computers are used for committing crime and fraud, and, thanks to the science of digital evidence forensics, law enforcement can now use computers to fight crime (NIJ, 2010). Digital evidence is information stored or transmitted in binary form. It can be found on computer hard drives, mobile phones, CDs, DVDs, flash drives, and cloud storage. Digital evidence is commonly associated with electronic crime, such as child pornography or credit card fraud (Digital Evidence and Forensics, 2010). Digital evidence is now used to prosecute all types of crimes, not just cyber crimes. In an effort to fight digital crime and to collect relevant digital evidence for all crimes, law enforcement agencies are incorporating the collection and analysis of digital evidence, also known as *computer forensics,* into their programs (James, Nordby, & Bell, 2009).

IMPRESSION AND PATTERN EVIDENCE

Impression evidence is created when two objects come in contact with enough force to cause an "impression." Impression evidence is either two-dimensional, (e.g., fingerprints) or three-dimensional (e.g., marks on a bullet caused by the barrel of a firearm).

Pattern evidence may be additional identifiable information found within an impression. As an example, a forensic examiner will compare shoe print evidence with several shoe-sole patterns to identify a particular brand, model, or size. If a shoe is recovered from a suspect that matches this initial pattern, the examiner can also identify unique characteristics that are common between the shoe and the shoe print, which can include wear, cuts, or nicks (James, Nordby, & Bell, 2009).

CONTROLLED SUBSTANCE EVIDENCE

Controlled substances are chemicals that have a legally recognized potential for abuse (NIJ, 2014a). They include "street drugs" such as heroin or ecstasy and prescription drugs such as oxycodone and other pain medications. Detecting and identifying controlled substances is a critical step in law enforcement's fight against drug-related crime and violence. Controlled substances present law enforcement and criminal justice professionals with many problems. New designer drugs emerge regularly, requiring crime laboratories to develop new analytical techniques and spend more time on analysis (NIJ, 2014a). Many drugs are similar in appearance and properties, creating a high degree of difficulty in distinguishing their exact identity. This is where regional poison control centers can assist law enforcement in identifying and characterizing certain drugs (Li, 2008).

ANTHROPOLOGY AND DENTAL EVIDENCE

Forensic anthropologists examine "skeletonized" or otherwise compromised human remains to assess age, gender, height, and ancestry (NIJ, 2014b). Forensic anthropologists can also identify injuries and estimate time of death. Examination of these remains may give information that can help investigators identify a victim from a missing person case and/or open death investigation. Forensic dentists, or odontologists, examine the development, anatomy, and any restorative dental corrections of the teeth, such as fillings, to make a comparative identification of a person (NIJ, 2014b). Bones and teeth are the most durable parts of the human body and may be the only recognizable remains in cases of decomposition, fire scenes, or mass fatalities, and they can be used to identify an individual in such cases (Bush, 2011).

ETHICS AND FORENSIC SCIENCE

Unfortunately, forensic science does not always guarantee the establishment of valid results in the end. The risk begins at the scene of the crime, where there is the possibility of evidence destruction or mishandling (Wecht & Rago, 2006). At the lab, evidence can be subject to contamination through poor testing methods, excess consumption, mislabeling, and even loss and/or destruction. After the analysis has been performed, those analyzing the evidence must then report on their findings. This is still a human reporting system and therefore at risk of human error (Dutelle, 2011).

Lab personnel must be accurate and honest when reporting their analysis results, even if errors have occurred. Errors, omissions, or fraudulent testimonies or reports are of particular concern due to the fact that forensic evidence that is testified to or reported on by "forensic science experts" is routinely given more weight and consideration by jurors. As a result, false testimony, inflated statistics, and laboratory fraud have led to wrongful conviction in many criminal cases, due to jurors' trust in the system (Dutelle, 2011).

There exists no single ethical code that applies to all disciplines of forensic science (Constantino & Crane, 2013). Two primary organizations have developed ethical codes relating to forensic testimony and the presentation of forensic analyses in court:

▪ **American Board of Criminalistics (ABC):** The ABC Code of Ethics requires all certified members to ensure that any opinions rendered with regard to their analyses are done so "only to the extent justified" by the evidence in question, and to also ensure that the testimony given is presented "in a clear, straightforward manner" that in no way misrepresents or extends "themselves beyond their field of competence." Testimony should be given "in such a manner so that the results are not misinterpreted" (ABC, 2010).

- **American Academy of Forensic Sciences (AAFS):** The AAFS Code states that members shall not "materially misrepresent data or scientific principles upon which his or her conclusion or professional opinion is based" (AAFS, 2010, Section 1C).

  An addition to the AAFS Code is a section that lists "Guidelines" for members and analysts. Under this section, it lists that analysts should "adopt good forensic practice guidelines, and that unlike attorneys, forensic scientists are not adversaries. Every reasonable effort should be made to ensure that others (including attorneys) do not distort the forensic scientist's opinions" (AAFS, 2010).

Garrett and Neufeld (2009) presented in the *Virginia Law Review* the first study undertaken to explore the relationship between forensic testimony and convictions ultimately leading to exonerations based upon post-conviction DNA analysis. The study sought out court transcripts and results for the 156 exonerees who had been identified at that time, with ultimately 137 being located for review. The testimony that was reviewed for the 137 exonerees primarily involved serological analysis testimony (100 cases) and testimony regarding microscopic hair comparison (65 cases), due to the majority of the cases being sexual assaults (Dutelle, 2011). Of those reviewed for this study, 82 of the cases, or approximately 60%, included invalid forensic testimony by prosecution experts, or "testimony with conclusions misstating empirical data or wholly unsupported by empirical data" (Garrett & Neufield, 2009, p. 15). According to the article, two basic categories of invalid scientific testimony were recurring themes within the cases reviewed, "the misuse of empirical population data, and conclusions regarding the probative value of evidence in the absence of empirical data" (Garrett & Neufield, 2009, p. 22).

Blood is the most common, and perhaps most important, form of evidence in forensic science today. Its presence will link a suspect and victim to one another and to the scene of the crime. Bloodstain patterns tell a great deal about position and movement during an attack, who struck whom first, in what manner, and how many times. In forensic cases, blood has always been considered the gold standard of evidence, and the potential exists for individualized blood typing. Forensic serologists can provide testimony with strong probability estimates linking a single individual, and that individual only, to a bloodstain at the scene of a crime.

CASE STUDY: THE BASICS OF FORENSIC SCIENCE

In this chapter, you reviewed the basics of forensic science and how science can impact a forensic case. As a nurse you should now have some understanding of how your practice can be impacted by forensic science. As you review the following case study, think about how the issues discussed can affect your practice.

You are a nurse practicing in an emergency department (ED). Kara, 32 years old, is admitted with stab wounds in the torso. She says that her boyfriend became violent and attacked her. Police restrained him outside the ED after he tried to enter the ED yelling that Kara is "crazy and says I tried to kill her...." Kara is bleeding profusely and will be taken to the surgical suite shortly. What, if anything, can the ED nurse do to help in this case?

Given the responsibilities of the ED nurse, what impact can her care have on the outcome of the case?

- How and what evidence can be collected that may be used in the court case should this case go to trial? Keep in mind that any blood found on her clothing may include the attacker's blood also. Think of the impact on the case if this should happen.

- What documentation will be most important from the perspective of the admitting nurse?

- What forensic principles need to be considered as the nurse cares for Kara during the intake in the ED?

SUMMARY

The science of forensics has evolved and will continue to do so exponentially in the years to come. Whether you are a forensic scientist or nurse, forensic science plays a large part of how you interpret and analyze different aspects of the criminal justice system (Sekula & Burgess, 2006). There is no doubt much has been learned from the science discovered, with new discoveries almost daily. It is imperative that the scientific community continues to uncover new methods while still relying on previous techniques in order to continue to grow in the scientific realm.

Forensic science is constantly changing, but hopefully this introduction to the field helps you understand how your work as a nurse fits into the analysis of evidence.

REFERENCES

American Academy of Forensic Sciences (AAFS). (2010). AAFS bylaws: Article II: Code of ethics and conduct. Retrieved from http://www.aafs.org/about-aafs/aafs-bylaws/article-ii-code-of-ethics-and-conduct/

American Board of Criminalistics (ABC). (2010). Rules of professional conduct. Retrieved from http://www.criminalistics.com/uploads/3/2/3/3/32334973/form_09-0001f_abc_rules_of_professional_conduct.pdf

Bevel, T., & Gardner, R. (2012). *Bloodstain pattern analysis with an introduction to crime scene reconstruction* (3rd ed.). Hoboken, NJ: Taylor and Francis.

Blackledge, R. (2007). *Forensic analysis on the cutting edge: New methods for trace evidence analysis.* Hoboken, NJ: John Wiley & Sons.

Bush, M. A. (2011). Forensic dentistry and bitemark analysis: Sound science or junk science? *Journal of The American Dental Association (JADA), 142*(9), 997–999.

Butler, J. (2012). *Advanced topics in forensic DNA typing methodology.* San Diego, CA: Elsevier Academic Press.

Constantino, R., & Crane, P. (2013). *Forensic nursing: Evidence-based principles and practice.* Philadelphia, PA: F. A. Davis Company.

Dutelle, A. (2011). *Ethics for the public service professional.* Boca Raton, FL: CRC Press.

Federal Bureau of Investigation (FBI). (2010). Combined DNA Index System (CODIS). Retrieved from http://www.fbi.gov/about-us/lab/biometric-analysis/codis

forensic. (n.d.). In Merriam-Webster online. Retrieved from http://www.merriam-webster.com/dictionary/forensic

Garrett, B. L., & Neufeld, P. J. (2009). Invalid forensic science testimony and wrongful convictions. *Virginia Law Review, 95*(1). Retrieved from http://ssrn.com/abstract=1354604

James, S., Nordby, J., & Bell, S. (Eds.). (2009). *Forensic science: An introduction to scientific and investigative techniques* (3rd ed.). Boca Raton, FL: CRC Press/Taylor & Francis.

Johnson, D., Peterson, J., Sommers, I., & Baskin, D. (2012). Use of forensic science in investigating crimes of sexual violence: Contrasting its theoretical potential with empirical realities. *Violence Against Women, 18*(2), 193–222. doi: 10.1177/1077801212440157

Li, R. (2008). *Forensic biology: Identification and DNA analysis of biological evidence*. Boca Raton, FL: CRC Press/Taylor & Francis.

Lynch, V., & Duval, J. (2011). *Forensic nursing science* (2nd ed.). St. Louis, MO: Mosby/Elsevier.

Maio, V., & Maio, D. (2001). *Forensic pathology* (2nd ed.). Boca Raton, FL: CRC Press/Taylor & Francis.

Meyers, T. C. (2006). Serology. In C. H. Wecht & J. T. Rago (Eds.), *Forensic science and law: Investigative applications in criminal, civil, and family justice* (pp. 409–417). New York, NY: CRC Press/Taylor & Francis.

National Institute of Justice (NIJ). (n.d.). What every law enforcement officer should know about DNA evidence brochure (#BC 000614). Washington, DC: Author.

National Institute of Justice (NIJ). (2010). Digital evidence and forensics. Retrieved from http://www.nij.gov/topics/forensics/evidence/digital/Pages/welcome.aspx

National Institute of Justice (NIJ). (2012a). DNA evidence basics. Retrieved from http://www.nij.gov/topics/forensics/evidence/dna/basics/Pages/welcome.aspx

National Institute of Justice (NIJ). (2012b). DNA evidence: Basics of analyzing. Retrieved from http://nij.gov/topics/forensics/evidence/dna/basics/pages/analyzing.aspx

National Institute of Justice (NIJ). (2012c). Evidence: Basics of identifying, gathering and transporting. Retrieved from http://nij.gov/topics/forensics/evidence/dna/basics/pages/identifying-to-transporting.aspx

National Institute of Justice (NIJ). (2014a). Controlled substances. Retrieved from http://nij.gov/topics/forensics/evidence/controlled-substances/Pages/welcome.aspx

National Institute of Justice (NIJ). (2014b). Forensic anthropology and forensic dentistry. Retrieved from http://nij.gov/topics/forensics/evidence/anthropology/pages/welcome.aspx

Riley, D. E. (2005). DNA testing: An introduction for non-scientists an illustrated explanation. *Scientific Testimony An Online Journal*. Retrieved from http://www.scientific.org/tutorials/articles/riley/riley.html

Saferstein, R. (2011). *Criminalistics: An introduction to forensic science* (10th ed.). Upper Saddle River, NJ: Prentice Hall.

Saferstein, R. (2013). *Forensic science: From the crime scene to the crime lab* (2nd ed.). Boston, MA: Pearson/Prentice Hall.

Sekula, L. K., & Burgess, A. W. (Eds.). (2006). *Forensic and legal nursing* (Vol. 1). Boca Raton, FL: CRC Press.

Shipley, S., & Arrigo, B. (2012). *Introduction to forensic psychology: Court, law enforcement, and correctional practices* (3rd ed.). San Diego, CA: Academic Press/Elsevier.

voiceprint (n.d.). Retrieved July 04, 2015. Dictionary.com Unabridged.

Wecht, C., & Rago, J. (Eds.). (2006). *Forensic science and law: Investigative applications in criminal, civil, and family justice.* Boca Raton, FL: CRC Press/Taylor & Francis.

Woods, P. (2006). Trace evidence examination. In C. H. Wecht & J. T. Rago (Eds.), *Forensic science and law: Investigative applications in criminal, civil, and family justice* (pp. 323–331). New York, NY: CRC Press/Taylor & Francis.

Neurobiology of Trauma

Julie Valentine, MS, RN, CNE, SANE-A; Linda Mabey, DNP, APRN, PMHCNS; and Leslie Miles, DNP, APRN, PMHNP

"Traumatic stress has a broad range of effects on brain function and structure, as well as on neuropsychological components of memory."
(Bremner, 2006, p. 455)

Key Points in This Chapter

- The neurobiology of trauma can affect the functioning of the brain with lasting consequences.

- The body's hormonal response to trauma affects the encoding of memory.

- Acute stress disorder (ASD) can result following trauma and can develop into post-traumatic stress disorder (PTSD) if symptoms last for more than 1 month.

- Trauma can cause immediate symptoms, such as tonic immobility and dissociation, and may lead to chronic symptoms of depression and anxiety.

- Exposure to trauma can cause physical health problems.

- Evidence-based psychotherapy treatment options following traumatic exposure are available.

- Providing compassionate, nonjudgmental care to victims of trauma helps their healing process.

Nurses work with many individuals who have suffered trauma as well as those who have inflicted trauma on others. Often, those who perpetrate crimes have been victims of trauma themselves. It is important to understand what occurs physiologically to the person who has experienced trauma and its aftermath. This chapter discusses the neurobiology of trauma, the repercussions of experiencing trauma, and interventions to improve the lives and functioning of traumatized individuals.

DEFINING TRAUMA

Trauma can be defined in a variety of ways, including bodily injury, a catastrophic occurrence, and psychological and physiological reactions to an overwhelmingly negative event. For the purposes of this chapter, *trauma* refers to an actual or threatened event that begins with the stress response but continues to negatively impact psychological and physiological functioning.

Exposure to traumatic events is common in the United States:

- The seminal National Comorbidity Study (NCS) reported that 60% of men and 51% of women experienced a traumatic event in their lifetime (Kessler, Sonnega, Bromet, Hughes, & Nelson, 1995).

- The most frequently encountered traumas involve a life-threatening accident, a natural disaster, or witnessing a traumatic event that happens to someone else.

- Over half of the individuals who experienced trauma reported more than one type of traumatic exposure.

Post-traumatic stress disorder (PTSD) is a mental disorder frequently associated with exposure to trauma. Although not all individuals exposed to traumatic events develop PTSD, a sizable proportion do, about 29% in the NCS sample. Of the various kinds of traumatic exposure surveyed by the NCS, individuals who faced assault, physical or sexual, were the most likely to develop PTSD (Kessler et al., 1995). Rape, a particularly violent form of assault, is a potent risk factor for PTSD (Ballenger et al., 2000; Tjaden & Thoennes, 2006). The higher incidence of rape and interpersonal violence in women may contribute to the higher prevalence of PTSD in women (American Psychiatric Association [APA], 2013).

Four neurobehavioral symptom clusters are characteristic of PTSD:

- Intrusive symptoms, including distressing memories and dreams

- Avoidance of reminders of the trauma

- Hyperarousal

- Negative alterations in cognition and mood

In addition, sufferers often experience flashbacks of the event, nightmares, increased startle reflexes, and emotional numbing. These symptoms are associated with "high levels of social, occupational, and physical disability, as well as considerable economic costs and high levels of medical utilization" (APA, 2013, p. 278). If individuals develop PTSD from trauma exposure, they are at high risk for developing an array of additional mental disorders, including depression, bipolar disorder, anxiety disorders, and substance disorders (APA, 2013).

DIAGNOSING TRAUMA'S EFFECT ON THE BRAIN

The ability to evaluate the effects of trauma has expanded in the past two decades. Prior to the 1990s, the impact of trauma could only be detected by observing the behaviors and psychological distress that resulted from it. Functional magnetic resonance imaging (fMRI) and positron emissions tomography (PET) now allow scientists to study what happens in the brain in response to trauma. Although individuals will have differing reactions and consequences from trauma, all responses are generated by brain activity. PET scans and fMRIs map the activity and brain circuitry involved in the central nervous system's traumatic response.

A nurse who is caring for a patient who has experienced significant trauma should remember that people are not only shaped by a lifetime of experiences (who they are) but also acutely impacted by the effect the current trauma has on their brain functioning (what has happened to them). This awareness helps the nurse accept each patient as a unique person doing the best he or she can to manage his or her distress.

The following sections explore various neurobiological factors that influence an individual's response to trauma, as well as how the brain reacts to traumatic events.

HOW GENES AND ENVIRONMENT INFLUENCE TRAUMA

In the normal day-to-day course of events, the brain processes experiences and retains information that is important to ensure not only survival but also growth and development as human beings. A significant amount of the information that contributes to the survival and development of human beings is transmitted through the collective human genome. In the process of transcription and translation, genes control the production of amino acids, the protein building blocks essential to human life.

It is beyond the scope of this chapter to discuss in detail how genes are constructed and function. However, it is important to know that gene expression—whether a gene is "turned on" to produce its amino acid product or "turned off" to not produce its product —is not a one-way process of genetic inheritance. Rather, unique personal experiences also influence how individual genes are expressed. How a person responds to trauma is not dependent upon a linear culmination of inherited factors, temperament, personality, and environmental influence; it is contingent upon the interaction of multiple environmental and genetic factors. For example, recent research examined how specific inherited forms of the serotonin transporter and corticotropin-releasing hormone receptor genes combined with a history of early childhood adversity to produce a greater susceptibility to depression when adults are faced with acute stress (Starr, Hammen, Conway, Raposa, & Brennan, 2014). Serotonin and cortisol are important players in mood and stress regulation, and a particular form—or allele—of their transporter genes affects their function negatively. Traumatic childhood experiences do not always produce depression in adults who face acute stress. A genetic vulnerability in the serotonin and cortisol systems appears to combine with two environmental insults, childhood adversity and adult stress, to confer a susceptibility to depression. Although not all stress can be classified as trauma, all trauma involves stress.

How Trauma Affects Brain Development

The human brain develops in an orderly sequence over time and is not mature until early adulthood. Even then, the brain remains quite "plastic"; that is, new connections between nerve cells continue to develop throughout life. This is both a blessing and a curse. It is a blessing because if the brain suffers a physical injury, such as a stroke, the brain can recruit undamaged areas to help the individual regain many functions that may have been lost due to the brain injury. It is a curse in the sense that when a trauma occurs, the individual may have the experience "etched" into his or her brain without psychological or physiological resolution. When this occurs, the experience is replayed, including all of its sensory aspects, when triggers ignite the trauma system. The same memory systems that help a person survive now turn against the person.

The brain develops in a bottom-up direction, with reptilian brain being the most primitive. Located in the brainstem, this is the part of the brain that regulates basic bodily functions, such as breathing, eating, and sleeping. Close in proximity to the reptilian brain is the limbic system. The *limbic system* is a series of structures whose functions include alerting us to danger; interpreting stimuli as frightening or fun, motivating or boring; as well as memory encoding. Together the reptilian brain and limbic system constitute what trauma specialist Bessel van der Kolk refers to as the "emotional brain" (2014, p. 57).

How the Limbic System and the Amygdala Contribute to Trauma

Certainly not all stress is a result of trauma. However, the stress response is an important initial reaction that can be triggered by a traumatic event. The limbic system is particularly important in how we respond to our environment and is constantly changing in response to internal and environmental stimuli, including threat. Yesterday you may have had no reaction to a picture of an alligator. However, after you encountered one on the golf course in Florida today, the same picture may now elicit sheer panic. This reaction is the result of a cascade of brain activity, including the activation of an almond-shaped limbic structure called the *amygdala*. It is part of the body's alert system and is stimulated when something noteworthy in the environment triggers its response. In a sense, the amygdala says, "I need to remember this!" Figure 3.1 depicts a model of the brain.

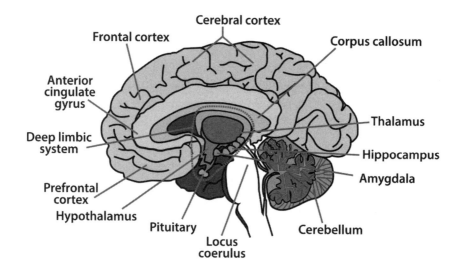

FIGURE 3.1 A DEPICTION OF A BRAIN MODEL.

The amygdala fires whether the experience is exquisitely lovely or decidedly dreadful and sets the process of encoding the memory in motion. Its firing can occur even before the brain is consciously aware of the significance of the stimulus. For example, when you startle because you see something in your path, your amygdala has sent the alert that the object may be a threat. A moment later, your frontal cortex, whose job is to evaluate and make reasoned judgments, sends the message back to the amygdala that "it is just a stick," and the amygdala ceases its threat alert. The experience of trauma can "over-sensitize" the amygdala, causing it to fire alert responses when there is no current danger, but instead activating memory traces of past trauma, often somatic or sensory in nature. This occurs because trauma memories are not stored in a discrete area of the brain but are encoded into neural networks connecting various emotions, body sensations, and cognitions associated with particular memories.

In the complex process of memory encoding, the amygdala plays a significant role, as do the hippocampus, hypothalamus, and anterior cingulate (Wheeler, 2014). The hippocampus is critical in inhibiting the amygdala, forming distinct memories and constructing the personal narrative that forms the autobiographical sense of self. The hypothalamus functions as a type of command center and exerts its influence through the hypothalamic-pituitary axis (HPA). It interacts with the amygdala and the endocrine system. A signal from the amygdala brings the hypothalamus on board to play the critical role of regulating the body's response, including blood pressure, pulse, and glucose availability. Additionally, the hypothalamus stimulates the release of cortisol through its discharge of corticotropin-releasing hormone (CRH). This hormone activates the pituitary gland to release cortisol from the adrenal glands. Cortisol stimulates glycogenolysis, releasing the glucose needed to respond to a threat.

Many of the mental and physical health problems associated with PTSD are in response to the overstimulation of the hypothalamic-pituitary axis (Wheeler, 2014). The anterior cingulate is involved not only in the regulation of the autonomic and neuroendocrine systems but also in the cognitive and emotional responses to stimuli. As explained by Wheeler, "This structure helps decide which emotional information to pay attention to and assists in processing emotion arising from the limbic system by recruiting other areas of the cortex to respond to emotions" (2014, p. 71). Although the limbic system is the key player in a person's response to stress and trauma, other brain structures, including the cerebellum, locus coeruleus, cerebral cortex, orbital medial prefrontal cortex, insula, corpus callosum, and right and left hemispheres, are also involved. In essence, trauma impacts the entire brain.

Understanding the Psychological and Physical Effects of Trauma

The majority of individuals do not develop PTSD following trauma, but experience short-term reactions. Time-limited trauma responses include:

- **Acute stress reaction:** An acute stress reaction occurs up to 48 hours after trauma exposure and may include symptoms such as nightmares, anxiety, aggression, and mood disturbances (Bryant, Friedman, Spiegel, Ursano, & Strain, 2011).

- **Acute Stress Disorder:** If the individual's symptoms are severe and remain after 2 days, the person may be experiencing Acute Stress Disorder (ASD).

ASD can develop from witnessing, directly experiencing, or even hearing about a trauma. First responders, including firefighters, police, and healthcare workers, are vulnerable to this disorder due to their job exposure to trauma. Recurrent and intrusive memories of the event, disturbing dreams, flashbacks, sleep disturbances, exaggerated startle response, and feeling "unreal" about one's environment or self are common manifestations of ASD. Individuals with ASD are often unable to recall aspects of the trauma.

ASD is a result of the same neurobiological cascade as PTSD, but in ASD the disorder is temporary and resolves within a month of the traumatic exposure. If ASD symptoms last for more than 1 month, the diagnosis changes to PTSD (APA, 2013). Approximately half of trauma survivors with ASD develop PTSD (Bryant, 2010).

It is important for nurses to understand and remember that there are no right or wrong reactions to trauma, as there is significant variability in behaviors. Some patients cry uncontrollably while others may become non-responsive or emotionally labile. During trauma, a hormonal flood is released, triggering the fight, flight, or freeze response. While some individuals fight or flee during trauma, others freeze, a response known as tonic immobility. Sexual assault victims often experience *tonic immobility,* causing an inability to run, fight, or yell (Campbell,

2012). Tonic immobility can be triggered when an individual experiences a terrifying, traumatic situation resulting in extreme fear (Abrams, Carleton, Taylor, & Asmundson, 2009; Campbell, 2012). Nurses should reassure patients who have experienced tonic immobility that their freezing or immobility reactions were normal, because many individuals blame themselves for not reacting to the trauma by taking action. The hormonal response to acute trauma may also result in peri-traumatic feelings of detachment, decreased awareness, hyper-awareness, or memory loss. Nurses must adopt a nonjudgmental attitude toward how patients respond to trauma, recognizing that trauma response is highly variable.

Exposure to trauma often results in physical manifestations. A large epidemiological study, the Adverse Childhood Experiences study (ACE), demonstrated that adult health outcomes were negatively affected by childhood trauma in a dose-dependent relationship; the more types of traumatic childhood events experienced, the more negative physical health outcomes reported by adults. The negative health outcomes included increased rates of cancer, liver disease, heart disease, and lung disease (Felitti et al., 1998). The ACE study findings have been replicated (Anda et al., 2006). More recently, Sledjeski, Speisman, and Dierker (2008) explored the relationship among PTSD, number of lifetime traumatic experiences, and adverse health outcomes. They found that the more traumatic events a person experienced, the more likely the individual was to self-report chronic medical problems, including chronic pain; cardiovascular, neurologic, and respiratory conditions; as well as diabetes, cancer, and ulcers.

The burden of accruing traumatic experiences shapes the function and structure of the central nervous system. Individuals, including children, who experience repeated trauma have a brain default setting of fear and distrust that plays out in many relationships, including with healthcare providers (van der Kolk, 2014). Children who have suffered serious abuse and neglect display a predictable pattern of behaviors, including the inability to regulate emotions, difficulty concentrating, and challenges in getting along well with others. The flood of stress hormones experienced by children facing multiple adversities is also associated with physical symptoms of headaches, sleep disturbances, self-harm, unexplained pain, and oversensitivity to touch or sound (van der Kolk, 2014).

COLLABORATIVE INTERVENTIONS FOLLOWING ACUTE TRAUMA

In the immediate aftermath of a trauma, primary attention should be on the physical and psychological safety of the patient.

First and foremost, the patient should be in a safe location where no further trauma can occur and basic physiological needs are met. Tell the patient that she is safe. Assessment of physical injuries and necessary medical care are priority interventions.

Following meeting basic needs and physical care, it is vitally important to address the psychological needs of the traumatized patient. During and after a traumatic event, individuals feel a loss of control. Help patients regain feelings of control by informing them of what will happen next and providing choices in their care. This helps patients feel an increased sense of control and aids in establishing a therapeutic relationship. Strive to establish a caring, compassionate relationship with traumatized patients without passing judgment on their choices or experiences. Fehler-Cabral, Campbell, and Patterson (2011) found that when nurses expressed compassion, believed victims, explained care, and provided choices to victims of sexual assault, the victims reported that the nurses' actions helped in their emotional recovery from the trauma.

To further instill a feeling of control in victimized patients, ask them permission before touching their bodies. Avoid the temptation to provide comforting touch unless the patient grants permission. It is best to ask as few questions as possible of patients immediately following trauma, as retelling the story may cause re-traumatization. Only ask necessary questions to guide healthcare delivery. Additionally, they may have impaired memory of the traumatic event, especially if it is a recent trauma. When individuals initially recount a traumatic experience, it is often in an emotionless and non-sequential way (Herman, 1997). The passage of time helps to solidify memories and ascribe feelings to the experiences (Campbell, 2012; Herman, 1997).

After establishing an atmosphere of safety and trust with the patient, complete a thorough assessment, noting the presence of the following symptoms (Veterans Health Administration [VHA]/Department of Defense [DoD], 2010):

- Physical (exhaustion, hyperarousal, somatic complaints)

- Emotional (anxiety, depression, guilt, hopelessness)

- Cognitive (amnesia, dissociation, hypervigilance, paranoia)

- Behavioral (avoidance, problematic substance use)

All trauma victims should be assessed for suicidal thoughts, self-harm, ASD, and PTSD from previous traumas. Feelings of guilt are highly prevalent in victims of trauma, especially in cases of sexual assault and interpersonal violence. Openly express to patients that they hold no responsibility for the actions of others; instead, they need to understand that they are victims of a crime. Support systems and coping resources should always be explored with patients. Hospitalization may be necessary if a victim is suicidal, psychotic, or unable to provide self-care.

TREATMENT OPTIONS

There are a variety of psychotherapy treatment options for traumatized individuals, including individual psychotherapy, group therapy, and support groups. It is important to recognize that treatment may also be required by significant others of a trauma victim, because they may experience secondary victimization. Different types of evidence-based treatment options are listed in Table 3.1. The goal of treatment is for the traumatized individuals to return to their previous or higher level of functioning.

TABLE 3.1 EVIDENCE-BASED TREATMENT OPTIONS

Type of Therapy	Brief Description of Therapy	Where to Find More Information
Trauma Focused-Cognitive Behavioral Therapy (TF-CBT)	Focus on altering trauma-related beliefs and behaviors. Teaches relaxation and breathing skills. Recommended for ASD treatment (Roberts, Kitchiner, Kenardy, & Bisson, 2009).	A web-based training course for TF-CBT: http://tfcbt.musc.edu/ TF-CBT Therapist Certification Program: https://tfcbt.org/
Eye Movement Desensitization and Reprocessing (EMDR)	Focus on teaching emotional stability skills and processing dysfunctionally stored emotions, body memories, and negative self-beliefs.	EMDR Institute, Inc.: http://www.emdr.com/ Trauma Recovery EMDR Humanitarian Assistance Program: http://emdrhap.org
Exposure Therapy	Focus on repeated confrontation with memories of the traumatic event. Gradually desensitizes the individual's reaction to trauma memories.	PTSD: National Center of PTSD, Prolonged Exposure Therapy: http://www.ptsd.va.gov/public/treatment/therapy-med/prolonged-exposure-therapy.asp Center for Deployment Psychology, Prolonged Exposure for PTSD (PE): http://www.deploymentpsych.org/treatments/prolonged-exposure-therapy-ptsd-pe

Psychotropic medications may be prescribed to help reduce patients' feelings of anxiety and depression. Although various medications, including hydrocortisone, have been trialed to attempt to ward off the development of PTSD, Amos, Stein, and Ipsen (2014) found insufficient evidence to recommend pharmacological intervention immediately following acute trauma.

INTERDISCIPLINARY RESOURCES AND REFERRALS

Because high levels of distress and anxiety make it difficult for victims to retain information, the nurse should provide a printed list of available community resources: legal aid advocacy center, local mental health center (Medicaid and

Medicare), local rape recovery center if a sexual assault occurred, and victim advocacy groups or contacts. If the victim has insurance, a referral to a mental health therapist certified in evidence-based trauma treatment should be provided. Therapists and advocacy groups can provide information on local resources such as group therapy or support groups. State laws vary regarding victims' compensation funds, which offer state financial assistance to victims, including healthcare and therapy programs. In addition to local resources, there are a number of additional resources for victims of trauma:

- National Sexual Assault Hotline sponsored by Rape, Abuse & Incest National Network (RAINN) (24/7): 1-800-656-HOPE

- National Sexual Assault Online Hotline sponsored by Rape, Abuse & Incest National Network (RAINN): https://ohl.rainn.org/online/

- Pandora's Project—Support and resources for survivors of rape and sexual assault and their friends and family: http://www.pandys.org/index.html

- Resources from the National Sexual Violence Resource Center: http://www.nsvrc.org/resources

- The National Domestic Violence Hotline (24/7): 1-800-799-SAFE (7233)

- National Center for PTSD: www.ptsd.va.gov/public/index.asp

- Disaster Distress Helpline (24/7): 1-800-985-5990

- National Center for Victims of Crime Resources: http://www.victimsofcrime.org/help-for-crime-victims/national-hotlines-and-helpful-links

CASE STUDY: TRAUMA

Pam, a 24-year-old woman, reports to her local emergency department (ED) to receive care following a rape. Pam is placed in an ED examination room, and a sexual assault nurse examiner (SANE) and rape recovery advocate are paged to respond. You are the ED nurse caring for Pam. You ask Pam what happened to her and if she was hurt. She makes little eye contact, speaks softly, and is curled up on her side on the hospital gurney. She tells you, "He raped me. I hurt all over, but mainly my arms and legs cause I think he held me down." After asking Pam's permission, you quickly examine Pam's arms and legs and notice scattered bruises on her upper arms and legs, but do not find any serious bodily injury. You tell Pam, "I'm so sorry this happened to you. A forensic nurse and a rape recovery advocate have been called in to see you. They should be here in a few minutes. When did this happen to you?" Pam responds, "Last night, around midnight." You inform Pam that it is best for evidence collection if she doesn't eat or drink anything, but you will get her food as soon as possible. You ask Pam if there is anything you can do to make her more comfortable. She shakes her head "no" and begins to cry softly. You give Pam a box of tissues and ask if she would like you to just sit with her until the SANE arrives. Pam shakes her head "yes." You ask if she would like a warm blanket. She indicates "yes" and you place a warm blanket on her.

■ Evaluate yourself as the first nurse responder.

■ You asked permission before touching Pam and asked only necessary questions as well as telling her what to expect. Was there anything else you could have done?

Within minutes the SANE (Mary) and the rape recovery advocate (Sue) arrive. They introduce themselves and you leave the room telling them to let you know if they want you to return to the room. Mary and Sue sit in chairs so that they are eye level with Pam, who remains curled up on her side. Mary says, "I'm so sorry this has happened to you. I don't know your story yet, but I know you are not to blame. You were a victim." Pam then tells Mary that she was to blame as she had gotten "really drunk on a first date." They tell her, "Just because you were drunk doesn't give anyone the right to hurt you." Pam begins to cry softly. Mary then says, "When you are ready I am going to tell you about the examination. It is important that you understand that you are in control of this examination. I won't do anything without telling you about it first and having your permission."

After a few moments, Pam says that she is ready. Mary explains the examination and interview process following a rape. Mary tells Pam that she would need to ask her specific questions about what happened to her. Pam signs the consent forms. Mary asks Pam to tell her what happened, and Pam states, "We were drinking at the bar and then went to his apartment. He seemed like a nice guy. He fixed me a drink at his apartment, but I was already feeling really drunk so I didn't want to drink it. After a few minutes, I asked him to take me home. He got mad and said that wasn't the plan. I started to get scared and just wanted to get out of there, but I couldn't find my purse. The next thing I remember, he grabbed my arms and pushed me down on the floor. At first I tried to get away, but then I froze. I couldn't even yell. After that, I only remember bits and pieces. He was on top of me and raped me. I felt like I wasn't connected to my body, like this was happening to someone else. I just wanted to get out of there." Pam tells most of the story with her eyes closed and a flat affect. When she is done, she cries softly. Mary asks Pam if anything like this had ever happened to her before. Pam nods "yes" and says, "When I was about 11 years old, my step-uncle held me down and touched my genitals. I told my mom, but she didn't do anything. She just told me not to be alone with him again."

What do you see reflected in Pam's story about the neurobiology of trauma?

- Tonic immobility: Pam reports feeling like she could not move or yell.

- Memory fragmentation: Pam reports remembering only portions of the rape.

- Dissociation: Pam reports feeling disconnected from her body. She also states that she was a victim of a prior sexual assault as a child. Disassociation is more common in victims of multiple traumas.

Following the forensic interview, examination, and evidence collection, Mary and Sue provide Pam with verbal and written information on the local rape recovery center, law enforcement victim advocate's contact information, follow-up healthcare information, and the state agency for payment of her examination as a victim. They ask Pam about her social support. Pam states that she has some good friends whom she might tell about the rape to help her through it. After the supportive response Pam receives at the hospital, she makes eye contact while speaking and no longer blames herself for what happened to her. Pam expresses interest in the group therapy sessions offered at the rape recovery center.

This case study highlights key points found in the neurobiology of trauma. By receiving compassionate nursing care by informed nurses on the immediate consequences of trauma, Pam is placed in a position to begin healing by seeking out appropriate resources.

SUMMARY

Nurses work with many individuals who have suffered trauma as well as those who have inflicted trauma on others. When they understand how the neurobiology of trauma can affect the functioning of the brain with lasting consequences, they can better help their patients. Patients may suffer immediate symptoms, such as tonic immobility and dissociation, which may lead to chronic symptoms of depression and anxiety, common aftermaths of sexual assault. They can develop Acute Stress Disorder or post-traumatic stress disorder, and may lose memory of the event. Patients can even experience physical health problems.

Nurses should adopt an evidence-based psychotherapy treatment to diagnose trauma and its effects. Providing compassionate, nonjudgmental care to victims of trauma helps in patients' healing process.

REFERENCES

Abrams, M. P., Carleton, N. R., Taylor, S., & Asmundson, G. J. (2009). Human tonic immobility: Measurement and correlates. *Depression and Anxiety, 26*(6), 550–556.

American Psychiatric Association (APA). (2013). *Diagnostic and statistical manual of mental disorders* (5th ed.). Washington, DC: Author.

Amos, T., Stein, D. J., & Ipsen, J. C. (2014). Pharmacological interventions for preventing post-traumatic stress disorder (PTSD). *Cochrane Database of Systematic Reviews, 7*, pp. 1–63. doi: 10.1002/14651858.CD006239.pub2

Anda, R. F., Felitti, V. J., Bremner, J. D., Walker, J. D, Whitfield, C., Perry, B. D. ... Giles, W. H. (2006). The enduring effects of abuse and related adverse experiences in childhood: A convergence of evidence from neurobiology and epidemiology. *European Archives of Psychiatry & Clinical Neuroscience, 256*, 174–186.

Ballenger, J. C., Davidson, J. R., Lecrubier, Y., Nutt, D. J., Foa, E. B., Kessler, R. C., ... Shalev, A. Y. (2000). Consensus statement on posttraumatic stress disorder from the International Consensus Group on Depression and Anxiety. *Journal of Clinical Psychiatry, 61*(Suppl. 5), 60–66.

Bryant, R. A. (2010). Acute stress disorder as a predictor of posttraumatic stress disorder: A systematic review. *Journal of Clinical Psychiatry, 72*(2), 233–239.

Bryant, R. A., Friedman, M. J., Spiegel, D., Ursano, R., & Strain, J. (2011). A review of acute stress disorder in DSM-5. *Depression and Anxiety, 28*(9), 801–817.

Bremner, J. D. (2006). Traumatic stress: Effects on the brain. *Dialogues in Clinical Neuroscience, 8*(4), 445–461.

Campbell, R. (2012, December). *The neurobiology of sexual assault* [transcript]. An NIJ Research for the Real World Seminar. Transcript retrieved from http://nij.gov/multimedia/presenter/presenter-campbell/Pages/presenter-campbell-transcript.aspx

Fehler-Cabral, G., Campbell, R., & Patterson, D. (2011). Adult sexual assault survivors' experiences with sexual assault nurse examiners (SANEs). *Journal of Interpersonal Violence, 26*(18), 3618–3639.

Felitti, V. J., Anda, R. F., Nordenberg, D., Williamson, D. F., Spitz, A. M., Edwards. V. ... Marks, J. S. (1998). Relationship of childhood abuse and household dysfunction to many of the leading causes of death in adults. *American Journal of Preventive Medicine, 14*(4), 245–258.

Herman, J. (1997). *Trauma and recovery.* New York, NY: Basic Books.

Kessler, R. C., Sonnega, A., Bromet, E., Hughes, M., & Nelson, C. B. (1995). Posttraumatic stress disorder in the national comorbidity survey. *Archives of General Psychiatry, 52,* 1048–1060.

Roberts, N. P., Kitchiner, N. J., Kenardy, J., & Bisson, J. I. (2009). Multiple session early psychological interventions for the prevention of post-traumatic stress disorder. *Cochrane Database of Systematic Reviews, 3,* pp.1–44. doi: 10.1002/14651858.CD006869.pub2

Sledjeski, E. M., Speisman, B., & Dierker, L. C. (2008). Does number of lifetime traumas explain the relationship between PTSD and chronic medical conditions? Answers from the National Comorbidity Survey Replication (NCS-R). *Journal of Behavioral Medicine, 31*(4), 341–349.

Starr, L. R., Hammen, C., Conway, C. C., Raposa, E., & Brennan, P. A. (2014). Sensitizing effect of early adversity on depressive reactions to later proximal stress: Moderation by polymorphisms in serotonin transporter and corticotropin releasing hormone receptor genes in a 20-year longitudinal study. *Development and Psychopathology, 26,* 1241–1254.

Tjaden, P., & Thoennes, N. (2006). *Extent, nature, and consequences of rape victimization: Findings from the National Violence Against Women Survey,* special report for National Institute of Justice and the Centers for Disease Control and Prevention. Washington, DC: U.S. Department of Justice, Office of Justice Programs.

van der Kolk, B. (2014). *The body keeps the score.* New York, NY: Viking.

Veterans Health Administration (VHA)/Department of Defense (DoD). (2010). *Clinical practice guidelines*. Retrieved from http://www.oqp.med.va.gov/cpg/PTSD/G/PTSD_about.htm

Wheeler, K. (2014). The neurophysiology of trauma and psychotherapy. In K. Wheeler (Ed.), *Psychotherapy for the advanced practice nurse* (pp. 53–93). New York, NY: Springer.

4

RESPONSE TO VICTIMIZATION

Angela F. Amar, PhD, RN, FAAN

KEY POINTS IN THIS CHAPTER

- Experiencing violence is associated with myriad short- and long-term physical and mental health symptoms and disorders.

- Violence is a common occurrence necessitating that nurses assess all patients for violence.

- Assessment for violence should also include assessment of health consequences.

Violence is an ever-present threat in society. Every day, the news media is full of stories about crime, murder, abuse, and violence. With violence comes victimization. Nurses need to understand common responses in the aftermath of violence and crime to be able to serve their patients. The range and types of victims a nurse will encounter vary; however, the prevalence and health effects of violence means that nurses will encounter victims in their practices.

- The Bureau of Justice Statistics reports that 6.1 million violent crime victimizations occurred in 2013 (Truman & Langton, 2014).

- Nearly 700,000 young people ages 10 to 24 are treated in emergency departments (EDs) each year for injuries sustained due to violence-related assaults (Centers for Disease Control [CDC], 2009).

- From 2006 to 2009, 112,664 visits made to United States EDs were for battering by a partner or spouse (Davidov, Larrabee, & Davis, 2014).

- The U.S. Department of Justice reported that 37% of all women treated in hospital EDs for violence-related injuries were injured by a current or former spouse, boyfriend, or girlfriend (Rand, 1997).

- In the National Violence Against Women Survey (NVAWS), only one-third of victims received healthcare (Tjaden & Thoennes, 2000). Further, individuals who reported the violence to the police were more likely to receive healthcare treatment than victims who did not report (Tjaden & Thoennes, 2000). Among 218 women presenting in a metropolitan emergency department with injuries due to violence, 28% required hospital admission and 13% required major medical treatment (Berrios & Grady, 1991). In general, victims of repeated violence experience more severe consequences than victims of one-time incidents experience (Johnson & Leone, 2005).

- In the United States, costs for interpersonal violence (IPV) reach 3.3% of the gross domestic product (Waters, Hyder, Rajkotia, Basu, & Rehwinkel, 2004). In 2003, costs for interpersonal violence exceeded $8.3 billion, and the annual healthcare costs for victims of IPV can continue for as many as 15 years after the abuse ends (Centers for Disease Control and Prevention [CDC], 2003; Rivara et al., 2007).

These serious mental and physical health effects and the prevalence of violence suggest that nurses in all aspects of healthcare will encounter victims of violence. The purpose of this chapter is to present the consequences of violence. It includes a discussion of physical- and mental-health consequences as well as behavioral, interpersonal responses, and healthcare utilization patterns. Finally, strategies and tools to identify survivors and health consequences are discussed.

OVERVIEW OF VICTIMIZATION

Experiencing violence and crime creates a sense of turmoil for the survivor and her loved ones. Trauma is a personal and often horrific event that profoundly affects a person and redefines her life. The experience of trauma has the potential to change ones' perceptions, worldview, and behavior. Trauma often leaves behind physical injury, emotional trauma, financial loss, and changes to the routines of daily life.

Violence and crime can also produce a crisis for the victim. *Crisis* is an intolerable situation in which one's usual coping strategies are not effective. It upsets the usual order of one's life, and often, after healing, a new sense of order and balance is created. Being unable to solve a problem can result in increased tension, anxiety, emotional unrest, and an inability to function (Caplan, 1964).

The two types of trauma one can experience are:

- **Acute trauma:** Trauma precipitated by a stressor that occurs one time. A crime committed by a stranger is an example of an acute trauma.

- **Chronic trauma:** Trauma that occurs over a period of time. Child, spousal, or elder abuse is considered a chronic stressor. These are also considered interpersonal violence as they occur within the context of a relationship. However, interpersonal violence can be both acute and chronic, as can trauma committed by a stranger.

Witnessing violence can also create a stress reaction and response (Reid-Quiñones et al., 2011). Chronic stressors continually upset one's equilibrium, and neurobiological changes occur, as discussed in Chapter 3, "Neurobiology of Trauma."

One of the earliest studies of victims of violence was that of Burgess and Holmstrom (1974) on rape survivors. Prior research on rape focused on perpetrators and specifically on identifying typologies of rapists. After interviewing numerous rape survivors at a Boston hospital, Rape Trauma Syndrome (RTS) was identified (Burgess & Holmstrom, 1974). RTS is a cluster of symptoms and reactions commonly experienced by rape survivors. Burgess and Holmstrom's definition of Rape Trauma Syndrome also outlines a process or phases that rape survivors go through toward reorganization. A key contribution of RTS is in identifying a range of responses and emotions experienced by survivors. Survivors may express their reactions in an expressed or controlled manner:

- The *expressed style* is the expected reaction and includes overt behaviors such as crying, hysteria, tenseness, confusion, and volatility. The response can be seen often as emotional and indicating a lack of control. Response to trauma can also be expressed in nontraditional ways such as laughing.

- The *controlled style* involves more ambiguous behaviors that are not frequently associated with trauma survivors. Controlled behaviors include calmness, shock, and subdued appearance. Some survivors appear distraught; others are quiet and reserved.

Individuals who dissociate during the attack may present as distant and withdrawn and may not be able to recall details related to the event. Immediate reactions to trauma are more dependent on individual coping styles than on the trauma experienced. The emotions of fear and anxiety begin during the assault; survivors' fear of rape and of being killed or hurt can continue for years after the assault. Scholars have built on the work of Burgess and Holmstrom and continue to identify health-related consequences of multiple types of violence. The next sections review physical and mental health consequences along with information about other indices of health.

IDENTIFYING RESPONSES TO VIOLENCE

Violence is an assault on the body, and the body reacts in a variety of ways. The most common consequence or response to victimization is injury, both physical and psychological.

Physical reactions include immediate consequences, such as injuries, and longer-term consequences, such as headaches, sleep disturbances, stomach pains, nausea, vaginal pain, or discomfort. The physical injury incurred depends on the type of violence:

- Sexual violence can result in vaginal, rectal, or perineal trauma. Common injuries include bruises, lacerations, abrasions, burns, fractured bones, and head injuries.

- Strangulation by an intimate partner is a particularly lethal form of violence that is also a risk factor for future violence (Glass et al., 2008). A person can become unconscious in seconds and death can occur in minutes.

  Strangulation is associated with substantial health consequences. These include physical symptoms such as dizziness, nausea, sore throat, voice changes, throat and neck injuries, breathing problems, ringing in ears, and vision change; neurological issues such as eyelid droop, facial droop, left or right side weakness, loss of sensation, loss of memory, and paralysis; and psychological symptoms such as PTSD, depression, suicidal ideation, and insomnia (McClane, Strack, & Hawley, 2001).

- Injuries from physical attacks can lead to long-term health consequences. For example, being hit in the head can result in hearing loss, vision impairment, and brain damage. Childhood abuse has been linked to health problems in adults, including ischemic heart disease, cancer, chronic lung disease, skeletal fractures, and liver disease, and health risk behaviors such as smoking, substance use, and risky sexual behavior (Felitti et al., 1998).

■ Sexual health concerns that are associated with victimization include repeated sexually transmitted diseases (STDs) and unwanted pregnancy (World Health Organization [WHO], 2013). Forced sex is associated with increased incidence of developing pelvic inflammatory disease and reoccurrence of STDs (Champion, Foley, Sigmon-Smith, Sutfin, & DuRant, 2008; Upchurch & Kusunoki, 2004). Fear of contracting a sexually transmitted disease is a factor that prompts individuals to seek healthcare after rape. Limited research documents occurrence of STDs; however, as many as 2% of women report contracting an STD as a consequence of sexual violence (Masho, Odor, & Adera, 2005).

Chapter 6, "Assessment of Wounds and Injury," provides a complete description of the types of injuries seen after violence.

LINKING BEHAVIORAL HEALTH CONSEQUENCES TO VIOLENCE

Behavioral responses to violence include aggressive and antisocial behavior, suicidal behavior, and substance abuse. Self-destructive behavior is the most frequent behavioral response to violence. For example, children may dart into traffic and take physical risks; adolescents and adults may eat, drink, or smoke excessively.

Self-destructive behaviors also include self-mutilation, suicide attempts, chronic suicidality, unprotected sex, reckless driving, and eating disorders. Abuse in any form affects the self-concept of the survivor. Emotional abuse often accompanies physical and sexual abuse. Harsh criticism, rejection, intimidation, and degradation can markedly alter or diminish the victim's self-worth.

RESPONSES TO INTERPERSONAL VIOLENCE

Exposure to interpersonal violence, both as victim and as a witness, increases the risk of substance abuse/dependence disorders (Kilpatrick et al., 2003). In situations of ongoing abuse, survivors may begin to use substances because their partners use or as a way to escape the reality of the abusive situation (Campbell, 2002). A study of adolescents in Belgium, Russia, and the United States found that exposure to violence was related to increased smoking, alcohol use, and marijuana use (Vermeiren, Schwab-Stone, Deboutte, Leckman, & Ruchkin, 2003).

Responses to interpersonal violence also include problems with intimacy, inability to trust, difficulties in interpersonal relationships, and revictimization. A history of abuse can create a disruption in the ability to form longstanding and healthy attachments (Anda et al., 2006). An abused person experiences abandonment, devaluation, and pain in the relationship with the abuser. This can make it difficult to trust and form intimate relationships.

RESPONSES TO SEXUAL ABUSE

Sexually abused children are more likely to exhibit sexualized behavior than those who were not. Sexualized behavior includes developmentally inappropriate or intrusive, coercive sexual behavior. Children who were abused at an early age, by a family member, and involving penetration are at greater risk of sexualized behavior (Kellogg, 2010). Sometimes, they may exhibit promiscuous behavior. Individuals who experience chronic sexual abuse may be conditioned to think that the only thing they are good for is sex.

Incest, rape, and sexual assault can create feelings of repulsion and a lack of enjoyment of sex. Children, adolescents, and adults who are abused sexually may feel dirty or different. They often feel that they are the only ones this is happening to. Sexual dysfunction can include lack of sexual desire, lack of orgasm, aversion to sexual contact, pain associated with sex, and difficulty with lubrication (Campbell, Lichty, Sturza, & Raja, 2006; Turchik & Hassija, 2014).

Revictimization is common among survivors of violence. For more information on this topic, see "The Cycle of Revictimization" later in this chapter.

Cataloguing Mental Health Responses to Violence

Mental health responses are all too common after experiencing violence. The experience of violence triggers the onset of intense emotions that can have a disintegrating effect on the mind. Each individual shows or conceals his emotional state using his unique response pattern.

Emotional Responses

Emotional responses to violence include depression, anxiety and fear, lowered self-esteem, anger, and guilt. Referrals to mental health or psychiatric services on an in- or out-patient basis may be necessary to facilitate healing and recovery from trauma. Depression is the most common emotional response in the aftermath of trauma and victimization. Individuals with abuse histories often have thoughts of suicide and feelings of guilt and blame. Members of society often promote victim blaming that can lead to lowered self-esteem and guilt. Perpetrators may tell survivors that the abuse is their fault or is because of the victim's perceived inadequacies. Blaming one's self for the incident can lead to lowered self-esteem. Survivors often feel anger against the perpetrator, fate, and society. This anger is unexpressed during the assault and may be expressed inappropriately or turned inwardly. Working through rage can be a critical factor in healing from trauma.

Psychiatric Disorders

Psychiatric disorders common after victimization include depression, post-traumatic stress disorder, acute stress disorder, anxiety, somatoform, and dissociative identity disorder. Depression is a common mental disorder, and it is a common consequence of violence. Symptoms of depression include significant weight loss or gain, sleep disturbances, increased or decreased motor activity, loss of energy, loss of pleasure in activities of life, decreased concentration, feelings of worthlessness, depressed mood most of the day, and recurrent thoughts of death or suicidal ideation (American Psychiatric Association [APA], 2013). Suicidal thoughts, plans, and behaviors are common in survivors (Campbell, 2002; Norman et al., 2012).

Symptoms of anxiety, such as restlessness, fear of going crazy, and panic, are common responses to victimization.

PSYCHOLOGICAL REACTIONS

The emotional trauma of victimization is often expressed through somatic disturbance. Common stress or anxiety related symptoms include sleep disorders, gastrointestinal concerns, muscle tension, headaches, palpitations, and chronic pain at an injury site. Unexplained chronic pain or conditions, such as pelvic pain, sexual problems, gastrointestinal problems, kidney or bladder infections, and headache, could give the clinician reason to suspect violence (WHO, n.d.).

General health effects abound following victimization. Survivors have been found to be disproportionately frequent users of healthcare services due to the acute and chronic physical, somatic, and psychological consequences of assault (Dichter, Cerulli, & Bossarte, 2011; Elhai, North, & Frueh, 2005; Schnurr & Green, 2004). Survivors have been found to have increased medical service usage even when perceptions of health and somatic symptoms are no longer elevated, reflecting the insidious and long-term effects of violence. Post-traumatic stress disorder (PTSD) appears to be a mediator that increases utilization of medical and mental health services after trauma (Rosendal, Mortensen, Andersen, & Heir, 2013). Survivors of trauma often report lower health-related quality of life (Schnurr & Green, 2004) and poorer physical and mental health outcomes (Coker et al., 2002; Ellsberg, Jansen, Heise, Watts, & Garcia-Moreno, 2008). Sleep and appetite disturbances are common in violence survivors.

POST-TRAUMATIC STRESS DISORDER

Post-traumatic stress disorder (PTSD) may be an immediate or chronic response to physical or sexual violence. PTSD is diagnosed in individuals who have experienced, witnessed, or were confronted with a traumatic event and have characteristic resulting symptoms. Resulting symptoms include persistent re-experiencing of the event, persistent avoidance of stimuli associated with the trauma, and symptoms of increased arousal (APA, 2013). The persistent re-living of the event creates an intrusion to daily functioning. Survivors may experience flashbacks, nightmares, or some experience in which the traumatic event is reenacted. They may also feel the need for safety rituals, such as extensive checking of locks.

Many people who experience traumatic events do not develop PTSD. Lifetime prevalence estimates suggest that about 8% of the general population have PTSD, with women being twice as likely as men to have PTSD at some point during their lifetimes (Kessler, Sonnega, Bromet, Hughes, & Nelson, 1995). A systematic review suggests that individuals who are exposed to intentional trauma are more likely than those exposed to unintentional trauma to be diagnosed with PTSD (Santiago et al., 2013).

Avoidance behaviors are efforts to avoid anything associated with the traumatic event. This can include efforts to avoid feelings, thoughts, activities, places, and people. Numbing behaviors, such as difficulty expressing feelings, lack of interest in pleasurable activities, or isolating from others, are another way to avoid the traumatic event. The restrictions may interfere with normal life functioning. Avoidance and numbing can lend itself to periods of dissociation. Dissociation provides a separation of feelings and thoughts and allows the person to disappear and feel as if the traumatic event did not happen to him. The person feels complete powerlessness and escapes the situation by dissociating. Alterations in memory after a traumatic event can be associated with dissociative symptoms. Other survivors may have symptoms of increased arousal. Hyperarousal symptoms include being extremely watchful of the environment, insomnia, anger, and rage. Individuals with arousal are constantly alert and on guard for signs of danger or trauma. Exposure to severe and uncontrollable stressors desensitizes a person to trauma. That is, the person is so used to being on edge that he may react to milder stressors with a major stress response. Intrusions, avoidance, and hyperarousal symptoms may persist for as long as 2 years, or longer, after the attack and usually cause some disruption in the individual's interpersonal, social, or occupational functioning.

Symptoms of PTSD often occur within 3 months of the stressor. However, symptoms may not emerge until years after an event. Acute Stress Disorder (ASD) is a more immediate response to a traumatic event. ASD usually occurs within 1 month after the traumatic event. The symptom profile of ASD is similar to PTSD. The main difference is that ASD has a shorter time of the onset of symptoms than does PTSD. Individuals with ASD may experience dissociative symptoms, persistent re-experiencing of the event, marked avoidance, and marked arousal (APA, 2013). Dissociative symptoms may occur during and after the trauma. They include numbing, detachment, reduced awareness of surroundings, depersonalization (feeling of lost identity), derealization (false perception that the environment is changed), and amnesia for important aspects of the trauma. These cognitive symptoms, during and after the trauma, provide an escape from the traumatic event by altering one's state of consciousness. The dissociative symptoms are not necessary for a diagnosis of PTSD. For a diagnosis of ASD to be given, the symptoms must cause significant distress or impair functioning. Most people recover from Acute Stress Disorder within a month; however, it is a significant predictor of PTSD (Brewin, Andrews, Rose, & Kirk, 1999). If the symptoms are unresolved, then the diagnosis is changed to PTSD.

THE CYCLE OF REVICTIMIZATION

Secondary revictimization occurs when survivors encounter victim-blaming attitudes in providers and other individuals whom they turn to for help. The experience of trauma results in a loss of control for survivors. They often turn to helpers looking for support and validation. When professionals or authorities respond in a distant manner, survivors feel rejected and not supported. This results in additional trauma. The treatment of victims of sexual assault is often found to be negative and upsetting to victims (Campbell, Wasco, Ahrens, Sefl, & Barnes, 2001).

As a society, we hold biases regarding victimization, victims, and certain crimes. For example, male rape survivors report negative treatment from authorities. Misbeliefs include that men cannot be raped or that men should be able to fight off rape. LGBT individuals face multiple levels of victimization and are likely to experience indifference, rejection, and stigmatization from police, healthcare personnel, and often family and friends.

Revictimization is common among survivors of violence. Multiple studies have identified prior victimization as a strong predictor of future victimization (Finkelhor, Ormrod, & Turner, 2007). Many survivors who were abused as children are revictimized later in life and sometimes on multiple occasions. It is thought that being abused negatively affects the ability to protect oneself. As discussed in Chapter 3, trauma can alter the development and function of the child and adolescent brain, which can elicit other consequences. Symptoms of PTSD, such as numbing and hyperarousal, may play a role in revictimization (Ullman, Najdowski, & Filipas, 2009). Increased levels of arousal can make the autonomic nervous system lose the ability to warn of impending danger. A lack of risk recognition predicts revictimization (Bockers, Roepke, Michael, Renneberg, & Knaevelsrud, 2014). In a study of victims of violence, exaggerated startle response, irritability, and outbursts of anger are related to revictimization (Kunst & Winkel, 2013). However, another study found that numbing symptoms and problem drinking are independent risk factors for revictimization (Ullman et al., 2009). Decreased self-esteem can create difficulty in setting boundaries, which can place survivors at risk for abuse and exploitation.

GENDER CONCERNS WITH VIOLENCE

Much of the research on partner violence and rape has been conducted using primarily female samples, often middle class and white samples. Men and boys are also victims of partner violence and rape at the hands of female and male perpetrators. However, in studies conducted by the Justice Department and Centers for Disease Control, the sample size of male survivors is too small to conduct meaningful analyses (Black et al., 2011; Tjaden & Thoennes, 2000, 2006). Despite this, on average, annually, 9,040 male victims experience completed rapes, and 10,270 male victims experience attempted rape (Rennison, 2001). More than 35% of women and 28% of men experience rape, physical violence, and/or stalking by an intimate partner in their lifetime (Black et al., 2011). Both men and women who experienced physical and sexual violence reported similar health effects (Black et al., 2011).

Society conceptualizes partner violence and rape as events that happen only to female victims. Societal perceptions can influence male responses to violence, causing them not to report partner or sexual violence to the police or seek healthcare due to fear of a negative reaction or of not being believed or taken seriously. Men who experienced rape reported psychological disturbance in response to being raped, specifically anxiety, depression, increased feelings of anger and vulnerability, loss of self-image, emotional distancing, self-blame, and self-harming behaviors (Walker, Archer, & Davies, 2005). Research specific to consequences of violence for men is limited.

CULTURAL IMPLICATIONS REGARDING VIOLENCE

One's cultural background exerts a strong influence on acceptable thoughts, behaviors, and attitudes. Culture also determines the values that a group uses to guide actions and decisions. Cultural values and norms provide a framework for roles, responsibilities, and behaviors related to behavior and relationships. Culture, race, and ethnicity can also affect the presentation of symptoms to a provider. For example, Italians often use words for drama to convey the emotional intensity of an experience. This is in contrast to Chinese culture, which avoids talking about problems, or Irish culture, in which it is embarrassing to discuss feelings with anyone (McGoldrick, Giordano, & Garcia-Preto, 2005).

Clearly, survivors will be best helped when the provider is able to provide culturally sensitive care. Cultural sensitivity would include behaviors that are open to diversity among individuals. It is important for you to recognize that there is no standard cookbook approach. There can be much diversity among members of the same ethnic or racial background. Assessment or intake tools can incorporate questions that uncover the cultural significance of events for clients. By asking clients about the meaning that this event may hold for their family, church, or social group, the healthcare or social service provider gains insight into the perspective of the survivor and may then implement a culturally sensitive plan of action.

ASSESSING INJURIES THAT OCCUR THROUGH VIOLENCE

Trauma assessment typically involves conducting a thorough history to identify all forms of traumatic events experienced directly or witnessed by the client. This background data is used to inform the choice of intervention. This history can be supplemented with trauma-specific standardized clinical measures. These measures help the nurse to identify the type and severity of symptoms the individual is experiencing. The National Center for PTSD has lists of surveys to measure traumatic exposure. The Trauma History Questionnaire, shown in Table 4.1, is a commonly used self-report measure that has 24 items and takes about 10 to 15 minutes to complete. The survey is established as a reliable and valid measure (Hooper, Stockton, Krupnick, & Green, 2011). Not all individuals who have experienced trauma need trauma-specific interventions.

TABLE 4.1   THE TRAUMA HISTORY QUESTIONNAIRE

The following is a series of questions about serious or traumatic life events. These types of events actually occur with some regularity, although we would like to believe they are rare, and they affect how people feel about, react to, and/or think about things subsequently. Knowing about the occurrence of such events, and reactions to them, will help us to develop programs for prevention, education, and other services. The questionnaire is divided into questions covering crime experiences, general disaster and trauma questions, and questions about physical and sexual experiences.

For each event, please indicate (circle) whether it happened and, if it did, the number of times and your approximate age when it happened (give your best guess if you are not sure). Also note the nature of your relationship to the person involved and the specific nature of the event, if appropriate.

| Crime-Related Events | Circle one | | If you circled yes, please indicate | |
			Number of times	Approximate age(s)
1 Has anyone ever tried to take something directly from you by using force or the threat of force, such as a stick-up or mugging?	No	Yes		

		Circle one		If you circled yes, please indicate	
2	Has anyone ever attempted to rob you or actually robbed you (i.e., stolen your personal belongings)?	No	Yes		
3	Has anyone ever attempted to or succeeded in breaking into your home when you were <u>not</u> there?	No	Yes		
4	Has anyone ever attempted to or succeeded in breaking into your home while you <u>were</u> there?	No	Yes		

General Disaster and Trauma	**Circle one**		**Number of times**	**Approximate age(s)**
5 Have you ever had a serious accident at work, in a car, or somewhere else? (**If yes**, please specify below) _____ _____	No	Yes		
6 Have you ever experienced a natural disaster such as a tornado, hurricane, flood or major earthquake, etc., where you felt you or your loved ones were in danger of death or injury? (**If yes**, please specify below) _____ _____	No	Yes		
7 Have you ever experienced a "man-made" disaster such as a train crash, building collapse, bank robbery, fire, etc., where you felt you or your loved ones were in danger of death or injury? (**If yes**, please specify below) _____ _____	No	Yes		

continues

TABLE 4.1 THE TRAUMA HISTORY QUESTIONNAIRE (CONTINUED)

General Disaster and Trauma	Circle one		If you circled yes, please indicate	
			Number of times	Approximate age(s)
8 Have you ever been exposed to dangerous chemicals or radioactivity that might threaten your health?	No	Yes		
9 Have you ever been in any other situation in which you were seriously injured? (**If yes**, please specify below) _____ _____	No	Yes		
10 Have you ever been in any other situation in which you feared you might be killed or seriously injured? (**If yes**, please specify below) _____ _____	No	Yes		
11 Have you ever seen someone seriously injured or killed? (**If yes**, please specify who below) _____ _____	No	Yes		
12 Have you ever seen dead bodies (other than at a funeral) or had to handle dead bodies for any reason? (**If yes**, please specify below) _____ _____	No	Yes		

13   Have you ever had a close friend or family   No   Yes
     member murdered, or killed by a drunk
     driver? (**If yes**, please specify relationship
     [e.g., mother, grandson, etc.] below)

     _____

     _____

14   Have you ever had a spouse, romantic   No   Yes
     partner, or child die? (**If yes**, please specify
     relationship below)

     _____

     _____

15   Have you ever had a serious or life-   No   Yes
     threatening illness? (**If yes**, please specify
     below)

     _____

     _____

16   Have you ever received news of a serious   No   Yes
     injury, life-threatening illness, or unexpected
     death of someone close to you? (**If yes**,
     please indicate below)

     _____

     _____

17   Have you ever had to engage in combat while   No   Yes
     in military service in an official or unofficial
     war zone? (**If yes**, please indicate where
     below)

     _____

     _____

continues

TABLE 4.1   THE TRAUMA HISTORY QUESTIONNAIRE   (CONTINUED)

Physical and Sexual Experiences	Circle one		If you circled yes, please indicate	
			Number of times	Approximate age(s)
18 Has anyone ever made you have intercourse or oral or anal sex against your will? (**If yes**, please indicate nature of relationship with person [e.g., stranger, friend, relative, parent, sibling] below) _____ _____	No	Yes		
19 Has anyone ever touched private parts of your body, or made you touch theirs, under force or threat? (If yes, please indicate nature of relationship with person [e.g., stranger, friend, relative, parent, sibling] below) _____ _____	No	Yes		
20 Other than incidents mentioned in Questions 18 and 19, have there been any other situations in which another person tried to force you to have unwanted sexual contact?	No	Yes		
21 Has anyone, including family members or friends, ever attacked you with a gun, knife, or some other weapon?	No	Yes		
22 Has anyone, including family members or friends, ever attacked you <u>without</u> a weapon and seriously injured you?	No	Yes		
23 Has anyone in your family ever beaten, spanked, or pushed you hard enough to cause injury?	No	Yes		

24	Have you experienced any other extraordinarily stressful situation or event that is not covered above? (**If yes**, please specify below)	No	Yes		
	_____ _____				

Source: Hooper et al. (2011)

Unfortunately, many individuals exposed to trauma lack natural support systems and need the help of trauma-informed care systems. Many people who do not meet the full criteria for PTSD still suffer significant post-traumatic symptoms that can strongly affect behavior, judgment, education/work performance, and ability to connect with family/caregivers. These individuals may benefit from a comprehensive trauma assessment to determine the most effective interventions.

Nurses can use screening tools that are covered in the following sections to assess and describe the violence.

THE ABUSE ASSESSMENT SCREEN (AAS)

The Abuse Assessment Screen (AAS) was developed and tested by nurses and has proven to be a reliable method of assessing violence (Laughon, Renker, Glass, & Parker, 2008). Its five items inquire about physical, sexual, and emotional abuse, in addition to asking about abuse during pregnancy. Male and female body maps are provided to document injuries. Respondents also identify the perpetrator. Direct questions and word choices are important to gather this information. While individuals may respond affirmatively to questions about kicking, punching, or hitting, they might not see themselves as battered, abused, or a victim. Similarly, individuals may respond affirmatively that someone made them have sex against their wishes but not see themselves as having been raped. It is important to frame violence assessment questions using behavioral terms rather than making judgments.

ASSESSMENT SCALES

The Beck Depression Inventory (BDI) is a widely used, self-report survey containing 21 items (Beck, Steer, & Carbin, 1988). It takes about 5 to 10 minutes to complete. The items are consistent with the diagnostic criteria for depression. Higher scores indicate higher levels of depression.

A shorter option is the Patient Health Questionnaire-9 (PHQ9). The nine-item assessment tool is also consistent with the diagnostic criteria for depression and takes less than 2 minutes to complete. The scores are interpreted into ranges or levels of depression (Kroenke, Spitzer, & Williams, 2001).

ANXIETY SCALES

Anxiety is often measured using the Hamilton Anxiety Scale. This 14-item scale is widely used by clinicians to determine the level of anxiety. Higher scores indicate more severe levels of anxiety (Maier, Buller, Philipp, & Heuser, 1988). The Beck Anxiety Inventory–Primary Care is a seven-item scale that measures anxiety and depression and screens for PTSD (Mori et al., 2003). The Impact of Events is a widely used, though longer measure of PTSD. The 22-item scale measures symptoms of intrusion, avoidance, and hyperarousal (Horowitz, Wilner, & Alvarez, 1979). Further information about these scales and others can be found at the National Center for PTSD website (http://www.ptsd.va.gov/index.asp).

SUMMARY

This chapter explained how experiencing violence can lead to short- and long-term physical- and mental-health symptoms and disorders, how nurses interact with patients who've experienced violence, and how to accurately assess injuries using verifiable scales of measurement.

The experience of violence can have profound effects on psychological and physical health and wellbeing of patients, as well as health utilization. Nurses routinely interact with individuals whose lives have been touched by violence. Each encounter represents an opportunity to provide teaching, referrals, and access to resources that can help individuals to manage and alleviate the consequences of violence. An understanding of the myriad ways that individuals respond to violence helps the nurse to identify individuals who have experienced violence and connect them to appropriate resources.

ADDITIONAL RESOURCES

Academy on Violence and Abuse: http://www.avahealth.org/

Futures Without Violence: http://www.futureswithoutviolence.org/

Georgetown University Center for Trauma and the Community: http://ctc.georgetown.edu/
toolkit

National Center for Injury Prevention & Control, Centers for Disease Control:
http://www.cdc.gov/injury/

National Center for PTSD, U.S. Department of Veterans Affairs: http://www.ptsd.va.gov/
index.asp

The Nursing Network on Violence Against Women International: http://nnvawi.org/

REFERENCES

American Psychiatric Association (APA). (2013). *Diagnostic and statistical manual of mental disorders (DSM-5)* (5th ed.). Arlington, VA: Author.

Anda, R. F., Felitti, V. J., Bremner, J. D., Walker, J. D., Whitfield, C. H., Perry, B. D., … Giles, W. H. (2006). The enduring effects of abuse and related adverse experiences in childhood. *European Archives of Psychiatry and Clinical Neurology, 256*(3), 164–186.

Beck, A. T., Steer, R. A., & Carbin, M. G. (1988). Psychometric properties of the Beck Depression Inventory: Twenty-five years of evaluation. *Clinical Psychology Review, 8*(1), 77–100.

Berrios, D. C., & Grady, D. (1991). Domestic violence. Risk factors and outcomes. *Western Journal of Emergency Medicine, 155*(2), 133–135.

Black, M. C., Basile, K. C., Walters, M. L., Merrick, M. T., Chen, J., & Stevens, M. R. (2011). *The National Intimate Partner and Sexual Violence Survey (NISVS)*. Atlanta, GA: National Center for Injury Prevention and Control, Centers for Disease Control and Prevention.

Bockers, E., Roepke, S., Michael, L., Renneberg, B., & Knaevelsrud, C. (2014). Risk recognition, attachment anxiety, self-efficacy, and state dissociation predict revictimization. *PLoS One, 9*(9), e108206.

Brewin, C. R., Andrews, B., Rose, S., & Kirk, M. (1999). Acute stress disorder and posttraumatic stress disorder in victims of violent crime. *American Journal of Psychiatry, 156*(3), 360–366.

Burgess, A. W., & Holmstrom, L. L. (1974). Rape trauma syndrome. *American Journal of Psychiatry, 131,* 981–986.

Campbell, J. C. (2002). Health consequences of intimate partner violence. *The Lancet, 359,* 1331–1336.

Campbell, R., Lichty, L. F., Sturza, M., & Raja, S. (2006). Gynecological health impact of sexual assault. *Research in Nursing and Health, 29*(5), 399–413.

Campbell, R., Wasco, S. M., Ahrens, C. E., Sefl, T., & Barnes, H. E. (2001). Preventing the "second rape": Rape survivors' experiences with community service providers. *Journal of Interpersonal Violence, 16*(12), 1239–1259.

Caplan, G. (1964). *Principles of preventive psychiatry.* New York, NY: Basic Books.

Centers for Disease Control and Prevention (CDC). (2003). *Costs of intimate partner violence against women in the United States.* Atlanta, GA: CDC, National Center for Injury Prevention and Control.

Centers for Disease Control and Prevention (CDC). (2009). *Youth risk behavioral surveillance-United States, 2009* (pp. SS–5).

Champion, H., Foley, K. L., Sigmon-Smith, K., Sutfin, E. L., & DuRant, R. H. (2008). Contextual factors and health risk behaviors associated with date fighting among high school students. *Women and Health, 47*(3), 1–22. doi: 10.1080/03630240802132286

Coker, A. L., Davis, K. E., Arias, I., Desai, S., Sanderson, M., Brandt, H. M., & Smith, P. H. (2002). Physical and mental health effects of intimate partner violence for men and women. *American Journal of Preventive Medicine, 23*(4), 260–268.

Davidov, D. M., Larrabee, H., & Davis, S. M. (2014). United States emergency department visits coded for intimate partner violence. *Journal of Emergency Medicine, 48*(1), 94–100. doi: 10.1016/j.jemermed.2014.07.053

Dichter, M. E., Cerulli, C., & Bossarte, R. M. (2011). Intimate partner violence victimization among women veterans and associated heart health risks. *Women's Health Issues, 21*(4), S190–S194. doi: 10.1016/j.whi.2011.04.008

Elhai, J. D., North, T. C., & Frueh, B. C. (2005). Health service use predictors among trauma survivors: A critical review. *Psychological Services, 2*(1), 3–19.

Ellsberg, M., Jansen, H. A., Heise, L., Watts, C. H., & Garcia-Moreno, C. (2008). Intimate partner violence and women's physical and mental health in the WHO multi-country study on women's health and domestic violence: An observational study. *The Lancet, 371*(9619), 1165–1172.

Felitti, V. J., Anda, R. F., Nordenberg, D., Williamson, D. F., Spitz, A. M., Edwards, V., ... Marks, J. S. (1998). Relationship of childhood abuse and household dysfunction to many of the leading causes of death in adults: The Adverse Childhood Experiences (ACE) Study. *American Journal of Preventive Medicine, 14*(4), 245–258.

Finkelhor, D., Ormrod, R. K., & Turner, H. A. (2007). Re-victimization patterns in a national longitudinal sample of children and youth. *Child Abuse and Neglect, 31*(5), 479–502.

Glass, N., Laughon, K., Campbell, J., Block, C. R., Hanson, G., Sharps, P. W., & Taliaferro, E. (2008). Non-fatal strangulation is an important risk factor for homicide of women. *The Journal of Emergency Medicine, 35*(3), 329–335.

Hooper, L. M., Stockton, P., Krupnick, J. L., & Green, B. L. (2011). Development, use, and psychometric properties of the Trauma History Questionnaire. *Journal of Loss and Trauma, 16*(3), 258–283.

Horowitz, M., Wilner, N., & Alvarez, W. (1979). Impact of Event Scale: A measure of subjective stress. *Psychosomatic Medicine, 41*(3), 209–218.

Johnson, M. P., & Leone, J. M. (2005). The differential effects of intimate terrorism and situational couple violence findings from the national violence against women survey. *Journal of Family Issues, 26*(3), 322–349.

Kellogg, N. D. (2010). Sexual behaviors in children: Evaluation and management. *American Family Physician, 82*(10), 1233–1238.

Kessler, R. C., Sonnega, A., Bromet, E., Hughes, M., & Nelson, C. B. (1995). Posttraumatic stress disorder in the National Comorbidity Survey. *Archives of General Psychiatry, 52*(12), 1048–1060.

Kilpatrick, D. G., Ruggiero, K. J., Acierno, R., Saunders, B. E., Resnick, H. S., & Best, C. L. (2003). Violence and risk of PTSD, major depression, substance abuse/dependence, and comorbidity: Results from the National Survey of Adolescents. *Journal of Consulting and Clinical Psychology, 71*(4), 692–700.

Kroenke, K., Spitzer, R. L., & Williams, J. B. (2001). The PHQ-9: Validity of a brief depression severity measure. *Journal of General Internal Medicine, 16*(9), 606–613.

Kunst, M. J., & Winkel, F. W. (2013). Exploring the impact of dysfunctional posttraumatic survival responses on crime revictimization. *Violence & Victims, 28*(4), 670–680.

Laughon, K., Renker, P., Glass, N., & Parker, B. (2008). Revision of the Abuse Assessment Screen to address nonlethal strangulation. *Journal of Obstetric, Gynecologic, and Neonatal Nursing, 37*(4), 502–507.

Maier, W., Buller, R., Philipp, M., & Heuser, I. (1988). The Hamilton Anxiety Scale: Reliability, validity and sensitivity to change in anxiety and depressive disorders. *Journal of Affective Disorders, 14*(1), 61–68.

Masho, S. W., Odor, R. K., & Adera, T. (2005). Sexual assault in Virginia: A population-based study. *Women's Health Issues, 15,* 157–166.

McClane, G. E., Strack, G. B., & Hawley, D. (2001). A review of 300 attempted strangulation cases Part II: Clinical evaluation of the surviving victim. *The Journal of Emergency Medicine, 21*(3), 311–315.

McGoldrick, M., Giordano, J., & Garcia-Preto, N. (Eds.). (2005). *Ethnicity and family therapy* (3rd ed.). New York, NY: Guilford Press.

Mori, D. L., Lambert, J. F., Niles, B. L., Orlander, J. D., Grace, M., & LoCastro, J. S. (2003). The BAI–PC as a screen for anxiety, depression, and PTSD in primary care. *Journal of Clinical Psychology, 10*(3), 187–192.

Norman, R. E., Byambaa, M., De, R., Butchart, A., Scott, J., & Vos, T. (2012). The long-term health consequences of child physical abuse, emotional abuse, and neglect: A systematic review and meta-analysis. *PLoS Med, 9*(11), e10011349. doi: 10.1371/journal. pmed.1001349

Rand, M. (1997). *Violence-related injuries treated in hospital emergency departments.* Washington, DC: Bureau of Justice Statistics.

Reid-Quiñones, K., Kliewer, W., Shields, B. J., Goodman, K., Ray, M. H., & Wheat, E. (2011). Cognitive, affective, and behavioral responses to witnessed versus experienced violence. *American Journal of Orthopsychiatry, 81*(1), 51–60.

Rennison, C. (2001). *Intimate partner violence and age of the victim: 1993–1999.* Washington, DC: United States Department of Justice.

Rivara, F. P., Anderson, M. L., Fishman, P., Bonomi, A. E., Reid, R. J., Carrell, D., & Thompson, R. S. (2007). Healthcare utilization and costs for women with a history of intimate partner violence. *American Journal of Preventive Medicine, 32*(2), 89–96.

Rosendal, S., Mortensen, E. L., Andersen, H. S., & Heir, T. (2013). Use of health care services before and after a natural disaster among survivors with and without PTSD. *Psychiatric Services, 65*(1), 91–97.

Santiago, P. N., Ursano, R. J., Gray, C. L., Pynoos, R. S., Spiegel, D., Lewis-Fernandez, R., ... Fullerton, C. S. (2013). A systematic review of PTSD prevalence and trajectories in DSM-5 defined trauma exposed populations: Intentional and non-intentional traumatic events. *PLoS One, 8*(4), e59236.

Schnurr, P. P., & Green, B. L. (Eds.). (2004). *Trauma and health: Physical health consequences of exposure to extreme stress.* Washington, DC: American Psychological Association.

Tjaden, P., & Thoennes, N. (2000). *Extent, nature, and consequences of intimate partner violence.* Washington, DC: National Institute of Justice and the Centers for Disease Control.

Tjaden, P., & Thoennes, N. (2006). *Extent, nature, and consequences of rape victimization: Findings from the National Violence Against Women Survey.* Washington, DC: National Institute of Justice.

Truman, J. L., & Langton, L. (2014). *Criminal victimization, 2013.* Washington, DC: Bureau of Justice Statistics.

Turchik, J. A., & Hassija, C. M. (2014). Female sexual victimization among college students: Assault severity, health risk behaviors, and sexual functioning. *Journal of Interpersonal Violence, 29*(13), 2439–2457.

Ullman, S. E., Najdowski, C. J., & Filipas, H. H. (2009). Child sexual abuse, post-traumatic stress disorder, and substance use: Predictors of revictimization in adult sexual assault survivors. *Journal of Child Sexual Abuse, 18*(4), 367–385.

Upchurch, D. M., & Kusunoki, Y. (2004). Associations between forced sex, sexual and protective practices, and sexually transmitted diseases among a national sample of adolescent girls. *Women's Health Issues, 14*(3), 75–84.

Vermeiren, R., Schwab-Stone, M., Deboutte, D., Leckman, P. E., & Ruchkin, V. (2003). Violence exposure and substance use in adolescents: Findings from three countries. *Pediatrics, 111*(3), 535–540.

Walker, J., Archer, J., & Davies, M. (2005). Effects of rape on men: A descriptive analysis. *Archives of Sexual Behavior, 34*(1), 69–80.

Waters, H., Hyder, A., Rajkotia, Y., Basu, S., & Rehwinkel, J. A. (2004). *The economic dimensions of interpersonal violence.* Geneva, Switzerland: World Health Organization.

World Health Organization (WHO). (n.d.). *Health care for women subjected to intimate partner violence or sexual violence: A clinical handbook.* Geneva, Switzerland: World Health Organization.

World Health Organization (WHO). (2013). *Responding to intimate partner violence and sexual violence against women: WHO clinical and policy guidelines.* Geneva, Switzerland: World Health Organization.

Theories of Violence: Victimization and Perpetration

Angela F. Amar, PhD, RN, FAAN

Key Points in This Chapter

- Theories are useful to describe, explain, and predict behaviors associated with victimization and perpetration.

- Causes of violence are multifactorial involving several perspectives to capture an accurate depiction.

- Many of the historical approaches to explore violence pathologize the offender and blame the victim.

Violence and crime have existed for as long as we can remember. The Bible, dating back to 1500 B.C., contains stories of genocide, fratricide, and other types of violence. Society grapples with issues related to prevention of violence, intervening with victims and offenders of violence, and maintaining public safety. Multiple factors can result in violence including, but not limited to, mental illness, racism, poverty, gangs, drugs, availability of guns, media influences, and family relations (Meadows, 2013). Criminologists, psychologists, social scientists, and healthcare providers are all interested in understanding victimization and perpetration and the factors that increase individuals' risk. An understanding of the factors that make an individual at risk for victimization and perpetration is essential to prevent violence from occurring. Theoretical perspectives allow a mechanism to link concepts and provide context for behaviors. *Theories* are organizing frameworks of interrelated concepts, facts, or tested hypotheses that systematically seek to describe, explain, and predict a phenomenon and the relationships among the constructs. Research rooted in theory is more effective in describing, explaining, and determining effective prevention and intervention strategies.

In every crime, there is a *victim*, the person who was harmed by a crime or unpleasant event, and a *perpetrator*, a person or persons who carry out a crime or deception. Victims are sometimes called *survivors*. Victim can be viewed as passive status whereby an individual lacks agency. Survivor connotes strength in living through a traumatic experience. This chapter provides nurses with theoretical information to understand violence, victimization, and perpetration. It includes historical and societal influences and perceptions of violence, victimization, and victims. Further, the chapter provides information to help clinicians to begin to understand the etiology and motivation of offender behavior.

UNDERSTANDING CRIME AND VICTIMIZATION

Much of the data on crime comes from two distinctly different sources: crime reports and research surveys.

Uniform Crime Reports

The Uniform Crime Reports (UCR), released by the Federal Bureau of Investigation (FBI), are annual reports that show the estimated crime rate for that year. The UCR program collects information reported by law enforcement agencies regarding the violent crimes of murder and non-negligent manslaughter, rape, robbery, and aggravated assault as well as the property crimes of burglary, larceny-theft, motor vehicle theft, and arson. In the latest available statistics, an estimated 11 million arrests were made in 2013 (FBI, 2013), most of which were for property crime rather than violent crime.

Arrest data describes offenders. Arrested persons were overwhelmingly male (73%). In 2013, over 68% of those arrested were White; 28% were Black, which is high in relation to the percentages of Blacks in the U.S.; and less than 3% were other races (FBI, 2014). Several factors limit the usefulness of the Uniform Crime Reports:

- Only eight types of crimes are tracked, and only the most serious is tracked if multiple offenses occurred at one time.

- The reports do not contain information regarding the victim, relationship of victim and offender, location, weapons, etc. (Hirschel, 2009).

- Crimes appear in this data only if victims report it to law enforcement. Research suggests that many individuals do not report criminal victimization to the police for reasons such as fear of reprisal, fear that police would not help, believing that the incident is not important enough to report, and choosing to deal with the incident alone rather than involve the authorities (Langton, Berzofsky, Krebs, & Smiley-McDonald, 2012).

National Crime Victimization Survey

The National Crime Victimization Survey (NCVS) offers a different perspective. Each year, a nationally representative sample of about 90,000 households participates in the survey. Researchers collect data from each household twice yearly to determine the frequency, characteristics, and consequences of crime victimization in the U.S. (Truman & Langton, 2014). Examination of socio-demographic correlates reveals that men, younger age people, and African Americans are most closely associated with being a victim. These individuals are at higher risk for violence than women, older age people, and Whites. The data from the NCVS is limited in that it only provides victims' perspectives on the crime experience. There is no mechanism to validate that the crime occurred or to gather the perceptions of the offender or law enforcement. However, the large sample and randomization are strengths of this survey.

UNDERSTANDING HOW VICTIMIZATION HAPPENS

The Uniform Crime Reports and National Crime Victimization Survey represent the major sources of data regarding crime and victimization. They provide descriptive data regarding crimes and victims. These sources do not provide any information on why people become victims or perpetrators. Theories provide a model for understanding influences and explanations for violence.

MENDELSOHN'S TYPES OF VICTIMS

Criminology perspectives attempt to understand what makes someone a victim and/or perpetrator so that the risk of victimization and perpetration can be decreased. Much of the early attempts to understand victimization centered on victim precipitation or contribution to his or her victimization. In other words, the typology attributes degrees of blame or causation to victims for the crime. Benjamin Mendelsohn is seen as the father of victimology (1956). As an attorney, he interviewed victims and identified six types (Mendelsohn, 1956):

- The completely innocent victim, or being in the wrong place at the wrong time

- The victim with minor guilt usually due to ignorance (For example, the victim unknowingly walks into a crime scene, such as the victim who is shot after entering a store during a robbery.)

- The victim who is as guilty as the offender or the voluntary victim (For example, two people are involved in a crime and one gets hurt.)

- The victim who is more guilty than the offender (For example, a person throws the first punch and is beaten.)

- The most guilty victim is a person who becomes a victim while being a perpetrator. (For example, a victim is shot while robbing someone.)

- Someone who falsifies victimization

A critique of this framework is that in only two categories is the victim innocent of guilt. Four of the six categories give more responsibility to the victim rather than giving all guilt and responsibility to the perpetrator. This victim-blaming theme continues in societal beliefs today. However, it was an early attempt at shifting our awareness to the victims of crime. Victimology is an important field today as victimologists use a scientific method to answer questions about victims. Victimology studies causes and consequences of victimization, how the criminal justice system assists victims, and how society responds to victims (Daigle, 2013).

FRAMEWORKS OF VICTIMIZATION

Other criminology frameworks include lifestyle-exposure theory and routine activities theory.

Lifestyle-exposure theory posits that victimization is a function of lifestyle (Hindelang, Gottfredson, & Garofalo, 1978). For example, high-risk behaviors, such as alcohol and drug use and gang participation, increase the chance of being involved in a crime. Certain professions, such as taxi drivers and police, and certain situations, such as nights and weekends, have a higher affinity for crime and victimization. The lifestyle-exposure theory is grounded in research and science. However, it still attributes blame for violence to victims by suggesting that victim activity, rather than perpetrator action, leads to victimization and crime.

Routine activities theory examines the context in which crimes occur and suggests that three things must be present for a crime to happen (Cohen & Felson, 1979):

- **A suitable target:** A suitable target is a person or object to which the offender has easy access.

- **Lack of a suitable guardian:** The suitable guardian is someone or something that presents a safeguard or serves as a deterrent to crime. For example, guard dogs, locks, and persons at home are all suitable guardians and deter crime.

- **The presence of a motivated offender:** Motivated offenders look for easy targets with limited protection.

Cohen and colleagues examined crime data from the 1960s and 1970s. They attributed increases in burglary to having men and women in the workforce and no suitable guardian at home. In addition, the increases in the workforce increased the availability of suitable targets for robbery on the streets. Decades of evidence support the association of target suitability, guardianship, and exposure with individual victimization, especially in property and street crimes (Wilcox, 2010). A limitation of this theory is in not discussing the motivations of offenders. Rather, the theory assumes that offender motivation is a given.

CAUSES OF VIOLENCE

The theoretical frameworks discussed in the previous section are limited by an emphasis on victims as somewhat culpable for their victimization. The following sections move beyond this early work to discussions of both victimization and perpetration.

SOCIAL THEORY

Social sciences perspectives view victimization and perpetration from the lens of the influences of societal structures. Social learning theory is a popular explanatory framework. The theory posits learning occurs in a social context and through the observation of others. Specifically, individuals learn knowledge and behavior by watching others within the context of social interactions. Individuals learn violence through both the experience of and exposure to violence. Violence is learned through the social experiences of the family. Witnessing and experiencing violence in one's family of origin can send the message that violence is an appropriate tactic for settling conflict and that the strong can prey on the weak. Bandura (1991) suggests that children learn about social interactions by observing and interacting with parents, adults, teachers, family members, etc. Children watch adults and develop scripts that are stored for future use in similar situations (Bandura, 1991).

Social cognitive theory is also used to explain the intergenerational transmission of violence. That is, social cognitive theory explains the link between witnessing interparental violence and subsequent intimate partner violence in adolescent and adult relationships (Stith et al., 2000). However, critics argue that the theory is insufficient because not everyone who was abused or witnessed abuse grows up to be violent. A meta-analytic review by Stith (2000) and colleagues found a weak to moderate relationship between growing up in an abusive family and subsequent perpetration of partner violence. Limited research explores and confirms the link between witnessing violence and subsequent victimization.

Exchange or social control theory assumes that most people are rational and engage in calculations of costs and benefits. Human behaviors and interactions are formed by this avoidance of costs and maximization of benefits (Lawson, 2012). When an individual is rewarded for a behavior, he or she tends to repeat the behavior. A perceived benefit to an action works as reinforcement for the behavior, and he or she would be more likely to use the behavior. If the costs of using violence are greater than the benefits, the individual is less likely to use violence. This perspective helps to understand why violence is more prevalent among those who are young in age. Younger individuals have fewer assets or resources (i.e., no established reputation or good standing and fewer economic assets) and less of a stake in conformity and society. In other words, a person who has more resources has more to lose from violence, and for a person with fewer resources, the benefits to violence would outweigh the costs. The more resources one has, the less likely one will use violence to achieve goals. Violence is a resource when all other avenues fail.

PSYCHOLOGICAL THEORY

Psychology explores individual and/or family pathology or dysfunction as a causative factor for violence (King, 2012). This theoretical perspective would suggest that individuals who are violence-prone and those who engage in violent acts have some sort of mental illness or personality disorder. Individual traits are thought to cause people to become criminals. Crime, then, is a result of individual adverse experiences or individual pathologies such as narcissistic personality disorder and psychopathy. This perspective aligns with criminology efforts that explore individual behavior to determine why certain people are more criminally inclined than others are. An unintended consequence of this approach is to consign violence to a rare experience engaged in by sick individuals who are different from other people. Focusing on personality characteristics of victims and abusers satisfies most people's need to view violence as a pathological behavior exhibited by someone who is different from most people. Emphasis on psychological conditions decreases abusers' responsibility for actions by blaming other factors. This approach adds context to our understanding of violence. However, it minimizes the contributions of social structure.

From a psychological perspective, the risk of violence may be understood in terms of four fundamental personality dimensions (Nestor, 2002):

- **Impulse control:** Someone who is unable to exert self-control exhibits poor impulse control. The individual is unable to avoid temptation or acting on urges. Poor impulse control makes an individual more likely to resort to violence as a means of getting one's way.

- **Affect regulation:** Affect regulation is a complex process whereby individuals are able to adapt their emotional state to reflect their situation. Most individuals are able to tolerate ranges and intensity of emotions. Individuals who are unable to demonstrate emotional control and to moderate their emotions are more likely to resort to violence in times of stress.

- **Narcissism:** Narcissism is a personality trait that is related to violence. It's an extreme sense of self-importance and an inability to identify and empathize with the perspectives of others. This excessive preoccupation with self can lead individuals to resort to violence when their needs aren't meet or admiration is not given.

■ **Paranoid cognitive personality style:** A paranoid cognitive personality style is characterized by extreme mistrust and feelings that others are out to get them. These individuals are constantly on the lookout for slights and wrongdoing by others. They often misperceive actions as hostile and respond in kind.

Some mental disorders increase the risk for violence, with higher rates of violence now firmly established most prominently for individuals with the diagnoses of substance abuse, followed by cluster B personality disorders, and to a lesser extent, schizophrenia spectrum disorders (Johnson et al., 2000).

Antisocial personality disorder and psychopathy are used to explain perpetration of violence. Antisocial personality disorder is clearly described in the psychiatric literature and the *Diagnostic and Statistical Manual (DSM-5)* (American Psychiatric Association [APA], 2013). Some scholars assert that psychopathy is a more extreme form of antisocial personality disorder (Coid & Ullrich, 2010). Psychopathic behavior is associated with violence and crime (Hare & Neumann, 2010). On the other hand, psychopathy describes a constellation of dysfunctional behaviors seen in individuals who commit criminal offenses. Persons diagnosed with psychopathy display a sense of entitlement. They appear unremorseful, apathetic to others, and affectively cold. These individuals are blameful of others, manipulative and conning, and nonconforming to social norms. They possess a disparate understanding of behavior and socially acceptable behavior and demonstrate disregard for social obligations. These individuals are not simply persistently antisocial individuals who meet DSM-5 criteria for ASPD; they are psychopaths—remorseless predators who use charm, intimidation, and, if necessary, impulsive and cold-blooded violence to attain their ends (Hare & Neumann, 2010). Antisocial personality is a mental disorder that begins in childhood and continues into adulthood, and involves the persistent violation of the rights of others and social norms in general. Deficits in emotional, motivational, and cognitive processes contribute to the development of the disorder (APA, 2013). Key differences in antisocial personality disorder and psychopathy include interpersonal traits such as an inflated notion of self-importance, and affective traits such as limited emotional responsiveness.

FEMINIST THEORY

Feminist theory uses the lens of male privilege to explain violence against women (Yllo, 1993). Victimization results from power differentials between victims and offenders. Expressions of violence stem from broader structural inequities such as age and gender. Particularly, crimes such as intimate partner violence and sexual assault are viewed as expressions of gender role socialization and maintaining the status quo (Warshaw & Koss, 1988). Historically and culturally, social structures are male-dominated. Women occupy subordinate positions within society. Society's institutions allow patriarchy to continue. Men have been privileged with power and control within a patriarchal society, and violence can be a tactic used to maintain power and control. Physical violence is a means of exerting and maintaining power and control. Boy and girl children are often socialized differently; specifically, boy children are socialized to be dominant (Kurz, 1989). Structural factors limit women's access to resources. Violence is then construed as a way to maintain social control and male power over women (Sokoloff & Dupont, 2005). A flaw of this perspective is its reliance on a single variable approach. It contains broad statements regarding male privilege and male dominance and ignores individual differences in men. For example, despite being in a culture dominated by patriarchy, only a small percentage of men use violence against women.

SUMMARY

No single theory can completely explain violence; rather, a multifactorial approach that includes biological, psychological, social, and environmental perspectives more accurately explains causes of violence. Theories help increase our understanding of the factors that influence victimization and perpetration of violence. Nursing has an important role in ensuring that all patients receive the healthcare that they need based on their presenting problems. It is important that patients receive treatment for injuries sustained. However, nurses are remiss if the other aspects of trauma and the medicolegal aspects of care are overlooked. Victims of crime or trauma and individuals accused or convicted of criminal activities are a unique subset of patients (Radzyminski, 2006). The nurse must understand the unique needs of these patients. Theoretical perspectives help the nurse to understand the dynamics of victimization and crime and to apply that knowledge to patient care.

References

American Psychiatric Association (APA). (2013). *Diagnostic and statistical manual of mental disorders (DSM-5)* (5th ed.). Arlington, VA: Author.

Bandura, A. (1991). Social cognitive theory of self-regulation. *Organizational Behavior and Human Decision Processes, 50*(2), 248–287.

Cohen, L. E., & Felson, M. (1979). Social change and crime rate trends: A routine activity approach. *American Sociological Review, 44*(588–608).

Coid, J., & Ullrich, S. (2010). Antisocial personality disorder is on a continuum with psychopathy. *Comprehensive Psychiatry, 51*(4), 426–433.

Daigle, L. E. (2012). *Victimology: The essentials.* Thousand Oaks, CA: SAGE Publications.

Federal Bureau of Investigation (FBI). (2013). *Uniform Crime Reports.* Washington, DC: Author.

Federal Bureau of Investigation (FBI). (2014). *Uniform Crime Reports.* Washington, DC: Author.

Hare, R. D., & Neumann, C. S. (2010). Psychopathy: Assessment and forensic implications. In L. Malatesti & J. McMillan (Eds.), *Responsibility and psychopathy: Interfacing law, psychiatry and philosophy* (pp. 93–123). New York, NY: Oxford University Press.

Hindelang, M. J., Gottfredson, M. R., & Garofalo, J. (1978). *Victims of personal crime: An empirical foundation for a theory of personal victimization.* Cambridge, MA: Ballinger.

Hirschel, D. (2009). *Expanding police ability to report crime: The National Incident-Based Reporting System.* Washington DC: Office of Justice Programs.

Johnson, J. G., Cohen, P., Smailes, E., Kasen, S., Oldman, J. M., Skodol, A. E., & Brook, J. S. (2000). Adolescent personality disorders associated with violence and criminal behavior during adolescence and early adulthood. *American Journal of Psychiatry, 157,* 1406–1412.

King, B. (2012). Psychological theories of violence. *Journal of Human Behavior in the Social Environment, 22*(5), 553–571.

Kurz, D. (1989). Social science perspectives on wife abuse: Current debates and future directions. *Gender & Society, 3*(4), 489–505.

Langton, L., Berzofsky, M., Krebs, C. P., & Smiley-McDonald, H. (2012). *Victimizations not reported to the police, 2006–2010.* Washington, DC: U.S. Department of Justice, Office of Justice Programs, Bureau of Justice Statistics.

Lawson, J. (2012). Sociological theories of intimate partner violence. *Journal of Human Behavior in the Social Environment, 22*(5), 572–590.

Meadows, R. J. (2013). *Understanding violence and victimization* (6th ed.). Upper Saddle River, NJ: Prentice Hall.

Mendelsohn, B. (1956). Une nouvelle branche de la science bio-psycho-sociale, la victimologie. *Etudes Internationales de Psycho-Sociologie Criminelle,* July–September, 95–109.

Nestor, P. G. (2002). Mental disorder and violence: Personality dimensions and clinical features. *American Journal of Psychiatry, 159*(12), 1973–1978.

Radzyminski, S. (2006). Population health as a framework for forensic nursing curriculum. *Journal of Forensic Nursing, 2*(1), 33–41.

Sokoloff, N. J., & Dupont, I. (2005). Domestic violence at the intersections of race, class, and gender challenges and contributions to understanding violence against marginalized women in diverse communities. *Violence Against Women, 11*(1), 38–64.

Stith, S. M., Rosen, K. H., Middleton, K. A., Busch, A. L., Lundeberg, K., & Carlton, R. P. (2000). The intergenerational transmission of spouse abuse: A meta-analysis. *Journal of Marriage and Family, 62*(3), 640–654.

Truman, J. L., & Langton, L. (2014). *Criminal victimization, 2013.* Washington, DC: Bureau of Justice Statistics.

Warshaw, R., & Koss, M. P. (1988). *I never called it rape.* New York, NY: Harper & Row Publishers.

Wilcox, P. (2010). Theories of victimization. In B. S. Fisher & S. P. Lab (Eds.), *Encyclopedia of victimology and crime prevention* (pp. 978–986). Thousand Oaks, CA: SAGE Publications.

Yllo, K. (1993). Through a feminist lens. In D. R. Loseke, R. J. Gelles, & M. M. Cavanaugh (Eds.), *Current controversies in family violence* (pp. 19–34). Thousand Oaks, CA: SAGE Publications.

6

ASSESSMENT OF WOUNDS AND INJURY

Mariah Eliza Smock, BA, BSN; and William S. Smock, MD

KEY POINTS IN THIS CHAPTER

- The nurse with forensic training is an asset to the patient, the hospital, and the criminal justice system.

- The determination of entrance versus exit wounds is made by examination of the wound's physical characteristics, not the wound size.

- Incised wounds have sharp wound margins and result from a sharp-edged implement (knife, glass, razor blade, or scalpel) being drawn across the skin.

- Superficial and/or parallel incisions should be assumed to be self-inflicted.

- A laceration has irregular wound margins and results from blunt-force trauma.

- The age of a contusion cannot be accurately determined from its color and appearance.

- A victim of strangulation can be rendered unconscious in less than 7 seconds without evidence of external trauma. The deprivation of oxygenated blood to the brain results in an anoxic brain injury.

- Physical injury, such as petechial hemorrhage, is not required to prove a patient was strangled. More than half of fatal strangulations have no visible external evidence of trauma.

Nurses providing patient care in acute care settings care for the young and the old, the sick and the injured. And they must do it without compromising valuable forensic evidence, jeopardizing the police investigation that may ensue, or reducing the patients' chances of getting justice in the court system if they seek it later. With the incorporation of forensic nursing into the hospital, the scope of the practice of nursing has been broadened (American Nurses Association [ANA], 2009). A nurse trained in forensics is one who can recognize traumatic conditions and evidence, document their presence, collect and preserve short-lived findings, and understand how the patient's illness or injury happened (Lynch & Duval, 2011).

When patients who are victims of assault, abuse, violent crimes, or even motor vehicle collisions present to the hospital, their wounds, clothing, and bodies may be ripe with forensic evidence (Darnell, 2011; Lynch & Duval, 2011). This forensic evidence can be used to connect perpetrators with their victims, to protect innocent parties, to help determine who was the driver versus the passenger in an automobile crash, and to ensure forensic questions regarding injury causation can be answered (Davis, Parks, Kaups, Bennink, & Bilello, 2003; Smock, 2007a). Unfortunately, forensic evidence is usually fragile (a dusting of soot, blood spatter patterns, biologic fluids, wound characteristics), and forensic evidence can be lost or contaminated while nurses and physicians provide care in the acute care setting (Eisert et al., 2010).

The purpose of this chapter is to provide a basic outline of the forensic examination of patients who present to the clinical setting with evidence on their person. It also explains how nurses can provide the highest standard of care without destroying or disposing of forensic evidence that presents on or in their patients.

PERFORMING THE PATIENT ASSESSMENT

When performing a patient assessment, it is essential that nurses are prepared to collect and document any and all forensic evidence discovered during their assessment (Darnell, 2011). Remember, forensic evidence is usually transitory. It is of the utmost importance that the nurse, performing the preliminary assessment, recognize the evidence and wound characteristics and preserve them descriptively and ideally photographically (Darnell, 2011; Lynch & Duval, 2011; Ryan & Houry, 2000; Smock, 2007a). A forensically trained nurse is a nurse first and foremost. However, in trauma centers and hospitals with forensic nurses, it's possible to provide the highest level of nursing care and simultaneously address the forensic needs of the patient without compromising care (Ryan & Houry, 2000). The joint provision of both nursing and forensic care is the standard nurses should strive to provide patients (Wiler, Bailey, & Madsen, 2007).

With any assessment where trauma is suspected, here's how to proceed:

1. **Remove the patient's clothes.**

   Do so in such a way as evidence is conserved, not destroyed. For example, if a bullet hole defect is present in the clothing, do not cut through it. All nurses and paramedics should cut around the defects in the clothing so as to preserve their characteristics and to avoid destroying trace evidence, which may be present around them (Darnell, 2011; Lynch, 2013).

2. **Accurately describe the physical characteristics of all wounds.**

   This should be done using appropriate terminology; for example, as a laceration, incision, soot, tattooing, abrasion collar, or stellate tears.

3. **Document all injuries.**

   The preferred method of documentation is photographic with the photographs electronically merged with the hospital chart. If the patient is capable of giving consent for photographs, secure consent before beginning a forensic assessment. If the patient is unconscious or not capable of providing consent, photographic consent is implied. It's always in the best interest of the patient that photographs are taken of any and all wounds with potential clinical or forensic significance, as their physical characteristics will be forever altered once care is provided (Smock, 2007b).

4. **As the clothes are removed from the patient, catalogue each piece of clothing in the nursing notes** (Eisert et al., 2010).

    Each article of clothing should be placed in a separate paper bag. Each bag should be identified with a patient label and then sealed (see Figure 6.1 on page 1 of the photo gallery). If the clothes have biological material (blood, semen, etc.) on them, it's important to place them in a paper bag. Plastic bags are acceptable short-term receptacles for blood-soaked clothing.

5. **Document who is taking charge of the clothes or forensic evidence, and document this exchange on the bag.**

    The documentation of who collected a piece of evidence and then transferred that evidence to another party establishes the chain of custody. The integrity of the chain is critical for any piece of evidence—be it blood sample, article of clothing, or bullet—and the chain of custody must be maintained for that evidence to be admissible in court. If the chain is not maintained, the defense will ask the court to exclude the forensic evidence at trial.

It is critical for justice and the patient's wellbeing that all evidence be properly collected (Carmona & Prince, 1989). The remaining sections in this chapter give specifics on how to properly collect evidence for the most common injuries.

GUNSHOT WOUNDS

There is a common misconception among healthcare providers that the size of a gunshot wound can determine whether a wound is an entrance or an exit wound. In truth, the size of a wound is no determinant of its etiology. Both entrance and exit wounds have characteristics unique to each type of wound (Dana & DiMaio, 2003; Smock, 2007b, 2014). These specific physical characteristics of the wounds distinguish one from the other; size is not one of them.

ENTRANCE WOUNDS

Entrance wounds are divided into four categories based upon the distance between the gun's muzzle and the victim, or *range of fire*.

Understanding how to differentiate among these types of wounds will help the nurse to provide the best patient care in the clinical setting and also support the gunshot-wound victim in the legal setting (Darnell, 2011; Lynch & Duval, 2011).

Contact Wounds

A *contact wound* occurs when the barrel or muzzle is in contact with the skin or clothing as the weapon is discharged. Contact wounds can be described in two ways:

- **Tight:** The muzzle is pushed hard against the skin.

- **Loose:** The muzzle is incompletely or loosely in contact with the skin or clothing.

Wounds sustained from tight contact with the barrel can vary in appearance from a small hole with seared, blackened edges (from the discharge of hot gases and an actual flame; see Figure 6.2 on page 1 of the photo gallery) to a gaping, stellate (triangle-shaped skin tears) wound (from the injection of hot gases causing the skin to stretch to the point of tearing; see Figure 6.3 on page 2 of the photo gallery).

Large stellate wounds are often misinterpreted as exit wounds. In a tight-contact wound, all materials—the bullet, gases, soot, and incompletely combusted gunpowder—are driven into the wound. If the wound is over thin or bony tissue, the hot gases cause the skin to expand to such an extent that it stretches and tears. These tears have a triangular shape, with the base of the tear overlying the entrance wound (see Figure 6.4 on page 2 of the photo gallery).

Stellate tears are not confined to contact wounds. Tangential wounds, wounds caused by ricocheting or tumbling bullets, and some exit wounds may also be stellate in appearance (see Figure 6.5 on page 3 of the photo gallery). These wounds are distinguished from tight-contact wounds by the absence of soot and powder within the wound. In some tight-contact wounds, expanding skin is forced back against the muzzle of the gun, causing a characteristic pattern contusion called a *muzzle contusion* (see Figure 6.6 on page 3 of the photo gallery). These patterns are helpful in determining the type of weapon (revolver or semiautomatic) used to inflict the injury and should be documented prior to wound debridement or surgery (Smock, 2007b, 2014).

Loose-contact wounds will display soot and seared skin as the byproducts of the burning gunpowder are spread across the surface of the skin. These wounds may also exhibit some degree of triangle-shaped tears if the gases of combustion are injected into the wound.

Close-Range Wounds

Close-range wounds happen at the maximum range at which soot is deposited on the clothing or wound; typically that's a muzzle-to-victim distance of 6 inches or less (see Figure 6.7 on page 4 of the photo gallery). On rare occasions, however, soot has been found on victims as far away as 12 inches from the offending weapon. The concentration of soot varies inversely with the muzzle-to-victim distance and the type of gunpowder and ammunition used. The barrel length, the caliber, and the type of weapon also affect its appearance.

Intermediate-Range Wounds

Intermediate-range wounds occur when the gun is as close as 6 inches to the victim, but can occur when the muzzle is as far away as 4 feet. "Tattooing" is the classic physical finding for an intermediate-range gunshot wound and presents as punctate abrasions. The skin marking is caused by impacts with partially burned or unburned grains of gunpowder (see Figure 6.8 on page 4 of the photo gallery). This tattooing cannot be wiped away and will disappear over the course of several days. Intermediate objects like clothing and hair may prevent the gunpowder

Figure 6.1
EACH ARTICLE OF
CLOTHING SHOULD BE
PLACED AND SEALED
IN A SEPARATE PAPER
BAG AND LABELED
WITH THE PATIENT'S
NAME, DATE, TIME
AND LOCATION OF
WHERE THE ITEM WAS
COLLECTED, AND BY
WHOM.

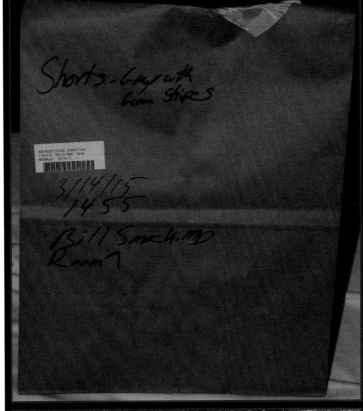

Figure 6.2
A CONTACT ENTRANCE
WOUND TO THE RIGHT
TEMPLE WITH SOOT
AND SEARED WOUND
MARGINS. THE WEAPON
WAS A .32 REVOLVER.

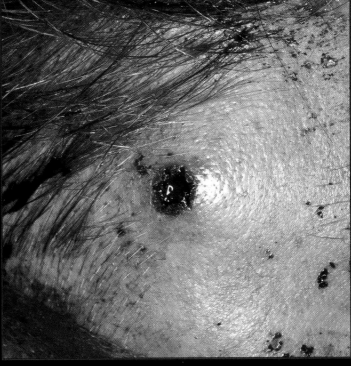

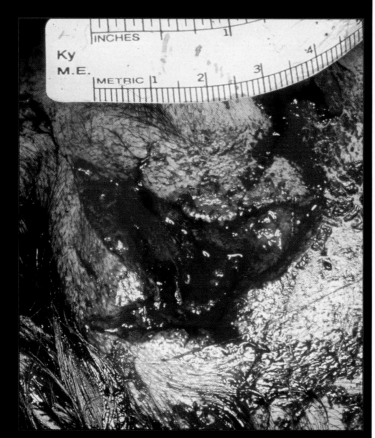

Figure 6.3
A CONTACT ENTRANCE WOUND TO THE RIGHT TEMPLE WITH LARGE TRIANGULAR-SHAPED TEARS CAUSED BY THE INJECTION OF GASES INTO THE SKIN.

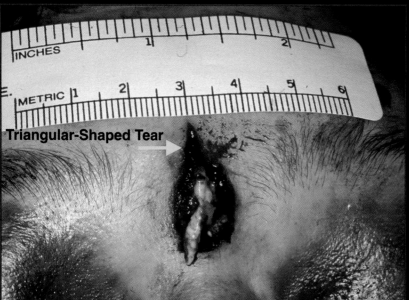

Triangular-Shaped Tear

Figure 6.4
THE "TRIANGULAR-SHAPED TEAR" ASSOCIATED WITH CONTACT WOUNDS HAS ITS BASE WHERE THE GASES WERE INJECTED AND ITS APEX POINTING AWAY FROM THE INJECTION SITE.

Figure 6.5

A TRIANGULAR-SHAPED
EXIT WOUND. EXIT
WOUNDS LACK THE
SOOT AND SEARED
SKIN ASSOCIATED
WITH A CONTACT
ENTRANCE WOUND.

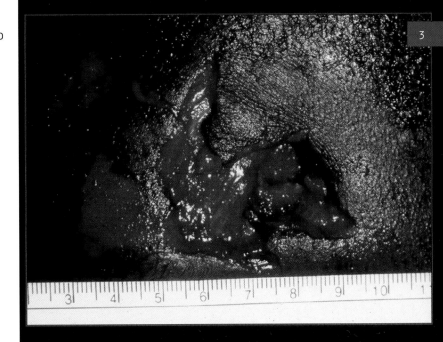

Figure 6.6

A MUZZLE CONTUSION
ASSOCIATED WITH A
CONTACT ENTRANCE
WOUND. THE MUZZLE
CONTUSION MAY
RESULT WHEN THE
GASES OF COMBUSTION
ARE INJECTED INTO
AND UNDER THE SKIN
CAUSING THE SKIN
TO RAPIDLY EXPAND.
THE DISTENDED SKIN
PUSHES AGAINST
THE GUN'S BARREL;
HENCE, THE CONTU-
SION.

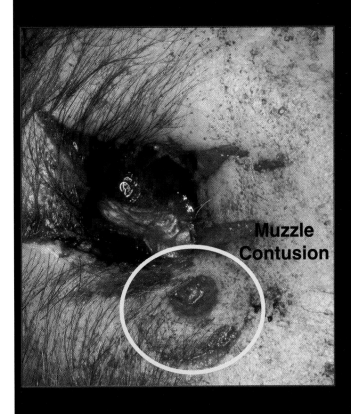

Muzzle
Contusion

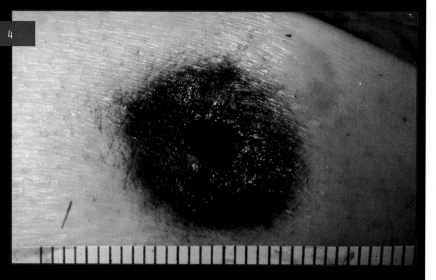

Figure 6.7
THE PRESENCE OF SOOT, THE CARBONACEOUS RES- IDUE FROM THE BURNING OF GUNPOWDER, INDI- CATES A CLOSE RANGE OF FIRE.

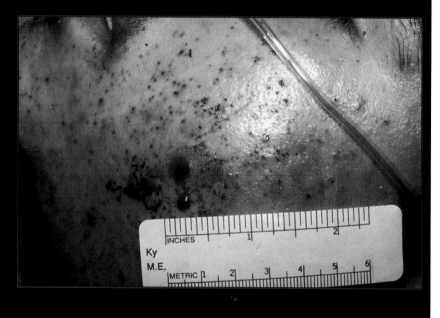

Figure 6.8
"TATTOOING" OR "STIP- PLING" ARE PUNCTATE ABRASIONS, WHICH OCCUR WHEN GRAINS OF UNBURNED GUNPOWDER IMPACT THE SKIN. TAT- TOOING OCCURS AT AN INTERMEDIATE RANGE OF FIRE, LESS THAN 48 INCHES.

Figure 6.9
THE ABRADED AREA
SURROUNDING AN
ENTRANCE WOUND IS
CALLED AN "ABRASION
COLLAR."

Figure 6.10
THE "COMET TAILED"
ABRASION COLLAR
INDICATES DIREC-
TIONALITY. IN THIS
CASE, THE BULLET IS
MOVING FROM RIGHT
TO LEFT.

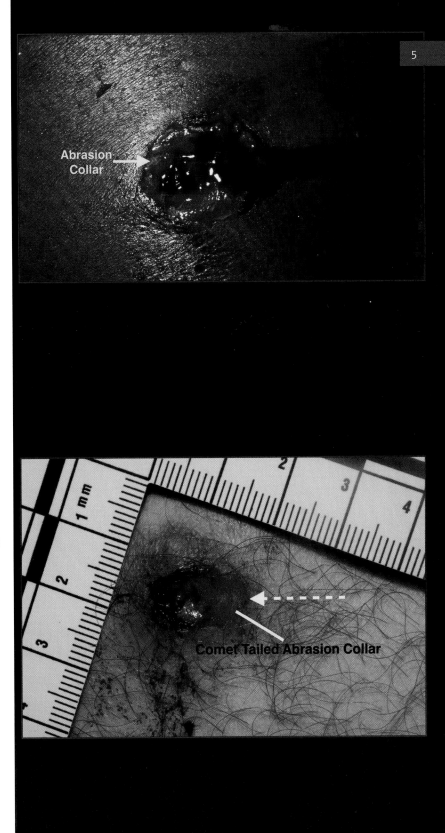

Abrasion Collar

Comet Tailed Abrasion Collar

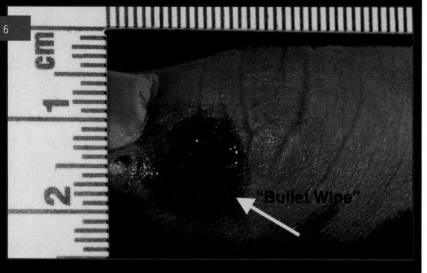

"Bullet Wipe"

Figure 6.11

"Bullet wipe" is a residue that can deposit around an entrance wound. The residue can be that of or a combination of lubricant, soot, lead from a soft nose lead bullet, primer residue, or dirt in the gun barrel.

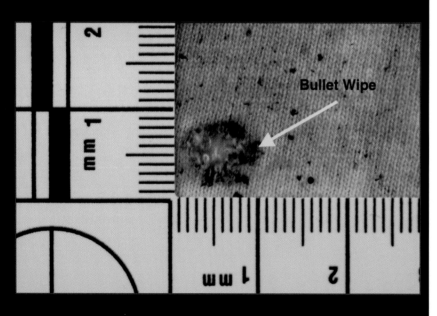

Bullet Wipe

Figure 6.12

"Bullet wipe" around the clothing defect from an entrance wound.

Figure 6.13

POST-INJURY SWELL-
ING OF THE UNDERLY-
ING TISSUE
INCREASED THE SIZE
OF THE EXIT WOUND.

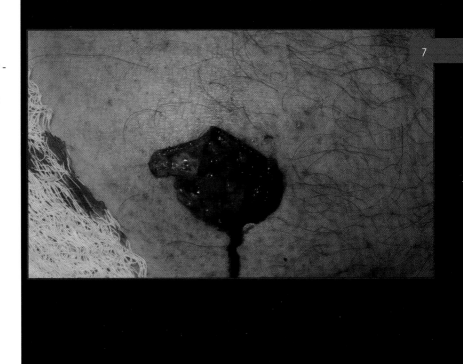

Figure 6.14

POST-INJURY SWELL-
ING OF THE UNDERLY-
ING MUSCLE REQUIRED
A FASCIOTOMY OVER
THE EXIT WOUND.

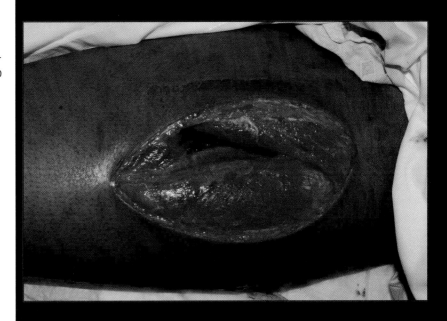

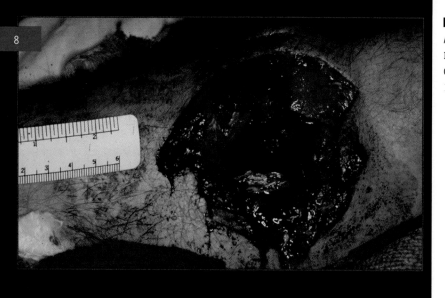

Figure 6.15
A GAPING EXIT WOUND
DUE TO THE TRANSFER
OF ENERGY TO UNDERLY-
ING BONE.

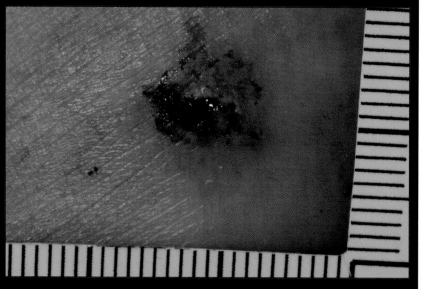

Figure 6.16
A SLIT-LIKE EXIT
WOUND, WHICH IS
SMALLER THAN ITS
ASSOCIATED ENTRANCE
WOUND.

Figure 6.17
LACERATIONS HAVE
IRREGULAR WOUND
MARGINS FROM TEAR-
ING OF THE SKIN.

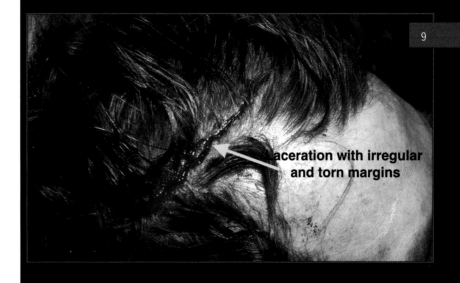

Laceration with irregular
and torn margins

Figure 6.18
A SINGLE-EDGED STAB
WOUND: A SHARP EDGE
AND A DULL EDGE.

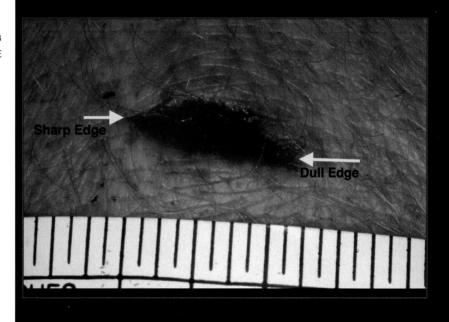

Sharp Edge

Dull Edge

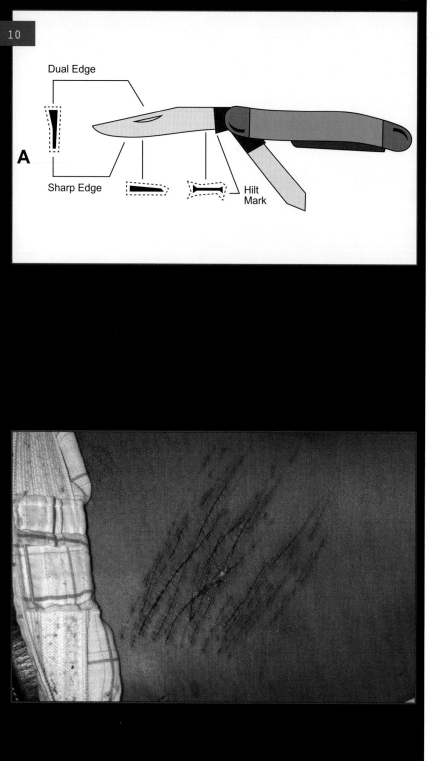

Dual Edge

Sharp Edge

Hilt Mark

A

Figure 6.19
DIAGRAM OF A SINGLE-
EDGED KNIFE.

Figure 6.20
MULTIPLE SUPERFICIAL
LINEAR AND PARALLEL
INCISIONS ARE SELF-
INFLICTED UNTIL PROV-
EN OTHERWISE.

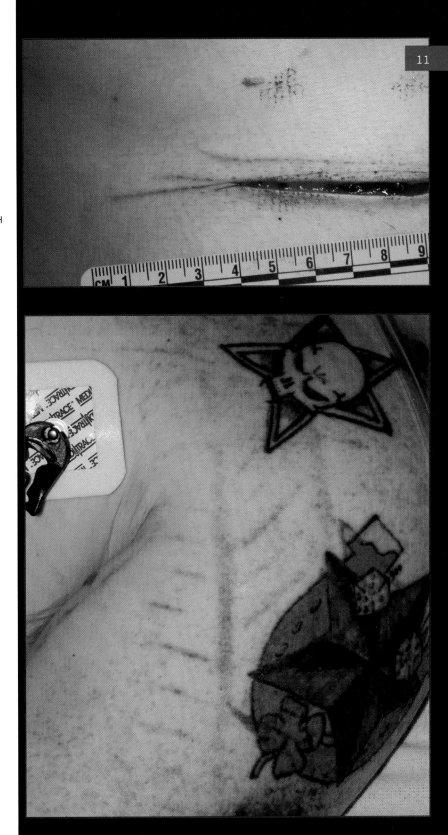

Figure 6.21

AN INCISION WITH MULTIPLE "HESITATION" MARKS ON THE WOUND MARGIN. THE PATIENT STATED THE INJURY OCCURRED WHEN THE ASSAILANT TOOK "ONE SWIPE" WITH A KNIFE. THE MULTIPLE INCISIONS ARE CONSISTENT WITH MULTIPLE INCISIONS, NOT A SINGLE SWIPE OF A KNIFE.

Figure 6.22

A TIRE MARK CONTUSION FROM BEING ROLLED OVER BY A CAR TIRE.

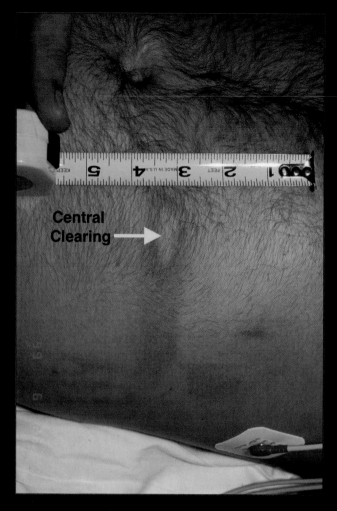

Central
Clearing →

Figure 6.23
A PATTERN CONTUSION
WITH CENTRAL CLEARING
FROM IMPACT WITH A
ROUNDED LINEAR
OBJECT.

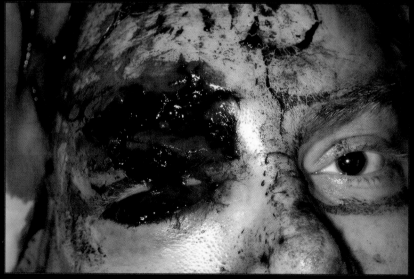

Figure 6.24
THE MARGINS OF THIS
PERI-ORBITAL LACERA-
TION ARE RIPPED AND
TORN FROM BLUNT-FORCE
TRAUMA ASSOCIATED
WITH AN AIR BAG
DEPLOYMENT.

Figure 6.25

PETECHIAL HEMOR-
RHAGE ON THE LOWER
LID CAUSED BY
INCREASED VENOUS
PRESSURE DURING A
STRANGULATION.

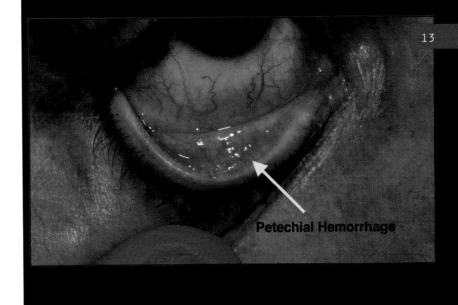

Petechial Hemorrhage

Figure 6.26

SCLERAL HEMORRHAGE
CAUSED BY INCREASED
VENOUS PRESSURE
DURING A STRANGULA-
TION.

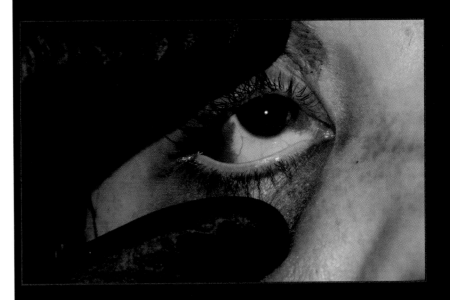

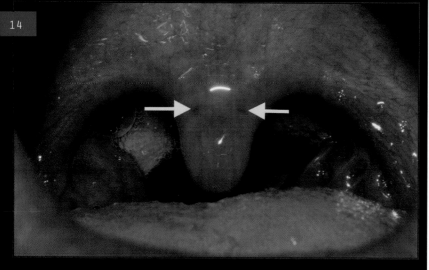

Figure 6.27
BILATERAL PETECHIAL
HEMORRHAGE ON THE
UVULA CAUSED BY
INCREASED VENOUS
PRESSURE DURING A
STRANGULATION.

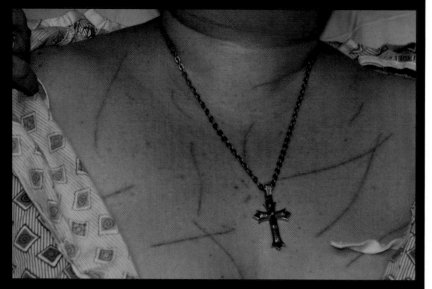

Figure 6.28
MULTIPLE SUPERFICIAL
LINEAR INCISIONS ON
THE ANTERIOR CHEST.
WOUNDS OF THIS NATURE
ARE ASSUMED TO BE
SELF-INFLICTED UNTIL
PROVEN OTHERWISE.

Figure 6.29

MULTIPLE SUPERFI-
CIAL LINEAR INCI-
SIONS ON THE RIGHT
FOREARM. WOUNDS OF
THIS NATURE ARE
ASSUMED TO BE SELF-
INFLICTED UNTIL
PROVEN OTHERWISE.

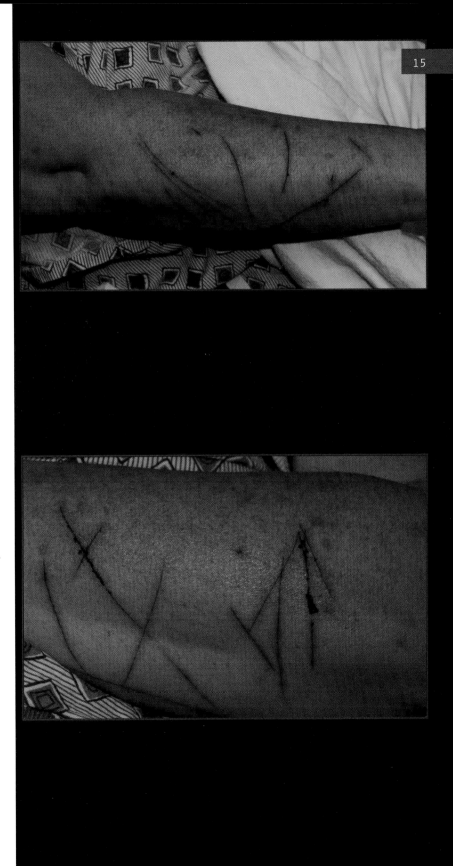

Figure 6.30

MULTIPLE SUPERFI-
CIAL LINEAR INCI-
SIONS ON THE LEFT
FOREARM. WOUNDS OF
THIS NATURE ARE
ASSUMED TO BE SELF-
INFLICTED UNTIL
PROVEN OTHERWISE.

grains from making contact with the skin. Rarely does tattooing occur on the palms and soles owing to the thickness of their epithelium.

Distant Wounds

A *distant wound* is inflicted from a distance sufficiently far enough that only the bullet reaches the skin. There is no tattooing or soot deposition associated with a distant entrance wound because they fall away before reaching the skin. As the bullet penetrates the skin, friction between it and the epithelium results in the creation of an *abrasion collar* (see Figure 6.9 on page 5 of the photo gallery). The width of the abrasion collar varies with the angle of impact. Elongated abrasion collars from projectiles that enter on an angle may produce a collar with a *comet tail* (see Figure 6.10 on page 5 of the photo gallery). Most entrance wounds have an abrasion collar. Gunshot wounds to the palms and soles will not; their entrance wounds appear slit-like. The skin on the palms and soles of the feet is very thick, and often callused, so there is no abrasion collar created by the bullet.

Nurses may note the presence of bullet wipe on the entrance wound or the clothing over the entrance wound (see Figures 6.11 and 6.12 on page 6 of the photo gallery). *Bullet wipe* is soot residue, soft lead, or lubricant, which may leave a gray rim or streak on the skin or clothing overlying an entrance wound (Smock, 2007b, 2014). This gray discoloration can also be found around the abrasion collar but is usually more prominent on clothing. Because bullet wipe can be deposited on skin or clothing at any range, it is important to differentiate between soot and bullet wipe. Bullet wipe is usually a thin, well-differentiated black ring deposited around the entrance wound, while soot is deposited in a more diffuse pattern around a close-range wound (refer to Figures 6.7 and 6.11).

EXIT WOUNDS

Exit wounds are differentiated from entrance wounds by their physical characteristics, not size. Three variables dictate the size and shape of the exit wound:

- The amount of energy transferred from the bullet to underlying tissue

- The orientation and size of the exiting bullet; i.e., yawed or deformed

- The post-injury swelling of underlying tissue (see Figures 6.13 and 6.14 on page 7 of the photo gallery)

If a bullet hits bone, bone fragments may be extruded from the wound. The potential for a large exit wound exists (see Figure 6.15 on page 8 of the photo gallery). If a bullet passes through soft tissue and does not impact bone, the exit wound will be small (see Figure 6.16 on page 8 of the photo gallery).

There are some characteristics a nurse will see present on an exit wound:

- No soot, seared skin, or tattooing

- Irregular, everted, and sharp edges

If a nurse is unsure about whether a wound is an exit wound, it is sometimes easier to tell if it is *not* an entrance wound.

SHARP-FORCE INJURIES

There are two types of sharp-force injuries:

- Incised wounds are longer than they are deep.

- Stab wounds are puncture wounds that are deeper than they are wide.

The wound margins of sharp-force injuries are clean and lack the abraded and torn edges of lacerations, which are caused by blunt-force trauma (see Figure 6.17 on page 9 of the photo gallery).

Forensic information can be gathered during the examination of a stab wound. Some characteristics of a knife's blade, whether it is single or double-edged for example, can be determined by visual inspection of the wound (see Figure 6.18 on page 9 and Figure 6.19 on page 10 of the photo gallery). Characteristics such as serrated versus sharp can be determined if the blade was drawn across the skin during insertion or withdrawal from the victim.

If a patient presents with superficial and/or parallel-incised wounds, the nurse should always assume that the wounds are self-inflicted (see Figure 6.20 on page 10 of the photo gallery) (Smock, 2014). A detailed history regarding exactly how the wounds were sustained should be documented and compared with the physical findings. Many patients claim these types of wounds were the result of an assault when in reality they were self-inflicted (see Figure 6.21 on page 11 of the photo gallery).

BLUNT-FORCE TRAUMA

The most common type of blunt-force trauma is a contusion. Contusions can present with or without a pattern. Some patterns are very specific. For example, if a person is run over by a car, pattern contusions of a tire tread may be present on the skin (see Figure 6.22 on page 11 of the photo gallery). Or, if the contusion is caused by a hand slap, the contusion may present with the pattern of the hand. A blow from a rounded linear object (like a bat) leaves a contusion that is characterized by a set of parallel lines separated by an area of central clearing (see Figure 6.23 on page 12 of the photo gallery) (Smock, 2000; Smock, 2014). The blood underlying the striking object is forcibly displaced to the sides, which accounts for the pattern's appearance.

When patients with blunt-force injuries present to the hospital setting, it is important to document all injuries that present on the person's body (Darnell, 2011; Lynch & Duval, 2011). This includes photo documentation and the use of correct and accurate terms describing the wounds. Blunt-force injuries that occur from abuse (or suspected abuse) are particularly important to document. This proper documentation is essential if the medical records are subpoenaed for court proceedings and the nurse is called to testify. Opinions regarding the cause of contusions without a distinct pattern can only be described as being caused by "blunt-force trauma."

The age of a contusion cannot be determined from its color or visual appearance (Vanezis, 2001). Red contusions may be an hour to 72 hours old, and brown rendering an opinion as to the age of a contusion based upon its color (Bariciak, Plint, Gaboury, & Bennett, 2003; Maguire, Mann, Sibert, & Kemp, 2005).

The laceration is also a form of blunt-force trauma. The edges of a lacerated wound are irregular, making it easy to distinguish it from a smooth-margined incised wound (see Figure 6.24 on page 12 of the photo gallery; refer to Figure 6.17). A laceration occurs when the skin is ripped or torn.

STRANGULATION

Victims of strangulation often seek treatment in the emergency department. *Strangulation* occurs when external pressure is applied to the neck resulting in either the blockage of oxygenated blood flow to the brain, the collapse of the trachea, or both. Brain cells suffer an anoxic injury and die when deprived of oxygen. Controlled strangulation studies conducted in the 1940s revealed that it takes an average of only 6.8 seconds of carotid occlusion to render an adult male unconscious (Rossen, Kabat, & Anderson, 1944). Victims usually report visual or auditory changes prior to the loss of consciousness. The loss of bladder control indicates a deep anoxic insult of at least 15 seconds in duration (Rossen et al., 1944).

Many victims of strangulation, including those fatally strangled, have no external evidence of trauma (Shields, Corey, Weakley-Jones, & Stewart, 2010). Therefore, evidence of trauma is not required to prove someone was strangled. The presence of petechial hemorrhage in victims of strangulation indicates an increase of pressure within the venous system (Faugno, Waszak, Strack, Brooks, & Gwinn, 2013). The most common locations for petechial hemorrhage are the conjunctiva, the sclera, and the soft palate (see Figures 6.25–6.27 on pages 13 and 14 of the photo gallery). Injuries to the trachea, larynx, and esophagus are also common. Patients with a history of unconsciousness or evidence of neck trauma should have their carotids evaluated with either a CTA or an MRA to rule out vascular injury.

CASE STUDY: WOUND ASSESSMENT

A 47-year-old woman presented to the emergency department with a history of being physically and sexually assaulted in her garage. She stated she went outside to let her dog in when she was grabbed by a hooded man who "threw me to the garage floor, cut my clothes off, and cut me." The emergency physician completed a sexual assault kit and notified the local police department. The detective, upon seeing the patient's "cuts," requested a consultation from a forensic nurse examiner. The nurse documented the presence of multiple superficial linear incisions (see Figures 6.28–6.30 on pages 14 and 15 of the photo gallery). When confronted with the characteristics of the incised wounds, the patient admitted the "cuts" were self-inflicted with a knife and the history of a sexual assault was fabricated.

The careful analysis of the wounds and recognition of the self-inflicted characteristics by the forensic nurse permitted the treating physician to have the patient admitted to the psychiatric unit. In addition, the detective did not need to spend time looking for a hooded suspect that did not exist. The use of a forensic nurse was clearly a benefit to the patient and the criminal justice system.

SUMMARY

The nurse with forensic training is an asset to the patient, the hospital, and the criminal justice system. The forensic nurse is in a unique position to properly assess and document wounds, while still providing a high degree of care to the patient. They can preserve fragile evidence on clothing or wounds that can be lost or contaminated during patient care. The trained forensic nurse can also identify and distinguish gunshot entrance wounds from exit wounds, differentiate incised wounds from lacerations, and determine when wounds are self-inflicted. They can also evaluate victims of strangulation for the appropriate history and document the possibly subtle physical findings. A nurse with forensic training is critical and necessary for complete patient care.

REFERENCES

American Nurses Association (ANA). (2009). *Scope and standards of clinical nursing practice.* Silver Spring, MD: American Nurses Publishing.

Bariciak, E. D., Plint, A. C., Gaboury, I., & Bennett, S. (2003). Dating of bruises in children: An assessment of physician accuracy. *Pediatrics, 112*(4), 804–807.

Carmona, R., & Prince, K. (1989). Trauma and forensic medicine. *J Trauma, 29*(9), 1222–1225.

Dana, S. E., & DiMaio, V. J. M. (2003). Gunshot trauma. In J. Payne-James, A. Busuttil, & W. Smock (Eds.), *Forensic medicine: Clinical and pathological aspects* (pp. 149–168). London, UK: Greenwich Medical Media.

Darnell, C. (2011). *Forensic science in healthcare: Caring for patients, preserving the evidence.* Boca Raton, FL: CRC Press.

Davis, J. W., Parks, S. N., Kaups, K. L., Bennink, L. D., & Bilello, J. F. (2003). Victims of domestic violence on the trauma service: Unrecognized and underreported. *Journal of Trauma, 54*(2), 352–355. doi: 10.1097/01.TA.0000042021.47579.B6

Eisert, P. J., Eldredge, K., Hartlaub, T., Huggins, E., Keirn, G., O'Brien, P., ... March, K. S. (2010). CSI: New York: Development of forensic evidence collection guidelines for the emergency department. *Critical Care Nursing Quarterly, 33*(2), 190–199. doi: 10.1097/CNQ.0b013e3181d913b4

Faugno, D., Waszak, D., Strack, G. B., Brooks, M. A., & Gwinn, C. G. (2013). Strangulation forensic examination: Best practice for health care providers. *Adv Emerg Nurs J, 35*(4), 314–327. doi: 10.1097/TME.0b013e3182aa05d3

Lynch, V. A. (2013). Forensic nursing science. In R. M. Hammer, B. Moynihan, & E. M. Pagliaro (Eds.), *Forensic nursing: A handbook for practice* (Vol. 1), (p. 518). Burlington, MA: Jones & Bartlett.

Lynch, V. A., & Duval, J. B. (2011). *Forensic nursing science* (2nd ed.). St. Louis, MO: Elsevier.

Maguire, S., Mann, M. K., Sibert, J., & Kemp, A. M. (2005). Can you age bruises accurately in children? A systemic review. *Archives of Disease in Childhood, 90*(2), 187–189.

Rossen, R., Kabat, H., & Anderson, J. P. (1944). Acute arrest of cerebral circulation in man. *Archives of Neuropsychiatry, 50*(5), 510–528.

Ryan, M. T., & Houry, D. E. (2000). Clinical forensic medicine. *Annals of Emergency Medicine, 36*(3), 271–273. doi: 10.1067/mem.2000.109266

Shields, L. B., Corey, T. S., Weakley-Jones, B., & Stewart, D. (2010). Living victims of strangulation: A 10-year review of cases in a metropolitan community. *American Journal of Forensic Medicine and Pathology, 31*(4), 320–325.

Smock, W. S. (2000). Recognition of pattern injuries in domestic violence victims. In J. A. Seigel, P. J. Saukko, & G. C. Knupfer (Eds.), *Encyclopedia of forensic sciences* (pp. 384–390). San Diego, CA: Academic Press.

Smock, W. S. (2007a). Forensic aspects of motor vehicle trauma. In J. S. Olshaker, M. C. Jackson, & W. S. Smock (Eds.), *Forensic emergency medicine* (2nd ed.), (pp. 72–84). Philadelphia, PA: Lippincott, Williams & Wilkins.

Smock, W. S. (2007b). Forensic photography in the emergency department. In J. S. Olshaker, M. C. Jackson, & W. S. Smock (Eds.), *Forensic emergency medicine* (2nd ed.), (pp. 53–71). Philadelphia, PA: Lippincott, Williams & Wilkins.

Smock, W. S. (2014). Forensic emergency medicine. In J. M. Marx (Ed.), *Rosen's emergency medicine, concepts and clinical practice* (8th ed.), (pp. 828–844). Philadelphia, PA: Elsevier.

Vanezis, P. (2001). Interpreting bruises at necropsy. *Journal of Clinical Pathology, 54*(5), 348–355. doi: 10.1136/jcp.54.5.348

Wiler, J. L., Bailey, H., & Madsen, T. E. (2007). The need for emergency medicine resident training in forensic medicine. *Annals of Emergency Medicine, 50*(6), 733–738. doi: 10.1016/j.annemergmed.2007.02.020

THEORIES OF CRIME PERPETRATION AND THE U.S. RESPONSE TO CRIME

Alison M. Colbert, PhD, PHCNS-BC; and
Lorie S. Goshin, PhD, RN

KEY POINTS IN THIS CHAPTER

- A nurse who understands the complexity of criminal behavior is better able to meet the unique care needs of this population.

- Violence and crime bring together the healthcare and criminal justice systems to ensure that the health and wellbeing of individuals and society are met.

- The application of criminal justice and social science theories to criminal behavior enhances the practice of nurses who care for offenders.

Most nurses rarely think about caring for patients involved in the criminal justice system. In our minds, experience in this area is limited to the occasional patient who presents to the acute care setting in the traditional orange jumpsuit, shackled and accompanied by an armed officer. The reality is that all nurses interact with people who are involved with the criminal justice system, though they might not be aware of it. Not acknowledging the broad reach of the criminal justice system or the unique needs of affected populations contributes to missed opportunities, incomplete care, and poorer health outcomes. Although it may not immediately appear relevant, a basic understanding of the criminal justice system—why patients might come into contact with that system, and the potential consequences of that contact for individuals, families, and communities—is critical to providing good nursing care. This is especially true for forensic nurses. According to *Forensic Nursing: Scope and Standards of Practice* (American Nurses Association [ANA], 2009), forensic nurses are charged with using the nursing process to diagnose and treat both victims and perpetrators. Forensic nurses are also expected to understand how the legal and healthcare systems intersect. This includes a comprehensive understanding of both the criminal justice and correctional systems.

This chapter begins by introducing some key concepts related to criminology and describes five of the prevailing theories to explain why people commit crimes in an effort to help all nurses understand more about the distinctive needs of this population. The chapter then provides a broad overview of the main parts of the U.S. criminal justice system, including important descriptive information regarding who is involved with the criminal justice system. The chapter concludes with a description of the current U.S. system of mass incarceration and the effect this has on public health, followed by a case study and questions to stimulate reflective practice. Chapter 15 goes into greater detail about the role of correctional nursing and healthcare, specific to the delivery of direct care to people involved in the criminal justice system.

THEORIES EXPLAINING PERPETRATION OF CRIME

Truly understanding the roots of how people come into contact with the criminal justice system is incredibly complex and requires an in-depth understanding of the myriad social, physiological, and behavioral factors related to crime and violence. Complicating things further is the reality that different cultures and societies define "crime" and "criminal" *differently*, thereby making the factors that contribute to perpetration heavily influenced by social constructs and norms. Additionally, the factors related to perpetration are dramatically different among the different offenses. For example, Peter Langman (2015), a psychologist who studies school shootings, identified three populations of people who perpetrate these crimes: psychopathic, psychotic, and traumatized. The people who commit these crimes may be dramatically different from people who commit drug crimes, sex offenses, or other interpersonal violence. According to Langman, each group has its own etiology, set of risk factors, and life circumstances, meaning that prevention and treatment are different for each. In order to think about how crime and violence can be prevented and treated, clinicians and researchers turn to theoretical frameworks that might explain the relationships between and among the variables related to perpetration.

VALUE OF THEORY

Taking some time to think deliberately about the application of theory to practice allows practitioners the opportunity to think beyond the task at hand and consider the broader picture, thereby potentially being able to focus on primary, secondary, and tertiary prevention of the dire health consequences related to crime and incarceration.

Theories are not just an academic exercise. They are an important and significant part of any discipline. In practice, theory may (among other things):

- Establish linkages between caring and forensic principles

- Provide the opportunity for self-evaluation to the public and profession

- Suggest appropriate and effective nursing strategies

- Allow for analysis of emerging care protocols

- Allow nurses to focus education and to set a research agenda

The following sections briefly describe some of the widely known theories. The list is not meant to be exhaustive but more to illustrate the complexity of the problem at hand. For the practicing nurse, a general understanding of how social, physical, and psychological factors contribute to perpetration provides some explanation about the relationships between and among the various factors related to crime, violence, and criminal behavior. In addition, we provide one or two research examples that have used the framework to try to explain perpetration or factors leading to perpetration. These are examples only, and they are not offered as definitive evidence in support of or against any particular theory; they simply provide an application of the theory in use.

STRAIN THEORY

Strain theory posits that social structures may put pressure on individuals to commit crimes. General Strain Theory (GST), an individual-level theory expanding on traditional strain theories, argues that negative interactions with others (acting as strains) create negative emotions, resulting in some kind of coping response (Agnew, 1992). This newer iteration of the theory expands the strains from economic and class-based to include other highly valued goals. The coping response becomes deviant when the strains are perceived as unjust, unfair, or severe.

For example, Watts and McNulty (2013) looked at the effect of childhood abuse on criminal behavior, using GST as the guiding framework. They found that childhood physical and sexual abuse (the strain) significantly increase self-reported offending in both males and females, and that those effects work through other factors such as depression, low self-control, and peers who are involved in illegal activity. They concluded that GST partially explained criminal behavior and that childhood abuse was a strain that increases the likelihood of offending in adolescence.

LABELING THEORY

Labeling theory suggests that an individual's behavior may be influenced by the labels and terms used by society to describe him or her. Coded language based on stereotypes may lead to stigma, thereby contributing more to the criminal behavior as the individual adopts the behaviors and attitudes ascribed to him or her through society's labels. Link and Phelan (2001) posit that stigma influences individual behavior when groups (such as those experiencing concentrated disadvantage) are living in marginalized communities and discriminated against, leaving individuals forced to function in society within the confines of those limiting definitions.

Much of the literature about labeling focuses on the impact of perceived labeling in adolescents. For example, Adams, Robertson, Gray-Ray, and Ray (2003) looked at the relationship between six descriptive adjectives/labels and delinquency, finding that labeling was a predictor of general and serious delinquency. Furthermore, there is significant research looking at the effect of perceived stigma on behavior and post-incarceration functioning, broadening the focus on labeling to the social response.

SOCIAL DISORGANIZATION THEORY

In an effort to explore violence and crime at a community level, theorists have explored many different versions of social disorganization theory, broadly defined as connecting crime to neighborhood characteristics. In 1942, Shaw and McKay (as cited in Walker, 2009) mapped patterns of crime in Chicago to particular areas in the city, often identified as economically disadvantaged areas, and the researchers posited that it was the neighborhood dynamics (consistent regardless of the racial group) that explained the higher rates of crime. This was not a direct connection between poverty and crime, but rather common characteristics such as high population turnover, weak traditional institutions of social support (churches, family, schools), and "criminal traditions" learned by young people in the community. This approach to explaining behavior (focusing on the community) has become less influential over time, as research exploring individual characteristics and other factors has become more common. Recent references to social disorganization in research is generally vague, with attention to the characteristics of the neighborhood but little fidelity to the original tenets of the theory (Walker, 2009).

Although this approach has become less influential over time, as opposed to those that look at individual or multilevel factors, researchers do still use the concept of social disorganization to try to explain criminal behaviors, such as aggression or drug use. For example, Karriker-Jaffe, Foshee, Ennett, and Suchindran (2009) looked at neighborhood socio-demographic disadvantage and social organization as they related to aggression in over 5,000 rural adolescents. Specifically, they wanted to know if social organization buffered the effect of neighborhood disadvantage on aggression; their findings said that it didn't, and further, that neighborhood disadvantage itself did not consistently predict aggression in this sample. In another study on social organization, drug activity, and violent crime, the authors studied the city of Miami using census and crime reports (Martínez, Rosenfeld, & Mares, 2008). They found that indicators for social disorganization, such as economic deprivation and instability, were associated with higher rates of aggravated assault and robbery. Conflicting findings across the literature suggest that social disorganization is difficult to clearly define between and among varying communities.

SOCIAL LEARNING THEORY

Social learning theory, originally conceptualized by Bandura (1971), focuses on the interaction among social, cognitive, and environmental factors to predict behavior. It was applied to criminal behavior in the 1970s by Ronald L. Akers (2009), who posited that individuals will commit crimes when they "differentially associate" with people who commit crimes, are exposed more to criminal models, are able to rationalize criminal behavior in certain situations, and perceive more benefits than risks in the behavior. This includes both direct and indirect exposure to others who commit crimes, and both real and anticipated consequences of criminal behavior. Akers contends that this theory can be applied to all criminal behavior, and all populations, with its focus on interaction in groups and peer associations that goes beyond social norms.

Social learning theory has been studied in the context of interpersonal violence, examining how models of behavior impact individual behavior. For example, Foshee et al. (2011) looked at whether models of perpetration in family, peer, school, and neighborhood contexts would predict dating and peer violence in adolescent boys and girls. They found that adolescents who were exposed to more models of aggression were more likely to use both types of violence (compared to neither).

BIOLOGY AND GENETIC THEORY

Recently, a great deal of attention has been focused on the genetic basis for explaining criminal behavior, as have genetic bases for all issues related to health, healthcare, and health behavior. Notably, biological theories were thought to be used in the early 1900s to offer scientific, rather than philosophical, explanations of crime. However, that focus was justifiably sidelined by the move to a more sociological paradigm, as work in the biological area seemed to be a justification for eugenics and other unethical pursuits (Rudo-Hutt, Portnoy, Chen, & Raine, 2015). The past 10 years have seen a resurgence in neuroscience research. It remains, however, highly problematic, due to the potential ethical, legal, and practical implications, and this line of research is often fraught with controversy. Current proponents have merged biological with social approaches to address the potential effects of both biology and environment.

Although this literature is still in its infancy, and the myriad facets are well beyond the scope of this book, biological-driven research explores all potential factors, from the physical structure of the brain, to hormones, to genetic variations. For example, studies have suggested that particular genes may have some effect on criminal behavior. Several studies in the past decade have focused on a version of the monoamine oxidase-A gene, recently called the warrior gene, a variant of which is thought to produce less MAO-A enzyme. "Low functioning" genotypes have been linked to increased aggression and antisocial behavior in men (Byrd & Manuck, 2014; Chester et al., 2015). Again, this work is still in the very beginning stages, and researchers are working hard to not only establish the potential link but also understand how and why the link may exist. Great caution is warranted, and significantly more research is needed, before any of these findings make their way into mainstream discussions around perpetration. Importantly, research in this area also includes studies exploring how individual factors like self-control might mediate the relationship (Barnes, 2012), which will help elucidate practical recommendations for prevention and treatment, bringing together biological and environmental factors.

THE CRIMINAL JUSTICE SYSTEM: STRUCTURE, COMPOSITION, AND IMPLICATIONS

In addition to understanding theoretical pathways to committing crime, it's also important for the practicing nurse to understand the basic building blocks of the system that has been developed to address crime and maintain public safety. In the United States, the criminal justice system is a loosely connected group of agencies tasked with maintaining public safety through the prevention, interdiction, and punishment of crime. The government most commonly operates criminal justice agencies, but functions can also be contracted out to private corporations, as in the case of private prisons and privatized correctional health services. Each agency works within a jurisdiction, which is a politically defined geographical area, such as a city, county, state, or the whole country. The criminal justice system can be broken down into three main parts, which the following sections describe in detail: the police, the courts, and corrections.

POLICE

The police represent the most visible face of the criminal justice system. The police officer's role is to enforce criminal laws. They do this by, among other things, responding to reports of criminal behavior, patrolling to prevent or identify criminal behavior, and investigating to determine the circumstances surrounding crimes. Police have the legal authority to physically detain or arrest people believed to have committed crimes. After arrest, the police officer brings the person to a police station for booking. *Booking* is when the officer makes a formal administrative recording of the arrest and the criminal charge. After booking, the other parts of the system begin to work. The police officer may later be called on to conduct further investigation into the crime, assist criminal prosecutors with the case, or testify in court.

THE CRIMINAL COURTS

The broad role of the criminal court system is to interpret and apply criminal laws. In addition to the accused person, there are three main actors within the criminal court system: prosecutors, defense attorneys, and judges:

- *Prosecutors* are lawyers who represent the government through the criminal court process. They have broad discretion to either bring or decline to bring formal criminal charges against accused persons, also known in the courts as *defendants*. After the decision to prosecute is made, these lawyers also decide the charges, which may be different from those for which the person was originally arrested. They also determine whether or not to offer the defendant a plea bargain. In a plea bargain, the prosecutor, defendant, and defense attorney agree on a particular sanction if the defendant pleads guilty instead of going to trial. Approximately 95% of all felony convictions in the United States result from plea bargains (Bohm & Haley, 2010).

- The *defense attorney* is a lawyer who represents the defendant. The Sixth Amendment of the U.S. Constitution establishes the defendant's right to an attorney. The state is required to provide an attorney at no cost to defendants who are unable to afford an attorney and are accused of crimes that may result in incarceration.

- *Judges* oversee the activities of the criminal courts and ensure that the law is followed. In addition to presiding over criminal trials, they also sign warrants, set or revoke bail, and accept guilty pleas.

The Juvenile Courts
The juvenile court system is unique and varies widely by state. These courts handle cases when young people at or below a specific age (set by each state) are

accused of crimes. This age is usually 17 years but can be as low as 15 years in some states (Office of Juvenile Justice and Delinquency Prevention [OJJDP], 2014). When the behavior is something an adult could be prosecuted for in the criminal courts, it is called a *delinquent offense.* These courts also handle cases for *status offenses,* certain behaviors that are prohibited under law for children but not for adults. These include, among other things, running away, truancy, and violating curfew. The cases of juveniles accused of very serious crimes, those who are close to the legal age of adulthood, or those who have repeatedly committed crimes may be moved to the adult criminal court system. Juvenile courts are more likely than criminal courts to order treatment or other community alternatives to formal correctional supervision. In particular, the federal Juvenile Justice and Delinquency Prevention Act uses grants to encourage states to keep youth adjudicated for status offenses out of detention facilities (OJJDP, n.d.).

CORRECTIONS

The correctional system has broad responsibilities for supervising people at multiple points in the criminal justice system, from those charged with crimes and remanded to those who have been convicted. This system can even supervise people in the community in lieu of incarceration. The following sections provide more information on community corrections, jails, and prisons, which represent the structures that supervise the majority of criminal justice–involved people. Some people are incarcerated in secure juvenile facilities, military prisons, immigration detention facilities, and civil commitment centers, which will not be described herein.

Community Corrections

In *community corrections,* the criminal justice system supervises people who have been convicted of a crime and allowed to remain in the community, as opposed to being placed in a locked correctional facility. This supervision can mean checking in with a community corrections officer in person or by telephone at regular intervals. Activities such as the following may also be mandated: paying fines, attending drug or alcohol treatment, obtaining employment, or attending school.

Probation, the most common type of community supervision, is a term of supervision that is usually granted instead of or after a brief period of time in jail. *Parole* refers to a conditional release from prison that allows people to serve the rest of their sentences in the community. In both probation and parole, not complying with the terms set out by the courts can result in being incarcerated.

Jails

Jails are secure correctional facilities that incarcerate people in multiple different phases of the criminal justice system. For example, jails can be used to confine people who have been arrested but not yet formally charged with a crime by a prosecutor. This group generally exits the jail within hours or days of admission. Jails also hold people awaiting trial or during the course of their trials. These two groups, who are both legally presumed innocent, account for approximately three out of five people in jail (Vera Institute of Justice, 2015). People who receive sentences of less than a year may also serve them in a jail. Jails may also incarcerate people who have violated a community corrections order. For example, if someone on parole has a positive urine toxicology screen indicating that she used an illicit substance, she may be sent to jail as a violation of parole conditions.

Local city or county law-enforcement authorities usually operate jails. Jails can be vastly different sizes. Los Angeles County in California has the largest jail system in the world (Vera Institute of Justice, 2011). On average, 18,000 people were incarcerated in Los Angeles jails on any given day in 2010 (Minton, 2011). In contrast, about half of U.S. jails hold fewer than 50 people (Bohm & Haley, 2010).

Prisons

Prisons incarcerate people who have been convicted of a crime and sentenced to over 1 year of detention. State and federal governments, as well as private corporations under government contract, operate prisons. Private corporations may also manage services inside prisons, such as healthcare, food, and telecommunications. Approximately half of the people incarcerated in U.S. state prisons are there for violent convictions, whereas the majority of people in federal prisons are there for drug possession or trafficking (Carson, 2014). Although some people do spend the rest of their lives in prison, most imprisoned people return to the community within 2 years. For people released from state prison in 2012, the median amount of time served was 28 months for violent convictions, 12 months for property crimes, and 13 months for drug crimes (Carson, 2014). There are wide variations in the sizes of state prison systems that are not completely attributable to population differences. For example, Texas holds 8% of the U.S. population but 12% of its state prisoners (U.S. Census Bureau, 2014).

HOW MANY PEOPLE ARE IN THE CRIMINAL JUSTICE SYSTEM?

According to the most recent federal estimates, approximately 6,899,000 people were being supervised by the U.S. adult criminal justice system at the end of 2013 (Glaze & Kaeble, 2014). This corresponds to 1 in every 35 adults, or approximately 3% of the U.S. adult population. Almost 70% of this group, or 4,751,400 people, were under community supervision. Approximately 731,200 people were incarcerated in local jails, and an additional 1,574,700 were in state and federal prisons. The state prison census includes 1,200 youth held in adult facilities (Carson, 2014). Just over 57,000 juveniles were being held in a secure placement facility at the time of the federal one-day count in 2012, the last year for which federal numbers are available (OJJDP, 2014).

Federal statistics, while shocking on their own, conceal the vast reach of the criminal justice system. These numbers are all single-day estimates of the number of people being supervised. Because people are constantly being admitted to and released from correctional facilities, the statistics underestimate the total number of people who are supervised over the course of a year. For example, jails in the U.S. admitted approximately 11.7 million people between June 2012 and June 2013 (Minton & Golinelli, 2014). Additionally, around half of people released from prison will return within 3 years, many of these for violations of parole (Durose, Cooper, & Snyder, 2014). Looking only at the numbers of incarcerated or otherwise supervised people also obscures the broader effects of the criminal justice system on families. Over half of state and federal prison inmates report having at least one minor child (Glaze & Maruschak, 2010). As of the last federal estimates taken in 2007, this meant an estimated 1,706,600 children, or 2.3% of all U.S. children less than 18 years of age, had a parent in state or federal prison (Glaze & Maruschak, 2010).

MASS INCARCERATION

The number of people incarcerated in the United States has grown dramatically over the past four decades. Figure 7.1 illustrates this rapid rise. Although rates have begun to stabilize somewhat since 2009 (Glaze, 2010), the U.S. continues to incarcerate more people than ever in its history and more people than any other country in the world. In 2013, the median imprisonment rate for Western European countries was 98 prisoners per 100,000 people in the country, whereas the U.S imprisonment rate was 716 per 100,000 (Walmsley, 2013). Social scientists have implicated multiple policy actions, including stepped-up drug-law enforcement (the "war on drugs") and laws establishing minimum amounts of time that had to be served for certain crimes (Garland, 2001). Crime rates have also fallen during this time; however, the effects of this "tough on crime" approach are estimated to account for a small proportion of the decrease (Western, 2007).

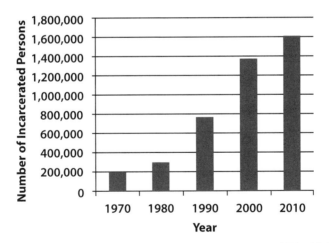

FIGURE 7.1 U.S. PRISON INMATES, 1970–2010.

SOURCE: BUREAU OF JUSTICE STATISTICS PRISON POPULATION COUNTS SERIES

The rapid rise and sheer number of people incarcerated in the U.S. since the 1980s has been labeled mass incarceration, mass imprisonment, and the prison boom (Garland, 2001; Western, 2007). In addition to the numbers of people affected, mass incarceration refers to the striking differences seen in incarceration rates between social groups, such that in many communities the experience of incarceration has become the norm (Garland, 2001). These disparities reflect racial disadvantages at each stage of the criminal justice system, as opposed to only reflecting differences in criminal behavior (Sentencing Project, 2015).

African Americans have been the most disparately affected by mass incarceration. An African-American male child born in 2001 has a 1 in 3 lifetime chance of being imprisoned compared to a 1 in 17 chance for a White male child (Sentencing Project, 2015). Mass incarceration also affects women. For example, the imprisonment rate for Black women (113 per 100,000) is over twice the rate for White women (51 per 100,000; Carson, 2014). For juveniles, African-American juveniles are almost five times more likely than White juveniles to be in the custody of a juvenile detention facility (OJJDP, 2013).

MASS INCARCERATION AS A PUBLIC HEALTH CRISIS

Mass incarceration has created a public health crisis across the U.S. Incarceration at the high levels at which it is currently seen destabilizes already vulnerable communities (Clear, 2007). It negatively affects critical social determinants of health in the areas of education, employment, and marriage, especially for young Black men (Western, 2007). Disproportionate incarceration by race has also been implicated in persistent African-American health disparities in the burden of infectious disease and stress-related health conditions, including cardiovascular disease (Lee, Wildeman, Wang, Matusko, & Jackson, 2014; Massoglia, 2008). It also partially explains U.S. Black-White gaps in both infant mortality and life expectancy (Wildeman, 2012). In these ways, mass incarceration, contrary to the core goal of the criminal justice system, reduces both public safety and public health.

CASE STUDY: CRIMINAL JUSTICE SYSTEM

For nurses working in the community, and those working in corrections, it's important to know upfront that you will encounter patients who are involved in the criminal justice system. Most of them will be poor, undereducated, or living with a lifetime history of traumatic adverse childhood events. They themselves may be victims of abuse, or dealing with a crippling substance abuse problem. Rarely, you may be asked to work with a patient who has been accused or convicted of what you view as truly unspeakable acts. The following case study illustrates the kind of patient the average practicing nurse may encounter in her practice.

You are a nurse at a primary healthcare clinic that serves an economically challenged community. Stephanie is a 23-year-old mother of a 2-year-old child who has been seen at the clinic for about 3 years for her and her child's healthcare needs. Both have frequent illnesses, although they are relatively minor, not requiring hospitalization. Over the time you've known her, you've slowly learned that Stephanie was a victim of childhood physical abuse, that she was with her daughter's father for several years starting in high school but he left right after the birth of their child, and that she has been struggling to make ends meet all her life. Her housing situation is unstable, as is her employment, due to her daughter's frequent illnesses and the need to take time off work to care for her and take her to appointments. She has no significant substance abuse history, but she has been treated for depression and anxiety since she was 13 years old, including a brief in-patient stay for suicidal ideation at 16 years old. At this visit, Stephanie reveals that she recently spent nearly a month at the county jail on retail theft charges. While talking about the experience, Stephanie says that she was tired of not being able to give her daughter the things she deserved and that she had only wanted to show her a good birthday. She is out on bail and working with a public defender on a plea deal. While she was at the jail, she stopped taking her psychiatric medications completely, and she has not been on them since. She has come to see you today with complaints of headaches and fatigue. You are seeing her before her visit with the nurse practitioner.

Taking what you've learned in this chapter, consider the following:

■ How might Stephanie's involvement in the criminal justice system influence her health and health status?

■ How relevant is this history in your plan of care?

■ How would you use General Strain Theory to think about Stephanie's past, present, and future, specific to her health, parenting, and behavior, and to organize your own thoughts about how you can contribute positively to her health and wellbeing?

Take a few minutes to reflect on your practice and how some of the theories of perpetration may influence your orientation to caring for people involved in the criminal justice system. Should nurses concern themselves with theories of perpetration when they are caring for individuals involved in the criminal justice system? Why or why not? Which of the described theories resonate most with you? How could healthcare providers use the explanatory mechanism described in that theory to design new interventions? Finally, what are the negative consequences of relying too much on theories like those to think about individuals in your care?

SUMMARY

Understanding theories related to perpetration and the general structure of the criminal justice system can offer insight and understanding for the clinician working with this population. However, some critics suggest that nurses need to concern themselves less with perpetration and focus more on the needs of the patient sitting right there in front of them. They might argue that if someone has committed a crime, the why is totally irrelevant and that all patients deserve the same level of care and respect, without attention to the mistakes of their past. On the other hand, as this chapter has demonstrated, involvement in the criminal justice system has distinct and serious health consequences, and the clinician must be able to contextualize that information as part of a patient's history, much like family medical history, smoking, diet, and exercise. The goal, we believe, is that the individual patient history, broad understanding of the system, and the potential explanatory theories of behavior should be used together to develop effective, evidence-based treatment plans that take the unique needs of the individual into account. All of this information should be used in the service of improved patient outcomes at the individual, community, and societal levels.

This chapter provided an introduction to some of the theories of perpetration most commonly discussed today, an overview of the criminal justice system, and the public health effects associated with the current U.S. system of mass incarceration. All nurses are asked to care for individuals involved with the criminal justice system, knowingly or unknowingly. We argue that this history has a demonstrable and significant effect on health, and it therefore is relevant to patient care. Additionally, nurses have a role to play in achieving public health goals—those specific to the health of populations, not just individuals—and that criminal justice involvement contributes to alarming health disparities in our country today.

REFERENCES

Adams, M. S., Robertson, C. T., Gray-Ray, P., & Ray, M. C. (2003). Labeling and delinquency. *Adolescence, 38*(149), 171–186.

Agnew, R. (1992). Foundation for a general strain theory of crime and delinquency. *Criminology, 30*(1), 47–88.

Akers, R. L. (2009). *Social learning and social structure: A general theory of crime and deviance.* New Brunswick, NJ: Transaction Publishers.

American Nurses Association (ANA). (2009). *Forensic nursing: Scope and standards of practice.* Silver Spring, MD: Author.

Bandura, A. (1971). *Social learning theory.* New York, NY: General Learning Press.

Barnes, J. C. (2012). Analyzing the origins of life-course-persistent offending: A consideration of environmental and genetic influences. *Criminology & Penology, 40*(5), 519–540.

Bohm, R. M., & Haley, K. N. (2010). *Introduction to criminal justice* (6th ed.). New York, NY: McGraw-Hill.

Byrd, A. L., & Manuck, S. B. (2014). MAOA, childhood maltreatment, and antisocial behaviour: Meta-analysis of a gene-environment interaction. *Biological Psychiatry, 75,* 9–17.

Carson, E. A. (2014). Prisoners in 2013. Washington, DC: Bureau of Justice Statistics.

Chester, D. S., DeWall, C. N., Derefinko, K. J., Estus, S., Peters, J. R., Lynam, D. R., & Jiang, Y. (2015). Monoamine oxidase A (MAOA) genotype predicts greater aggression through impulsive reactivity to negative affect. *Behavioral Brain Research, 283,* 97–101.

Clear, T. R. (2007). *Imprisoning communities: How mass incarceration makes disadvantaged neighborhoods worse.* New York, NY: Oxford University Press.

Durose, M. R., Cooper, A. D., Snyder, H. N., Chadha, J., & Jaggers, J. W. (2014). Recidivism of prisoners released in 30 states in 2005: Patterns from 2005–2010. Washington, DC: Bureau of Justice Statistics.

Foshee, V. A., McNaughton Reyes, H. L., Ennett, S. T., Suchindran, C., Mathias, J. P., Karriker-Jaffe, K. J., & Benefield, T. S. (2011). Risk and protective factors distinguishing profiles of adolescent peer and dating violence perpetration. *Journal of Adolescent Health, 48,* 344–350.

Garland, D. (2001). Introduction: The meaning of mass imprisonment. In D. Garland (Ed.), *Mass imprisonment: Social causes and consequences* (pp. 1–3). London, UK: Sage.

Glaze, L. E. (2010). Correctional population in the United States, 2009. Washington, DC: Bureau of Justice Statistics.

Glaze, L. E., & Kaeble, D. (2014). Correctional populations in the United States, 2013. Washington, DC: Bureau of Justice Statistics.

Glaze, L. E., & Maruschak, L. M. (2010). Parents in prison and their minor children (NCJ 222984). Washington, DC: Bureau of Justice Statistics.

Karriker-Jaffe, K. J., Foshee, V. A., Ennett, S. T., & Suchindran, C. (2009). Sex differences in the effects of neighborhood socioeconomic disadvantage and social organization on rural adolescents' aggression trajectories. *American Journal of Community Psychology, 43,* 189–203.

Langman, P. (2015). *School shooters: Understanding high school, college, and adult perpetrators.* New York, NY: Rowman & Littlefield Publishers.

Lee, H., Wildeman, C., Wang, E. A., Matusko, N., & Jackson, J. S. (2014). A heavy burden: The cardiovascular health consequences of having a family member incarcerated. *American Journal of Public Health, 104,* 421–427.

Link, B. G., & Phelan, J. C. (2001). Conceptualizing stigma. *Annual Review of Sociology, 27,* 363–385.

Martínez, R., Rosenfeld, R., & Mares, D. (2008). Social disorganization, drug market activity, and neighborhood violent crime. *Urban Affairs Review, 43,* 846–874.

Massoglia, M. (2008). Incarceration, health, and racial disparities in health. *Law & Society Review, 42,* 275–306.

Minton, T. D. (2011). Jail inmates at midyear 2010: Statistical tables (NCJ 233431). Washington, DC: Bureau of Justice Statistics.

Minton, T. D., & Golinelli, D. (2014). Jail inmates at midyear 2013: Statistical tables. Washington, DC: Bureau of Justice Statistics.

Office of Juvenile Justice and Delinquency Prevention (OJJDP). (n.d.). *Legislation/JJDP Act.* Washington, DC: Author. Retrieved from http://www.ojjdp.gov/about/legislation.html

Office of Juvenile Justice and Delinquency Prevention (OJJDP). (2013). *Custody data (1997–Present).* Washington, DC: Author. Retrieved from http://www.ojjdp.gov/ojstatbb/ corrections/qa08203.asp

Office of Juvenile Justice and Delinquency Prevention (OJJDP). (2014). *Jurisdictional boundaries.* Washington, DC: Author. Retrieved from http://www.ojjdp.gov/ojstatbb/ structure_process/qa04101.asp?qaDate=2013

Rudo-Hutt, A. S., Portnoy, J., Chen, F. R., & Raine, A. (2015). Biosocial criminology as a paradigm shift. In M. DeLisi & M. G. Vaughn (Eds.), *The Routledge international handbook of biosocial criminology* (pp. 22–31). New York, NY: Routledge.

Sentencing Project (2015). Black lives matter: Eliminating racial inequity in the criminal justice system. Washington, DC: Author. Retrieved from http://sentencingproject.org/doc/ publications/rd_Black_Lives_Matter.pdf

U.S. Census Bureau (2014). Annual estimates of the resident population: April 1, 2010 to July 1, 2013. Washington, DC: Author.

Vera Institute of Justice. (2011). *Los Angeles County Jail overcrowding reduction project: Final report: Revised.* New York, NY: Author. Retrieved from http://www.vera.org/sites/default/ files/resources/downloads/LA_County_Jail_Overcrowding_--_Executive_Summary.pdf

Vera Institute of Justice. (2015). *Incarceration's front door: The misuse of jails in America.* New York, NY: Author. Retrieved from http://www.vera.org/pubs/incarcerations-front-door-misuse-jails-america

Walker, J. (2009). Social disorganization theory. In J. Miller (Ed.), *21st century criminology: A reference handbook* (pp. 312–323). Thousand Oaks, CA: SAGE Publications, Inc. doi: 10.4135/9781412971997.n36

Walmsley, R. (2013). *World prison population list* (10th ed.). London, UK: International Centre for Prison Studies. Retrieved from http://www.apcca.org/uploads/10th_Edition_2013. pdf

Watts, S. J., & McNulty, T. L. (2013). Childhood abuse and criminal behavior: Testing a general strain theory model. *Journal of Interpersonal Violence, 28*(15), 3023–3040.

Western, B. (2007). *Punishment and inequality in America.* New York, NY: Russell Sage.

Wildeman, C. (2012). Imprisonment and infant mortality. *Social Problems, 59,* 228–257.

CHAPTER 8

MURDER, ASSAULT AND BATTERY, STRANGER DANGER

Paul Thomas Clements, PhD, APRN-BC, CGS, DF-IAFN

KEY POINTS IN THIS CHAPTER

- Murder, assault, and battery are all violent crimes that greatly impact the victim and surviving loved ones.

- Education about violence should dispel myths regarding stranger danger and provide strategies to avoid violence.

- Resources exist at the federal and state level to provide compensation and assistance to victims and their survivors of crime.

Murder and assault and battery represent crimes that are significantly traumatic for both the victims and surviving family members and friends. According to the Office for Victims of Crime (n.d.), in 2010, an estimated 725,189 incidents of aggravated assault and 2.4 million cases of simple assault occurred in the United States. In 2010, incidents of assault accounted for 63% of violent crime in the United States. In both simple and aggravated assaults, firearms were the most common weapons used, followed by knives. During a 1-year period, 47% of youth ages 14 to 17 experienced a physical assault. In 2010, an aggravated assault occurred every 41 seconds (Office for Victims of Crime, n.d.).

Further, the nature of the relationship of the offender to the victim can have a significant impact on the recovery of the victim. Although most of American society focuses on "stranger danger," research consistently shows that most victims do know their offenders (Finklehor, 2013). Specifically, according to the Federal Bureau of Investigation (FBI, 2015a), in 2011, in incidents of murder for which the relationships of murder victims and offenders were known, 54.3% were killed by someone they knew (acquaintance, neighbor, friend, boyfriend, etc.); 24.8% of victims were slain by family members. Additionally, according to the National Center for Missing and Exploited Children (NCMEC, 2015), more than 200,000 children were abducted by family members.

The damaging impact of crimes such as murder and assault and battery are traumatic both physically and emotionally, and this trauma is often compounded by the fact that someone (the offender) has "taken" something—whether it be a life, property, or a sense of safety in daily life. According to an analysis of reported crimes in the United States from 2009 to 2012, the U.S. Department of Justice reported that the majority (91%) of violent crime victims with socio-emotional problems experienced one or more emotional symptoms for a month or more. Most (61%) experienced one or more physical symptoms for a month or more. Further, a greater percentage of female than male victims experienced socio-emotional problems, regardless of the type of violence or victim-offender relationship (Langton & Truman, 2014).

Subsequently, it's important for nurses to be aware of the foundational facets relative to these criminal activities and related psychosocial impact toward prevention efforts and the ability to conduct targeted yet sensitive assessments and determine appropriate interventions toward adaptive coping and mental health in survivors (Clements et al., 2015; International Association of Forensic Nurses, 2015).

MURDER

Murder is an overarching term for the multiple legal categorizations of homicide. *Homicide* is the intentional killing of one human being by another, and in most cases, includes a specific motive accompanied with pre-meditated intent. The state of mind differentiates murder from other types of criminal homicide like *voluntary manslaughter* (intentional killing in which the offender had no prior intent to kill, such as a killing that occurs in the "heat of passion") and *involuntary manslaughter* (unintentional killing that results from recklessness or criminal negligence, or from an unlawful act that is a misdemeanor or low-level felony, such as driving while intoxicated/DWI) (Manslaughter, 2015).

To constitute premeditated murder, a period of time actually has to elapse between the formulation of a plan to commit murder and its being carried out. The courts consider four different states of mind foundational facets of murder (FBI, 2015b):

- An intent to kill

- An intent to commit grievous bodily injury

- A reckless indifference to the value of human life

- The intent to commit certain dangerous felonies, such as armed robbery

The FBI's Uniform Crime Reporting (FBI, 2015b) Program defines murder and non-negligent manslaughter as the willful (non-negligent) killing of one human being by another. The classification of this offense is based solely on police investigation as opposed to the determination of a court, medical examiner, coroner, jury, or other judicial body. The UCR Program doesn't include the following situations in this offense classification: deaths caused by negligence, suicide, or accident; justifiable homicides; and attempts to murder or assaults to murder, which are classified.

The scope and various facets of homicide based on the most current information from the Uniform Crime Reports (FBI, 2015b) is:

- Of the estimated number of murders in the United States, 43.8% were reported in the South, 21.4% were reported in the Midwest, 21.0% were reported in the West, and 13.8% were reported in the Northeast.

- In 2013, the estimated number of murders in the nation was 14,196. This was a 4.4% decrease from the 2012 estimate, a 7.8% decrease from the 2009 figure, and a 12.1% drop from the number in 2004.

- There were 4.5 murders per 100,000 people. The murder rate fell 5.1% in 2013 compared with the 2012 rate. The murder rate was down from the rates in 2009 (10.5%) and 2004 (18.3%).

You can also assess the nature of the relationship between murderer and victim. Some murderers are motivated by rage or anger and the expressiveness is seen in the murder. For example, a person is having an argument with a neighbor. The argument has been escalating over several weeks. The last confrontation leads to murder. Others are instrumental, resulting in some gain. For example, a murder occurs during a robbery or drug deal. Gender can also play a role. Men commit more murders; however, women are more likely to kill someone they know (Siegel, 2011).

Legally speaking, murders are classified as:

- First degree: Planned or pre-meditated

- Second degree: While not pre-meditated was planned

- Manslaughter: An act done without intent that deserves blame

Serial killers are persons who kill three or more people in separate events. The most common form of serial murder is motivated by sadism or a need for dominance. Mass murder involves killing four or more individuals by one or more perpetrators in a single event (Siegel, 2011).

Knowledge of the scope and prevalence of homicide helps nurses to develop strategies to enhance recognition, intervention, and prevention. Turn to Chapter 18, "Community Violence Intervention Programs," for more information when dealing with offenders in a nursing practice. For more information on how to deal with victims and their families, see "Navigating the Chaotic Aftermath of Victimization," later in this chapter.

ASSAULT AND BATTERY

In most states, assault and/or battery is committed when someone (FBI, 2015c):

- Tries to or does physically strike another

- Acts in a threatening manner to put another in fear of immediate harm

Many states declare that a more serious or "aggravated" assault/battery occurs when someone (FBI, 2015c):

- Tries to or does cause severe injury to another

- Causes injury through use of a deadly weapon

Assault and battery often are related to bar fights, gang warfare, riots at sports events, and similar mayhem-based encounters. Some states combine the two offenses; however, the terms are actually two separate legal concepts with distinct elements. In short, an assault is an attempt or threat to injure another person, while battery would be actually contacting another person in a harmful or offensive manner (Aggravated battery, n.d.). By examining the two offenses, comparing and contrasting their foundational elements, we can see how these two offenses are so closely tied together. Subsequently, some jurisdictions have combined assault and battery into a single offense because the two offenses are so closely related and often occur together.

ASSAULT

The definitions for assault vary from state to state, but *assault* is an attempt to cause injury to someone else, and in some circumstances can include threats or threatening behavior against others. One common definition would be an intentional attempt, using violence or force, to injure or harm another person. Another straightforward way that assault is sometimes defined is as an attempted battery. Indeed, generally the main distinction between an assault and a battery is that no contact is necessary for an assault, whereas an offensive or illegal contact must occur to meet the definition of battery (FBI, 2015c; Holt, 2015).

Even though contact is not generally necessary for an assault offense, a conviction for assault still requires a criminal "act." The types of acts that fall into the category of assaults can vary widely, but typically an assault requires an overt or direct act that would put the reasonable person in fear for his or her safety. Spoken words alone are not enough of an act to constitute an assault unless the offender backs the words up with an act or actions that put the victim in reasonable fear of imminent harm.

In order to commit an assault, an individual need only have "general intent." This means that although someone can't accidentally assault another person, it's enough to show that an offender intended the actions that make up an assault. So, if an individual acts in a way that's considered dangerous to other people, that can be enough to support assault charges, such as wielding a broken beer bottle as a weapon or throwing rocks in a person's direction, even if the person didn't intend a particular harm to a particular individual. Ultimately, the intent to scare or frighten another person can be enough to establish assault charges.

The FBI Uniform Crime Reporting Program (FBI; 2015c) defines *aggravated assault* as an unlawful attack by one person upon another for the purpose of inflicting severe or aggravated bodily injury. The UCR Program further specifies that this type of assault is usually accompanied by the use of a weapon or by other means likely to produce death or great bodily harm. Attempted aggravated assault that involves the display of—or threat to use—a gun, knife, or other weapon is included in this crime category because serious personal injury would likely result if the assault were completed. When aggravated assault and larceny-theft occur together, the offense falls under the category of robbery.

The following FBI statistics (FBI, 2015c) provide an overview of aggravated assaults in the United States:

- In 2011, there were an estimated 751,131 aggravated assaults in the nation.

- Of the aggravated assault offenses in 2011 for which law enforcement agencies provided expanded data, 26.9% were committed with personal weapons such as hands, fists, or feet.

- Slightly more than 21% (21.2%) of aggravated assaults were committed with firearms, and 19.1% were committed with knives or cutting instruments. The remaining 32.8% of aggravated assaults were committed with other weapons.

- In 2011, the estimated rate of aggravated assaults was 241.1 offenses per 100,000 inhabitants.

- The estimated number of aggravated assaults in 2011 declined 3.9% when compared with data from 2010 and 15.7% when compared with the estimate for 2002.

An understanding of the scope of assault helps nurses to identify affected individuals they encounter in their practice. Turn to Chapter 18, "Community Violence Intervention Programs," for more information when dealing with offenders in a nursing practice. For more information on how to deal with victims and their families, see "Navigating the Chaotic Aftermath of Victimization" later in this chapter.

BATTERY

Although the statutes defining battery vary by state and other jurisdictions, a typical definition for *battery* is the intentional offensive or harmful touching of another person without that person's consent. Under this general definition, a battery offense requires all of the following (Aggravated battery, n.d.):

- Intentional touching

- The touching must be harmful or offensive

- No consent from the victim

Of note, battery does not explicitly require that the offender have intent to harm the victim (although such intent often exists in battery cases). Instead, a person need only have intent to contact or cause contact with an individual. Additionally, if someone acts in a criminally reckless or negligent manner that results in such contact, it may constitute an assault. As a result, accidentally bumping into someone, offensive as the "victim" might consider it to be, doesn't constitute a battery. Conversely, purposefully shoving the victim, causing a fall that results in a blunt-force injury to the head from hitting a brick wall or sidewalk curb, does constitute battery.

The most important element to keep in mind is that battery requires an offensive or harmful contact. This can range anywhere from the obvious battery where a physical attack such as a punch or kick is involved, to even minimal contact in some cases. Although it isn't required that a victim be injured or harmed for a battery to have occurred, offensive contact must be involved. In a classic example, spitting on an individual doesn't physically injure the person, but it nonetheless can constitute offensive contact sufficient for a battery. Within the court system, determining if an act is "offensive" in nature is determined by the perceptions and interpretation of the "ordinary person."

Simple battery is the least serious form of battery and usually involves only minor injury, if any, and usually is a petty misdemeanor. Aggravated battery, however, involves circumstances that make the crime more serious and usually is charged as a full misdemeanor or as a felony. Examples of aggravated battery include:

- Striking a person with a weapon or dangerous object

- Shooting a person with a gun

■ Battery resulting in temporary disfigurement

■ Battery resulting in permanent disfigurement or other serious physical injury

■ Battery against a member of a protected class, such as a police officer, health-care provider, social services worker, or developmentally disabled or elderly person

See "Navigating the Chaotic Aftermath of Victimization" later in this chapter for more information on how to deal with victims and their families. Turn to Chapter 18, "Community Violence Intervention Programs," for more information when dealing with offenders in a nursing practice.

STRANGER DANGER

We live in a world where trust is necessarily instilled as a foundation for daily function. In essence, we trust in the social appropriateness of strangers on a regular basis. For example, school bus drivers safely navigating children to school and back; a pilot flying a plane; the preparer at the fast food restaurant ensuring the standards for sanitation while cooking our order; the day-to-day safety of walking on the street. Without this inherent trust of society-at-large, it would be impossible for children to maintain an on-time trajectory of psychosocial growth and development and would ultimately result in an inability to navigate daily life as they grow.

Specifically, children come into contact with strangers every day and everywhere, including the park, the walk home from school, people walking by when playing in the front yard at home, in the aisles of a grocery or department store, and in their community-at-large. Most of these strangers are nice, normal people; however, a few may not be. It's important to educate children about foundational approaches, cues, and clues to make a determination of those strangers who could represent danger. Nurses, as one of the consistently trusted professionals in the nation (Riffkin, 2015), are in a strategic position to educate children and parents and promote safety by teaching about strangers and suspicious behaviors, and also to expose the myths and realities regarding "stranger danger."

DETERMINING WHO IS A STRANGER

The National Crime Prevention Council (NCPC, 2015) defines a stranger as "anyone that your family doesn't know well." It is not uncommon for adults and children to think of "bad" strangers as being "scary looking," dressed in a very disheveled manner, and either lurking in the shadows or trailing behind them as they walk across a parking lot, down an empty street, or in the woods on a short-cut on the way home from school. These images are easy to visualize; however, not only are they inaccurate but they can be dangerously misleading to both children and parents. "Bad" strangers can be (and are typically) very charming, engaging, attractive, and nicely dressed. When educating children about strangers, it is very important to stress that no one can tell whether strangers are nice or not nice just by looking at them, and that they should be careful around all strangers. Simultaneously, it's important to avoid making it seem like all strangers are bad, because this can have a significant impact on the development of their worldview. Further, this could be lifesaving if children need help when they're lost, being threatened by a bully, or being followed by a stranger; the safest thing for them to do in many cases is to ask a stranger for help. This can be made easier for children by showing them which strangers are okay to trust (NCPC, 2015).

FINDING SAFE STRANGERS

When educating children regarding stranger danger, identify strangers who are "safe," indicating that these are people who can be asked for help when needed. For example, police officers and firefighters are two examples of very recognizable safe strangers. Teachers, principals, school nurses, and librarians are adults children can trust too, and they are easy to recognize when they're at work. It's very important to emphasize that whenever possible, children should go to a public place to ask for help (i.e., "go to where there are lots of people and look for someone you can trust," like a policeman). Nurses can educate parents to point out examples of safe strangers to their children when doing errands, shopping, walking in public places, etc. This is also a good opportunity to show children safe places to go to if they need help, such as local stores, a school (for example, an elementary-school child may be hesitant to enter a high school, yet, the school's main office will be filled with adults who can help), restaurants, and the homes of family and parent-approved neighbors.

WHAT TO DO WHEN A CHILD IS SCARED OR IN TROUBLE

It is best to teach children about potentially dangerous situations when the environment is calm and casual. It allows them to focus on the information being provided, to ask questions of the parent, and to process the information in a non-anxietal manner (which aids recall when needed). Such primary prevention efforts will help them when dealing with strangers as well as with known adults who may not have good intentions (remember that a significant number of victimized children know the offender).

Case scenarios should be presented in a matter-of-fact manner to increase awareness but not to cause significant anxiety. The goal should be to teach children to recognize the warning signs of inappropriate adult behavior, such as when an adult asks them to do something without their parents' permission, asks them to keep a secret, or makes them feel uncomfortable in any way (such as being "too friendly," hugging or touching, or asking them to sit on their lap). One of the most significantly important tenets to teach and reinforce to children is that an adult should never ask a child for help, and if one does ask for the child's help (for example, to find a lost puppy or help carry something), the child should leave immediately and find a trusted adult right away to tell what happened and ask that adult to call the child's parents.

Some dangerous situations require more overt responses; specifically, when the child is in imminent danger from an adult who persists with attempts at inappropriate behavior or tries to coerce or force the child to do something or come with him. The National Crime Prevention Council (2015) suggests teaching the *No, Go, Yell, Tell* method. If in a dangerous situation, children should say *no*, run away (*go*), *yell* as loud as they can, and *tell* a trusted adult what happened right away. Make sure that the children know that it is okay to say *no* to an adult in a dangerous situation and to yell to keep themselves safe, even if they are indoors. It's good for parents to practice this with children using different situations as examples so that children will feel confident in knowing what to do. A few possible scenarios for educating children as recommended by the National Crime Prevention Council (2015) are:

- A nice-looking stranger approaches your child in the park and asks for help finding the stranger's lost dog.

- A woman who lives in your neighborhood but that the child has never spoken to invites your child into her house for a snack.

- A stranger asks if your child wants a ride home from school.

- Your child thinks he or she is being followed.

- An adult your child knows says or does something that makes him or her feel bad or uncomfortable.

- While your child is walking home from a friend's house, a car pulls over and a stranger asks for directions.

NAVIGATING THE CHAOTIC AFTERMATH OF VICTIMIZATION

The FBI (2015d) stresses the importance of dispelling myths and stereotypes regarding crime in the nation; specifically, that crime does not discriminate based on age, race, gender, economic status, or geographic location (urban, suburban, or rural). Anyone can become a victim of a crime (National Center for Victims of Crime, 2008). When working with victims of crime toward regaining a sense of control and reinvestment in daily life, nurses can offer important points as they navigate the often-chaotic wake of what has happened to them.

Being a victim of a crime is typically a very difficult and stressful experience. Although most people are naturally resilient and over time find ways to cope and adjust, there can be a wide range of after-effects to a trauma. One person may experience many, few, or no effects at all. In some people the reaction may be delayed days, weeks, or even months. Some victims may think they are "going crazy," when they are having a normal reaction to an abnormal event. Getting back to normal can be a difficult process after a traumatic experience, especially for victims of violent crime and families of murder victims. Learning to understand and feel more at ease with their intense feelings can help victims better cope with what happened. Subsequently, victims may need to seek help from friends, family, a member of the clergy, a counselor, or a victim-assistance professional.

HEALTH AND HELP

Although often difficult for victims to consider, it's significantly beneficial to find a family member or friend (an "anchor for safety") to talk over thoughts, feelings, and daily challenges. Remind victims that there will be good days and bad days and that backsliding is normal. Recovery from traumatic events can be a roller coaster—there may be highs, lows, significant climbs, and scary falls—but in the end the safety and stability of the "station" will be reached and one can finally get off of the ride.

There are some simple, yet highly beneficial, tips that promote a less chaotic journey through the traumatic aftermath. Some of these include (FBI, 2015d; National Center for Victims of Crime, 2012; Office for Victims of Crime, 2015a):

- Keep the phone number of a good friend nearby to call when you feel overwhelmed or feel panicked.

- Allow yourself to feel the pain. It will not last forever.

- Keep a journal—to record not only current experiences, sensations, and fear, but to also write down positive thoughts and memories prior to the event and goals for accomplishing recovery in the weeks and months ahead.

- Spend time with others, but make time to spend time alone.

- Take care of your mind and body. Rest, sleep, and eat regular, healthy meals.

- Re-establish a normal routine as soon as possible, but don't overdo.

- Make daily decisions, which will help to bring back a feeling of control over your life.

- Exercise, though not excessively, and alternate with periods of relaxation.

- Undertake daily tasks with care. Accidents are more likely to happen after severe stress.

- Recall the things that helped you cope during trying times and loss in the past and think about the things that give you hope. Turn to them on bad days. (This helpful hint can be extremely useful during the many holidays, occasions, and anniversary dates that occur within each calendar year, particularly the first year following the traumatic event.)

Things to avoid:

- Be careful about using alcohol or drugs (illicit or prescription) to relieve emotional pain. Becoming addicted not only postpones healing but also creates new problems.

- Make daily decisions, but avoid making life-changing decisions in the immediate aftermath; judgment may be temporarily impaired.

- Don't blame yourself—it wasn't your fault.

- Your emotions need to be expressed. Try not to bottle them up.

VIOLENCE AND CRIME ARE A FAMILY MATTER

For victims and families of victims, life is forever changed. Many will say, "I just want to forget about the entire thing." However, such a goal is unrealistic, always results in failure to do so, and typically perpetuates the traumatic response pattern. Although the victim's life may feel "empty" and does not "feel like it used to," a significant part of adaptive coping and reintegrating and reinvesting in daily life is redefining the future. What seemed important before may not be important now. Most victims find new meaning in their lives as a result of their experience. It's important to remember that emotional pain is not endless and that it will eventually ease. Although it's not possible to undo what has occurred, it is possible to integrate what happened in a way that life can be good again in time. It is eloquently described in a Native American proverb that states, "What is past and cannot be prevented should not be grieved for."

It is not uncommon for family and friends to want to provide help and support, yet they often feel uncertain about how best to go about this. Frequently, attempts to console, placate, or even avoid the situation can result in perpetuating the traumatic responses in the victim. Because nurses provide education to not only the victim but also the family and friends who are a part of the victim's life, you can use some helpful hints as guidelines for providing support:

- Listen actively; avoid diverting your attention or engaging in distractions.

- Offer your support and assistance, even if they haven't asked for help; many victims may see asking for help as a form of failure or weakness or feel guilty and ashamed for what has happened to them.

- Some of the most powerful ways to provide support are to help with everyday tasks like cleaning, cooking, caring for the family, and minding the children. Victims are often overwhelmed with the amount of activities and responsibilities that come with daily life while now simultaneously feeling a lack of energy, focus, or desire to complete them.

- Be respectful of private time; this must be balanced with not allowing the victim to move into a state of significant isolation.

- Don't take their anger or other feelings personally.

- Don't tell them they are "lucky it wasn't worse"—traumatized people are not consoled by such statements.

- Tell them that you are sorry such an event has happened to them and you want to understand and help them.

NATIONAL RESOURCES FOR HELPING VICTIMS

There are many resources for victims of crime and their families. The Office for Victims of Crime, a facet of the Office of Justice Programs (Office for Victims of Crime, 2015b), offers a significantly useful online interactive: U.S. Resource Map of Crime Victim Services & Information: http://ojp.gov/ovc/map.html. Victims of crime or family members can click on their state or territory to find the following resources:

- Victim compensation and assistance

- Victim notification programs

- Other victim assistance programs through the online directory

- Information on reporting crime victims' rights violations

For nurse providers or community leaders, the site allows you to point and click on the appropriate state or territory to find:

- Conferences and events

- Victims' rights legal provisions

- Statistics

- Statewide performance reports

CASE STUDY: VIOLENT CRIME

You are a nurse in a suburban emergency department. You are just about to go with the ED physician to let Mrs. Willis and her family know that her 23-year-old son, Charles (whom they call "Chip"), has died from a stray gunshot wound to the head that occurred as he was walking out of the local fast food restaurant with takeout for dinner. His family has been required to remain in the ED waiting room and there has not been time, until now, to provide any information, as the code has been in progress for the past 25 minutes. In the interim, the police have been speaking to Mrs. Willis regarding her son's activities that afternoon. Mrs. Willis is simultaneously terrified about the loss of her son and angry that the police seem to be insinuating that Chip was in some way responsible for what has happened to him.

Because Mrs. Willis and her family are in the public waiting room, you find a room in the ED or nearby where the family can have more privacy to process this information. You ask Mrs. Willis which two people she would like to join her for the meeting with the physician. As the physician provides the death notification, you are carefully watching the family's response. Upon hearing the news, Mrs. Willis cries out loudly, clutches her chest, and falls to the floor. You catch her falling from the chair and help lower her gently to the floor. On the floor, she can't fall any further and injure herself. After she regains composure, you assist her back to the chair.

You then let the family talk and provide support using a soft yet deliberate tone when speaking and allowing for periods of silence and pauses. You try to keep your composure and avoid trying to soften the blow. A simple, "I am sorry for your loss" and some periods of silence can be very therapeutic. The nurse will ensure that there is a designated driver before the family departs. For example, Mrs. Willis may have driven herself to the hospital but may be too distraught to drive home. Finally, provide support group information (or other support services) for your area. This should include any crisis hotline numbers, families of murder victims support agencies, and grief support groups.

Because the death has criminal justice implications, it's important to educate the family on differences from the usual hospital protocols. The body contains evidence of a murder that must be preserved. The family can view the body but will not be permitted to touch or approach it closely. The personal items will accompany the body to the medical examiner's/coroner's office instead of being returned to the family. Certain items (jewelry, wallet, etc.) may be returned to the family; however, this must be approved by a representative from the medical examiner's/coroner's office and should be clearly documented in the chart that permission was given.

Other follow-up includes providing the location and phone number of the medical examiner's/coroner's office and letting the family know that all pro-cedural questions regarding the investigative follow-up should be directed there.

Summary

Murder, and assault and battery, represent crimes that are significantly traumatic for both the victims and surviving family members. The damaging impact of such crimes can be very traumatic, both physically and emotionally, and is often described as being compounded by the fact that someone (the offender) has taken away something—whether a life, property, or a sense of safety in daily living—that can never be given back. Subsequently, it's important for nurses to be aware of the foundational facets relative to these criminal activities and the related psychosocial impact toward prevention efforts, and to conduct targeted yet sensitive assessments and determine appropriate interventions toward adaptive coping and mental health in survivors.

Additional Resources

The website for the Office for Victims of Crime in the Department of Justice includes an online directory of victim assistance programs: http://ovc.ncjrs.gov/findvictimservices/

Anti-Defamation League: www.adl.org

Battered Women's Justice Project: (800) 903-0111; www.bwjp.org

Bereaved Parents of the USA: http://www.bereavedparentsusa.org/

Bureau of Indian Affairs, Indian Country Child Abuse Hotline: (800) 633-5155

Futures Without Violence: (415) 678-5500; www.futureswithoutviolence.org/

International Association of Forensic Nurses: http://www.forensicnurses.org/

Mothers Against Drunk Driving: (800) 438-6233; www.madd.org

National Center for Missing and Exploited Children: (800) 843-5678; www.missingkids.com

National Center for Victims of Crime: (800) 394-2255; www.ncvc.org

National Organization of Parents of Murdered Children: (888) 818-7662; www.pomc.com

National Resource Center on Domestic Violence: (800) 537-2238; www.nrcdv.org

Parents of Murdered Children: http://www.pomc.com/

Rape, Abuse & Incest National Network: (800) 656-4673; www.rainn.org

REFERENCES

Aggravated battery. (n.d.). In *Wex, a free legal dictionary from Cornell University Law School.* Retrieved from https://www.law.cornell.edu/wex/aggravated_battery

Clements, P. T., Pierce-Weeks, J., Holt, K. E., Giardino, A. P., Seedat, S., & Mortiere, C. M. (2015). *Violence against women: Contemporary examination of intimate partner violence.* St. Louis, MO: STM Learning.

Federal Bureau of Investigation (FBI). (2015a). *Crime in the United States 2011: Expanded homicide data.* Retrieved from http://www.fbi.gov/about-us/cjis/ucr/crime-in-the-u.s/2011/crime-in-the-u.s.-2011/offenses-known-to-law-enforcement/expanded/expanded-homicide-data

Federal Bureau of Investigation (FBI). (2015b). *Uniform crime reports: Murder.* Retrieved from http://www.fbi.gov/about-us/cjis/ucr/crime-in-the-u.s/2013/crime-in-the-u.s.-2013/violent-crime/murder-topic-page/murdermain_final

Federal Bureau of Investigation (FBI). (2015c). *Uniform crime reports: Aggravated assaults.* Retrieved from http://www.fbi.gov/about-us/cjis/ucr/crime-in-the-u.s/2011/crime-in-the-u.s.-2011/violent-crime/aggravated-assault

Federal Bureau of Investigation (FBI). (2015d). *Victim assistance: Coping with crime victimization.* Retrieved from http://www.fbi.gov/stats-services/victim_assistance/coping

Finklehor, D. (2013, May 10). Five myths about missing children. *The Washington Post.* Retrieved from http://www.washingtonpost.com/opinions/five-myths-about-missing-children/2013/05/10/efee398c-b8b4-11e2-aa9e-a02b765ff0ea_story.html?hpid=z2

Holt, A. (2015). Winning in court: Maximizing protection through prosecution. In P. T. Clements, J. Pierce-Weeks, K. E. Holt, A. P. Giardino, S. Seedat, & C. M. Mortiere (Eds.), *Violence against women: Contemporary examination of intimate partner violence* (pp. 139–154). St. Louis, MO: STM Learning.

International Association of Forensic Nurses. (2015). *What is forensic nursing?* Retrieved from http://www.forensicnurses.org/?page=WhatisFN

Langton, L., & Truman, J. (2014). *Socio-emotional impact of violent crime.* Special report for the U.S. Department of Justice. Retrieved from http://www.bjs.gov/content/pub/pdf/sivc.pdf

Manslaughter. (2015). *FindLaw legal dictionary.* Retrieved from http://dictionary.findlaw.com/definition/manslaughter.html

National Center for Missing and Exploited Children (NCMEC). (2015). *Key facts.* Retrieved from http://www.missingkids.com/KeyFacts

National Center for Victims of Crime. (2008). *The trauma of victimization.* Retrieved from http://www.victimsofcrime.org/help-for-crime-victims/get-help-bulletins-for-crime-victims/trauma-of-victimization

National Crime Prevention Council (NCPC). (2015). *What to teach kids about strangers.* Retrieved from http://www.ncpc.org/topics/violent-crime-and-personal-safety/strangers

Office for Victims of Crime. (n.d.). *The facts about assault.* Retrieved from http://www.ovc.gov/pubs/helpseries/pdfs/HelpBrochure_Assault.pdf

Office for Victims of Crime. (2015a). *OVC HELP series for crime victims.* Retrieved from http://www.ovc.gov/pubs/helpseries/index.html

Office for Victims of Crime. (2015b). *U.S. resource map of crime victim services & information.* Retrieved from http://ojp.gov/ovc/map.html

Riffkin, R. (2015, December 18). Americans rate nurses highest on honesty, ethical standards. *Gallup.* Retrieved from http://www.gallup.com/poll/180260/americans-rate-nurses-highest-honesty-ethical-standards.aspx

Siegel, L. J. (2011). *Criminology* (11th ed.). Independence, KY: Cengage Learning.

INTIMATE PARTNER VIOLENCE

Angela F. Amar, PhD, RN, FAAN

"Domestic violence causes far more pain than the visible marks of bruises and scars. It is devastating to be abused by someone that you love and think loves you in return."

–Dianne Feinstein (http://www.stopdatingviolence.org/
quotes/violence-quotes.htm)

KEY POINTS IN THIS CHAPTER

- Intimate partner violence is a pattern of coercive, controlling, and abusive behaviors inflicted by one partner in an intimate relationship.

- IPV is associated with multiple long- and short-term physical and mental health consequences.

- Nurses should screen for violence and its related consequences and provide counseling and referrals to IPV survivors.

Intimate partner violence (IPV) is a pattern of assaultive and coercive behaviors, including physical, sexual, and psychological abuse and violence, that adults or adolescents use against their intimate partners. Often referred to as domestic violence, IPV occurs between current or former dating, married, and cohabitating relationships of individuals of all sexual orientations. Violence-related injuries lead as a cause of death in the United States and cost more than $406 billion in medical care and lost productivity each year (Centers for Disease Control and Prevention [CDC], 2013). Globally, 5.8 million people of all ages and economic groups die each year from both unintentional and violence-related injuries (World Health Organization [WHO], 2010). This chapter provides the nurse with an overview of intimate partner violence.

OVERVIEW OF INTIMATE PARTNER VIOLENCE

Each year, women experience 4.8 million intimate partner–related physical assaults and rapes; men are victims of about 2.9 million intimate partner–related physical assaults (Black et al., 2011). Gender and age increase susceptibility to IPV. Women report more IPV than men and are more likely to sustain injuries (Archer, 2000). Younger individuals, ages 16 to 24, have the highest risk of non-fatal violence; women ages 35 to 49 have the highest risk of fatal violence (Rennison, 2001). Research documents the increased incidence of health problems such as injury, chronic pain, gastrointestinal problems, gynecological signs including sexually transmitted diseases, depression, and post-traumatic stress disorder in survivors of IPV (Campbell, 2002).

Because IPV is a leading cause of injury, many survivors seek care in the emergency departments of hospitals and clinics. However, violence also leads to long-term physical- and mental-health consequences; survivors seek ongoing health-care in primary care, pre- and post-natal areas, labor and delivery, pediatricians' offices, mental health services, and other areas within most hospitals and clinics (Laughon, Amar, Sheridan, & Anderson, 2010). Each of these encounters provides nurses and other healthcare providers with opportunities to assess and intervene for IPV and health-related consequences (Sharps et al., 2001).

Intimate partner violence takes many forms (Amar, 2007):

- Physical violence inflicts pain or bodily harm. It includes actions such as hitting, punching, kicking, choking, pushing, burning, and throwing things.

- Emotional violence causes mental anguish and can include threatening, humiliating, intimidating, degrading, and controlling behaviors.

- Sexual violence includes any form of sexual contact or exposure without consent or by force.

- Economic abuse includes withholding of financial support, failing to provide for the needs of the victim, and controlling resources.

- Stalking is a pattern of willful, malicious, and repeated following or harassing of another person that would cause a reasonable person to feel fear; stalking frequently occurs as a part of intimate partner violence.

An understanding of the dynamics of abuse is crucial for effective intervention. IPV is a combination of assaultive and coercive behaviors. The assaultive behaviors are easier manifestations of abuse to conceptualize. We grasp the significance of being hit, punched, or kicked. We see bruises, cuts, or broken bones and are able to appreciate the pain of the injuries.

The coercive behaviors are more difficult to understand. The hurtful nature of words is subjective. Words that are insulting or offensive to one person might not be offensive to another. Emotional injuries damage the soul or spirit of an individual and are not readily apparent. These behaviors are the mechanism for maintaining control over another human. Forced sexual activity, isolating the survivor from others, and controlling finances and resources all exemplify coercive behaviors. Some violent or harmful behaviors can be normalized. For example, extreme jealous behavior is coercive and controlling; however, jealousy is often viewed as a sign of love.

Another common manifestation of control is the abuser making all decisions for the partner and the family. This includes finances and even things like attire, and with whom the family socializes. For instance, a partner may exert control by deciding that only she can open mail. This would mean that even a child's acceptance letter to college would have to wait for the abusive partner to open it. Threats of violence and stalking behaviors also demonstrate the abuser's power. These behaviors can create a terrorizing environment.

Understanding the context of an abusive relationship enables the nurse to be supportive and to offer appropriate help to the survivor.

TYPOLOGIES OF PERPETRATORS

Intimate partner violence is a significant issue with implications for public health, criminal justice, healthcare, and social services. Further, this crime is pervasive and affects many relationships and families. Scholars have attempted to provide typologies for perpetrators and survivors of IPV. These efforts have been more successful for describing perpetrators than for describing survivors. Reasons posited for why abusers are violent include violence in the family of origin, alcohol and drug use, and mental illness or character defects. Thus far, these hypotheses have not been proven (Edleson, Eisikovits, & Guttmann, 1985). A meta-analytic review identified increased anger and hostility as more common with abusers than nonabusers (Norlander & Eckhardt, 2005). Risk factors for perpetrators of partner homicide include previous IPV, being a childhood victim of abuse, drug and alcohol abuse, sexual jealousy, threat of separation, stalking behavior, and personality disorder (Aldridge & Browne, 2003).

CYCLE OF VIOLENCE

The cycle of violence, shown in Figure 9.1, is a common explanation of the dynamics of IPV relationships, usually depicting men as perpetrators and women as victims; however, it can apply to both genders. The relationship begins pleasantly and without violence. Gradually, tension begins to builds until it erupts in a violent episode. During the violent episode, the perpetrator is unpredictable and the victim feels helpless. After the violent episode, the perpetrator is contrite and attentive and the couple returns to a honeymoon period. The perpetrator is sorry for the episode and tries to make amends. The victim feels torn between the dichotomous presentations of the abuser. Soon, however, the tension builds, the victim attempts not to trigger a violent episode until the tension erupts and the same cycle repeats (Walker, 2009). This cycle of violence helps to explain the dynamics of the relationship and each partner's behavior. Most outsiders only see the violence and have difficulty understanding and responding to the relationship.

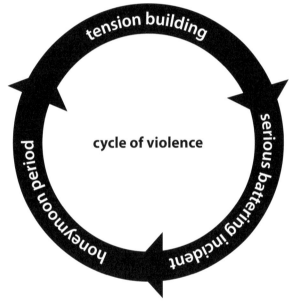

FIGURE 9.1 THE CYCLE OF VIOLENCE.

CONTRIBUTING FACTORS TO IPV

Many factors make it difficult to respond appropriately and end intimate partner violence. As a society, the United States is conflicted regarding violence. We categorically reject violence while at the same time making excuses for perpetrators and keeping violence secret. Discussions of intimate partner violence often center more on issues related to survivors rather than the perpetrator. We ask why does he/she stay rather than asking why did he/she hit a partner. This approach blames victims and makes them responsible for controlling another person's behavior. Another predominant narrative regarding violence is a preoccupation with stranger danger, despite evidence to support that individuals are more likely to be harmed or killed by someone they know rather than a stranger (Harrell, 2012). Many violence-prevention programs focus on crimes perpetrated by strangers. An inadvertent consequence of this approach is reinforcing the hidden nature of crimes by intimate partners. Families and intimate relationships reside in a private zone that makes witnesses reluctant to intervene and prevents conversations regarding violence. For example, parents prepare their children for dating, but these discussions seldom include information regarding violence or an abusive partner. The secretiveness extends even within the scholarly world with the scarcity of funding for violence-related research.

Institutions within society often lend support for violence through historical interpretations, various customs, and social mores. Religion is a major societal institution that is used to support violence and to make it difficult to end violent relationships. For example, the biblical notions of women submitting to their husbands and what God has joined let no man put asunder are used to support and normalize violence in relationships. A historical patriarchal structure lends support to societal factors such as gender roles and inequality, normalization of violence, and objectification of women. Traditional gender role beliefs that support patriarchy and male dominance are associated with violence against women (Sokoloff & Dupont, 2005). Violence against women occurs in many countries in the world; however, the prevalence of violence is higher in rural areas as compared to industrialized areas. Further, more severe violence is higher in rural areas as compared to industrialized areas (Moreno-Garcia, Jansen, Ellsberg, Heise, & Watts, 2009). Media portrayals of violence and control as signs of a loving relationship help to normalize violence and make it difficult for survivors to come forward. Misogynistic media that portray women as sexual objects negatively affect perceptions of gender equality. These societal and cultural influences make it difficult to have frank conversations about violence and for survivors to report violence to authorities and to seek help.

Nurses are not immune to the societal influences regarding violence and victimization. These attitudes and beliefs can affect the care given. Because violence is common, many nurses have had prior experience as victims and witnesses. Nurses may feel a range of emotion regarding violence. A "blame the victim" mentality can make it difficult and frustrating to provide nursing care for survivors. It can lead to feeling embarrassed for the survivor and feeling confused and helpless about how to respond. A significant factor that keeps providers from inquiring about violence is a fear of how to assess, intervene, and respond (Rhodes et al., 2007). Nurses may also feel anger regarding IPV. The nurse can feel anger directed toward the person responsible, those who allowed it to happen, and toward society for condoning violence through attitudes, traditions, and laws. Discouragement can set in, particularly if the violence is chronic and the nurse wants the survivor to end the relationship. Survivors who present for care are often afraid of the response from caregivers and particularly attuned to the nonverbal and verbal cues of the provider (Amar, Sutherland, Laughon, Bess, & Stockbridge, 2012). The provider's frustration is often transmitted to the survivor and results in revictimization. It is important for nurses to understand their own beliefs and the potential effects on the care given.

ASSESSING AND DOCUMENTING INTIMATE PARTNER VIOLENCE

In clinical practice, nurses routinely encounter survivors of IPV. Providers should ask patients of all ages about current and past experiences of violence at every visit (Amar, Laughon, Sharps, & Campbell, 2013). Women ages 16 to 24 years old are at greatest risk of nonfatal violence, while women ages 35 to 49 are most vulnerable to fatal violence (Rennison, 2001). Routine screening should extend to men of all ages. Survivors may seek healthcare due to injuries; however, inquiries about violence should occur at every visit, regardless of the absence or presence of abuse indicators (Groves, Augustyn, Lee, & Sawirds, 2002). Nurses should suspect abuse when the health visit is for ongoing emotional issues, drug or alcohol misuse, repeated sexually transmitted diseases, unexplained chronic pain, or repeated health consultations with no clear diagnosis (WHO, 2013). Screening can occur at annual visits, new patient visits, new presenting complaints, and pedi-atric well and sick child visits (Amar et al., 2013; Falsetti, 2007).

The nurse must build rapport while assessing for violence. Verbal and nonverbal communication is a key component. It is important for the nurse to be direct, hon-est, and professional while using language that the patient understands. Technical medical terms might be misinterpreted. For example, the nurse should ask the survivor about bruises rather than using the technical term of abrasions. Further, individuals may answer affirmatively that they have experienced abusive behaviors yet not identify themselves as abused, battered, or raped. Sample questions include, "Has your partner ever hit, shoved, or otherwise physically hurt you? Is your part-ner very jealous or controlling? Has your partner made you have sex when you didn't want to?" These questions are direct, gender-neutral, and useful for identifying IPV (Rhodes & Levinson, 2003).

INTERVIEW TECHNIQUES FOR IPV

Due to the dynamics of abuse and concern for safety, it's important to interview the patient alone, separate from his or her partner (Falsetti, 2007). Interviews with an abusive partner present can result in the partner dominating the interview and the victim fearful of retaliation. One large urban hospital evaluated the use of a computerized screening protocol for patients, filled out during the wait for services in the emergency department. As compared to face-to-face, screening for IPV using the computerized tool had a higher detection rate of IPV (Trautman, McCarthy, Miller, Campbell, & Kelen, 2007).

The World Health Organization recommends the Listen, Inquire, Validate, Enhance Safety, and Support (LIVES) technique (WHO, 2013):

- **Listen (L):** The nurse listens to the survivor closely, using empathy and without judgment. Silence can be an effective technique to encourage communication and demonstrate active listening. The nonverbal communication conveys a man-ner of understanding and attentiveness.

- **Inquire (I):** Inquiring about needs and concerns allows the nurse to respond to emotional, physical, social, and practical issues. It is important not to display horror, shock, anger, or disapproval or place blame or try to prove abuse occurred by making accusations or demands.

- **Validate (V):** Validation shows the survivor that you understand and believe what is being said. The therapeutic techniques of reflection and restatement convey understanding.

- **Enhance Safety (E):** Enhance safety by discussing a plan to prevent harm in future violence.

- **Support (S):** Support is provided by giving the survivor referrals to services, information, and support.

Building rapport and a therapeutic relationship enables the nurse to work with the survivor to meet health and psychosocial needs.

Verbal communication is important; however, nonverbal communication is equally important to assess. Behavioral clues from the survivor can be indicative of exposure to violence. Factors such as response, appearance, and history of present injury can be indications that abuse has occurred. For example, if a person cowers or flinches in response to touch, the nurse would suspect violence. Hair, makeup, and clothing can be used to conceal injuries. For example, large sunglasses worn inside could be concealing a black eye, just as long sleeves on a warm day could be concealing bruises. Multiple injuries in various stages of healing could also raise suspicion and prompt the nurse to assess further. Another potential indicator of abuse is a mismatch between the injury and the story of how it happened (WHO, n.d.). For example, being told that multiple injuries to the chest and face resulted from a fall.

It's useful for the nurse to be able to distinguish between accidental and purposive injury. Accidental injuries tend to be located on the peripheral extremities and bony prominences. They also tend to occur on one area or side of the body. For instance, when we fall we tend to put out our hands, forearms, or knees to break the fall. People do not usually fall face or chest first. When a perpetrator intentionally inflicts an injury, it is purposive. Usually, this type of injury happens on the upper arms, head (especially face and neck), upper lateral and medial thighs, and the rectal and perineal region. Purposive injuries tend to be more proximally located and often involve more than one plane of the body (Sheridan & Nash, 2007).

TOOLS FOR IDENTIFYING IPV

Scholars in the field have developed and tested several validated tools for identifying intimate partner violence in a variety of settings. Screening tools are available and clearly described on the Futures Without Violence and Nursing Network on Violence Against Women International websites (www.futureswithoutviolence.org & www.nnvawi.org). The Abuse Assessment Screen (AAS), partly shown in Figure 9.2, is a quick, easy-to-use measure that is effective in identifying intimate partner violence (Laughon, Renker, Glass, & Parker, 2008). This widely used questionnaire contains four questions on a range of violent behaviors, one of which asks about abuse during pregnancy. A body map is available to document injuries. In addition to assessing for past-year intimate partner violence, it assesses for sexual violence from any person and asks, "Are you afraid of anyone right now?" which would include current stalking threats.

For women who screen positive for intimate partner violence, the 20 items of the Danger Assessment (DA) help the provider to determine the woman's risk of lethality or homicide in intimate partner violence (Campbell, Webster, & Glass, 2009). The provider needs to know the risk of homicide to determine the urgency and types of referrals to make. In particular, high DA scores are associated with a greater risk of lethal violence. Low scores do not mean "no risk." Rather, "unknown risk" is a better interpretation of low scores. The nurse and survivor should review the findings together. It's important that survivors are aware of and appreciate the lethality risk of their partner's behavior. Significant factors to consider in determining the patient's safety are any increases in frequency and severity of the violence, threats of homicide or suicide, presence of firearms weapons in the home, increased drug or alcohol use, and attempts to separate from or plans to leave the partner (Campbell et al., 2009). Subsequent discussion centers on resources and strategies to protect oneself and stay safe or end the relationship.

ABUSE ASSESSMENT SCREEN

1. WITHIN THE LAST YEAR, have you been pushed, shoved, slapped, hit, kicked, choked, or otherwise physically hurt by your partner or ex-partner?

If yes, by whom? _____

Total number of times _____

2. SINCE YOU'VE BEEN PREGNANT, have you been hit, slapped, kicked, or otherwise physically hurt by someone?

If yes, by whom? _____

Total number of times _____

3. WITHIN THE LAST YEAR, has anyone forced you to have sexual activities that you did not want?

If yes, by whom? _____

Total number of times _____

4. Are you afraid of anyone?

Who? _____

FIGURE 9.2 THE ABUSE ASSESSMENT SCREEN: ONE TOOL TO IDENTIFY IPV.

RELEVANT LAWS AND STATUTES FOR IPV

The main federal law in the United States is the Violence Against Women Act (VAWA), which provides states with funding for investigation and prosecution efforts, protection of victims, and training to create a coordinated response. Key services include the federal rape shield law, violence prevention programs, funding for victim assistance programs, and legal aid for survivors. State laws determine definitions and legal remedies for IPV. Most state laws provide a measure for civil protective or restraining orders. Protective orders are designed to increase safety by mandating no contact and providing stipulations that an abuser stay a certain distance away from someone and the person's home, workplace, or school. In many states, violating civil protective orders can put the violator at risk of being arrested and charged with a crime. Federally, it is illegal for a person to possess a firearm while subject to a court-ordered restraining order for IPV. Nurses do not have to be experts in issues related to protective orders but should be able to refer patients for assistance in obtaining them.

The federal U.S. Family Violence Prevention and Services Act offers funding to provide shelter and other help to victims of domestic violence and their dependents. It financially supports prevention programs and the National Domestic Violence Hotline, a 24-hour confidential resource. Domestic violence advocates are another resource provided by police stations, courts, crisis centers, and domestic violence programs. Advocates can accompany victims to court, find helpful resources, and help with completing paperwork and safety planning. Nurses can ensure that survivors are educated about and connected to the available resources.

In Canada, there are no laws specific to family violence. Rather, acts of family violence are covered under the Criminal Code. Provisions made for family violence include release conditions such as no contact or peace bonds. Provinces may have laws related to family violence in their jurisdictions.

INTERVENTIONS AND STRATEGIES FOR INTIMATE PARTNER VIOLENCE

Routine screening must be followed by focused intervention. Patients who present for treatment after an IPV episode should receive immediate attention and care to treat their physical injuries. It is important that the nurse use a nonjudgmental approach. Because abuse can negatively affect one's sense of self, it is important that the nurse take care to boost the survivor's self-esteem. Examples of this include telling the survivors it is not their fault and that no one deserves abuse. A critical area for assessment is determining the survivor's level of safety and planning strategies to maintain safety (Amar et al., 2013). Assessing and planning for safety is an ongoing process rather than a one-time event. Each visit represents an opportunity to reevaluate safety. The nurse determines the immediate risk of future harm. If it is currently not safe for a survivor to return home, the nurse will discuss options. Safe housing choices include domestic violence shelters, or even the homes of friends and family. It's also useful to talk about the necessity of involving the police. If the survivor does not wish to leave the relationship, the nurse would help her think about her safety at home. A discussion of an escape plan to be used for rapid escape in a crisis is essential. Questions such as, "If you need to leave your home in a hurry, where would you go?" can be helpful.

Safety plans are used to help a survivor plan to leave the abusive partner. Safety plans are important because leaving an abusive partner increases the risk of being killed by the partner (Campbell, 2001). The nurse would make sure that the survivor understands that the risk of injury necessitates careful planning before leaving an abusive relationship. All patients in violent relationships should be engaged in a discussion of options and in the creation of a safety plan. Together, the nurse and survivor might consider options of places and people she can go to for help. For example, the survivor might keep spare keys, clothes, money, and important papers in a safe place with easy access after leaving. The nurse could provide referrals, phone numbers, and websites for external services and information (Dienemann, Campbell, Wiederhorn, Laughon, & Jordan, 2003). While face-to-face interviews can be effective in planning for safety, the use of a computerized aid can improve the safety decision-making process related to IPV (Glass, Eden, Bloom, & Perrin, 2009).

Most women eventually leave an abusive partner; however, most women make multiple attempts before they successfully leave (Campbell, 2001). Leaving is a process, and survivors need time to prepare emotionally for ending the relationship. Some women are not interested in leaving their partner; they only want the abuse to stop. It's important that the nurse respects the woman's choices and does not assume she will leave. The nurse can ask direct questions to determine the woman's needs and what forms of help she perceives to be most useful. Providing information on domestic violence and resources with each visit helps to prepare the woman. It's also important to be careful with handouts. Leaving a visit with pamphlets and handouts related to IPV can alert the partner to the disclosure and prompt retaliatory violence and increased controlling behavior. A phone number on a prescription pad can be safe and effective.

Referrals to advocacy and counseling are beneficial. These services can link survivors with resources and have documented results in decreasing re-abuse and increasing quality of life (Wathen & MacMillan, 2003). Referrals are an important mechanism to connect the survivor with resources for health, safety, and social support (WHO, 2013). Examples include crisis lines, shelters, support groups, legal aid, and mental health programs. From a legal perspective, good documentation of injuries using body maps, photographs, and descriptions help with a court case. Referral to community resources includes notifying law enforcement and a hospital social worker as well as providing numbers of the domestic violence hotline, IPV shelter, and IPV legal advocate (Glass, Dearwater, & Campbell, 2001).

IPV coexisting with pregnancy is associated with late entry in prenatal care, low-birth-weight babies, premature labor, fetal trauma, and unhealthy maternal behavior (Jasinski, 2004; Shah & Shah, 2010). Screening for IPV should occur at each prenatal visit. The nurse should advise women about the risks and educate them about available resources. Evidence suggests that community worker visits and counseling can be effective in decreasing physical violence (McFarlane, Groff, O'Brien, & Watson, 2006; O'Reilly, Beale, & Gillies, 2010).

REHABILITATION OF OFFENDERS

IPV is a crime that enables the court system to determine legal recourse, including punishment for abusers. Court-mandated batterer intervention programs are the most commonly used option. Most programs use the Duluth model, which focuses on power and control (Paymar & Pence, 1993). Group therapy, psychoeducation, and a pro-feminist approach are common elements of most programs (Price & Rosenbaum, 2009). Group therapy enables perpetrators to offer and receive mentorship, peer feedback and confrontation, and to share experiences. Psychoeducation provides information regarding the dynamics of abuse and the short- and long-term consequences. The perpetrator needs an intellectual understanding of IPV to make sustained behavioral changes. The effectiveness of batterer intervention programs is modest from the perpetrator perspective and zero when victim perspective is considered (Feder & Wilson, 2005). Problems of these programs include the lack of non-English language programs and a one-size-fits-all approach (Price & Rosenbaum, 2009). Other research has shown benefits to including substance-abuse treatment as part of batterer intervention (Stover, Meadows, & Kaufman, 2009). The court-mandated approach is appropriate insofar as IPV is a misdemeanor that does not indicate incarceration. However, this approach does not ensure that perpetrators are emotionally committed to the effort required to make and sustain behavioral change.

EDUCATION

Despite the profound consequences of intimate partner violence, nurses and other providers receive limited education and training in this area. The following are educational resources that can be used in nursing schools, continuing education, and patient education:

- **Power and Control: Domestic Violence in America** (http://www. powerandcontrolfilm.com/): This website contains educational films; information for survivors, medical providers, educators, and law enforcement officials; interviews with experts; and other information.

- *Telling Amy's Story* (http://telling.psu.edu/): A documentary film that follows the timeline of a domestic violence homicide.

- **One Love Foundation** (https://joinonelove.org/who-we-are/#body-mission): An organization whose mission is to stop relationship violence in young people and offer education and resources.

- **Duluth Model** (http://www.theduluthmodel.org/index.htm): This website contains information, DVDs, books, curriculum, and training opportunities, including resources for working with perpetrators.

CASE STUDY: INTIMATE PARTNER VIOLENCE

You're working in the emergency department (ED) when the police bring in a 30-year-old woman named Kennedy after her husband beat her. People saw a man driving a car with a woman hanging out of the passenger door being dragged and called the police. Kennedy also has bruises to her face and chest, and fingermarks on her neck. Kennedy cries while being treated by the medical personnel. She refuses to provide any additional information about the causes of her injuries but consents to forensic photography of her injuries. Kennedy sits slumped in the bed, her hands in her lap, head hanging down, and has tears in her eyes. You say, "It seems like things are overwhelming right now. Is that how you're feeling?" Kennedy begins to sob, saying she can't do this. You sit quietly for a while and then encourage Kennedy to tell you what she can't do so that you can solve it together. Kennedy says that her partner gets angry easily and that when he drinks it's worse. She says that he doesn't mean to hurt her and she knows he loves her. However, she doesn't know how much longer she can take this but is afraid to leave because she "knows he'll find me and make me pay." Despite not feeling safe at home, she's not sure that she can leave. She tells the nurse that she doesn't have a close relationship with her family, doesn't have a job, and has no money of her own.

Once Kennedy has identified all of the issues and emotionally vented, you discuss her options. Kennedy continues to verbalize feelings of shame and doubt. She questions whether she is exaggerating the effects of violence and if she should give him another chance. Even as she verbalizes these doubts, Kennedy is able to tell you that she has left before. Each time, her husband stalked, harassed, and threatened her until she came home. Each time, he is apologetic and nice for a short period of time, and then the abuse starts back up. You remind Kennedy that she does not deserve to be abused and that nothing she did caused the abuse. Because Kennedy lives on the outskirts of the city, you call the local domestic violence hotline to learn of the resources in Kennedy's area.

SUMMARY

Intimate partner violence (IPV) is a pattern of coercive, controlling, and abusive behaviors inflicted by one partner in an intimate relationship. IPV is an important public health and societal issue that requires major effort to eradicate. IPV affects the psychological and physical health of survivors, which increases the likelihood of contact with nurses in varied areas of healthcare. Nurses' understanding of the societal norms and attitudes regarding violence and the dynamics of abuse is crucial to provide the needed care. They should screen for violence and its related consequences and provide counseling and referrals to IPV survivors.

ADDITIONAL RESOURCES

National Coalition Against Domestic Violence: http://www.ncadv.org/

National Health Resource Center on Domestic Violence—Futures Without Violence: http://www.futureswithoutviolence.org/health/national-health-resource-center-on-domestic-violence/

National Resource Center on Domestic Violence: http://www.nrcdv.org/

Nursing Network on Violence Against Women International: http://nnvawi.org/pages/Tools.cfm

REFERENCES

Aldridge, M. L., & Browne, K. D. (2003). Perpetrators of spousal homicide: A review. *Trauma, Violence, & Abuse, 4*(3), 265–276.

Amar, A. F. (2007). Behaviors that college women label as stalking. *Journal of the American Psychiatric Nurses Association, 13*(4), 210–220.

Amar, A., Laughon, K., Sharps, P., & Campbell, J. (2013). Screening and counseling for violence against women in primary care settings. *Nursing Outlook, 61*(3), 187–191.

Amar, A. F., Sutherland, M., Laughon, K., Bess, R., & Stockbridge, J. (2012). Peer influences within the campus environment on help seeking related to violence. *Journal of the National Black Nurses Association, 23*(1), 1–7.

Archer, J. (2000). Sex differences in aggression between heterosexual partners: A meta-analytic review. *Psychological Bulletin, 126*(5), 651–680.

Black, M. C., Basile, K. C., Walters, M. L., Merrick, M. T., Chen, J., & Stevens, M. R. (2011). *The National Intimate Partner and Sexual Violence Survey (NISVS)*. Atlanta, GA: National Center for Injury Prevention and Control, Centers for Disease Control and Prevention.

Campbell, J. C. (2001). Safety planning based on lethality assessment for partners of batterers in intervention programs. *Journal of Aggression, Maltreatment, and Trauma, 5*(2), 129–143.

Campbell, J. C. (2002). Health consequences of intimate partner violence. *The Lancet, 359*, 1331–1336.

Campbell, J. C., Webster, D. W., & Glass, N. (2009). The danger assessment validation of a lethality risk assessment instrument for intimate partner femicide. *Journal of Interpersonal Violence, 24*(4), 653–674.

Centers for Disease Control and Prevention (CDC). (2013). *Injury prevention & control: Key data and statistics.* Retrieved from http://www.cdc.gov/injury/overview/data.html

Dienemann, J., Campbell, J., Wiederhorn, N., Laughon, K., & Jordan, E. (2003). A critical pathway for intimate partner violence across the continuum of care. *Journal of Obstetric, Gynecologic, and Neonatal Nursing, 32*(5), 594–603.

Edleson, J. L., Eisikovits, Z., & Guttmann, E. (1985). Men who batter women: A critical review of the evidence. *Journal of Family Issues, 6*(2), 229–247.

Falsetti, S. A. (2007). Screening and responding to family and intimate partner violence in the primary care setting. *Primary Care: Clinics in Office Practice, 34*(3), 641–657.

Feder, L., & Wilson, D. B. (2005). A meta-analytic review of court-mandated batterer intervention programs: Can courts affect abusers' behavior? *Journal of Experimental Criminology, 1*(2), 239–262.

Glass, N., Dearwater, S., & Campbell, J. (2001). Intimate partner violence screening and intervention: Data from eleven Pennsylvania and California community hospital emergency departments. *Journal of Emergency Nursing, 27*(2), 141–149.

Glass, N., Eden, K. B., Bloom, T., & Perrin, N. (2009). Computerized aid improves safety decision process for survivors of intimate partner violence. *Journal of Interpersonal Violence, 25*(11), 1947–1964.

Groves, B. M., Augustyn, M., Lee, D., & Sawirds, P. (2002). *Identifying and responding to domestic violence: Consensus recommendations for child and adolescent health.* San Francisco, CA: Family Violence Prevention Fund.

Harrell, E. (2012). *Violent victimization committed by strangers, 1993–2010.* Washington, DC: Bureau of Justice Statistics.

Jasinski, J. L. (2004). Pregnancy and domestic violence: A review of the literature. *Trauma, Violence, & Abuse, 5*(1), 47–64.

Laughon, K., Amar, A. F., Sheridan, D. J., & Anderson, S. (2010). Legal and forensic nursing responses to family violence. In J. Humphreys & J. C. Campbell (Eds.), *Family violence and nursing practice* (2nd ed.), (pp. 367–380). New York, NY: Springer Publishing Company.

Laughon, K., Renker, P., Glass, N., & Parker, B. (2008). Revision of the Abuse Assessment Screen to address nonlethal strangulation. *Journal of Obstetric, Gynecologic, and Neonatal Nursing, 37*(4), 502–507.

McFarlane, J. M., Groff, J. Y., O'Brien, J. A., & Watson, K. (2006). Secondary prevention of intimate partner violence: A randomized controlled trial. *Nursing Research, 55*(1), 52–61.

Moreno-Garcia, C., Jansen, H. A. F. M., Ellsberg, M., Heise, L., & Watts, C. (2009). *WHO multi-country study on women's health and domestic violence against women.* Geneva, Switzerland: World Health Organization.

Norlander, B., & Eckhardt, C. (2005). Anger, hostility, and male perpetrators of intimate partner violence: A meta-analytic review. *Clinical Psychology Review, 25*(2), 119–152.

O'Reilly, R., Beale, B., & Gillies, D. (2010). Screening and intervention for domestic violence during pregnancy care: A systematic review. *Trauma, Violence, & Abuse, 41,* 128–133.

Paymar, M., & Pence, E. (1993). *Education groups for men who batter: The Duluth Model.* New York, NY: Springer.

Price, B. J., & Rosenbaum, A. (2009). Batterer intervention programs: A report from the field. *Violence and Victims, 24*(6), 757–770.

Rennison, C. (2001). *Intimate partner violence and age of the victim: 1993–1999.* Washington, DC: United States Department of Justice.

Rhodes, K. V., Frankel, R. M., Levinthal, N., Prenoveau, E., Bailey, J., & Levinson, W. (2007). "You're not a victim of domestic violence, are you?" Provider–patient communication about domestic violence. *Annals of Internal Medicine, 147*(9), 620–627.

Rhodes, K. V., & Levinson, W. (2003). Interventions for intimate partner violence against women: Clinical applications. *JAMA, 289*(5), 601–605.

Shah, P. S., & Shah, J. (2010). Maternal exposure to domestic violence and pregnancy and birth outcomes: A systematic review and meta-analyses. *Journal of Women's Health, 19*(11), 2017–2031.

Sharps, P. W., Koziol-McLain, J., Campbell, J., McFarlane, J., Sachs, C., & Xu, X. (2001). Health care providers' missed opportunities for preventing femicide. *Preventive Medicine, 33*(5), 373–380.

Sheridan, D. J., & Nash, K. R. (2007). Acute injury patterns of intimate partner violence victims. *Trauma, Violence, & Abuse, 8*(3), 281–289.

Sokoloff, N. J., & Dupont, I. (2005). Domestic violence at the intersections of race, class, and gender: Challenges and contributions to understanding violence against marginalized women in diverse communities. *Violence Against Women, 11*(1), 38–64.

Stover, C. S., Meadows, A. L., & Kaufman, J. (2009). Interventions for intimate partner violence: Review and implications for evidence-based practice. *Professional Psychology: Research and Practice, 40*(3), 223–233.

Trautman, D. E., McCarthy, M. L., Miller, N., Campbell, J. C., & Kelen, G. D. (2007). Intimate partner violence and emergency department screening: Computerized screening versus usual care. *Annals of Emergency Medicine, 49*(4), 526–534.

Walker, L. E. (2009). *The battered woman syndrome* (3rd ed.). New York, NY: Springer Publishing.

Wathen, C. N., & MacMillan, H. L. (2003). Interventions for violence against women: Scientific review. *JAMA, 289*(5), 589–600.

World Health Organization (WHO). (n.d.). *Health care for women subjected to intimate partner violence or sexual violence: A clinical handbook.* Geneva, Switzerland: World Health Organization.

World Health Organization (WHO). (2010). *Injuries and violence: The facts.* Geneva, Switzerland: World Health Organization.

World Health Organization (WHO). (2013). *Responding to intimate partner violence and sexual violence against women: WHO clinical and policy guidelines.* Geneva, Switzerland: World Health Organization.

SEXUAL VIOLENCE

Carolyn M. Porta, PhD, MPH, RN, SANE-A; Di Fischer, MN, RN, PHN; and Emily Ruth Johnson, MN, MA, RN, SANE-A

"I think there is a socialization that goes where violence becomes acceptable. You have to change that and say, 'No, that's not acceptable, rape is not acceptable' … We must not be ambiguous about violence. The greatest war is fought inside our own hearts, a war of anger and resentment and greed. So we start within ourselves and then with our families and our communities."

–Mairead Maguire, Nobel Peace Laureate

KEY POINTS IN THIS CHAPTER

- Anyone can be a victim of sexual violence.

- Sexual violence often occurs in conjunction with other perpetrator-initiated crimes and risk behaviors (e.g., burglary, intimate partner violence, substance use, prostitution/ trafficking).

- Sexual assault nurse examiners (SANEs) fulfill a key role in the care of victims of sexual violence.

- Care includes health assessment and treatment as well as forensic assessment, specimen collection, and documentation to maintain the proper legal chain of custody processes.

- Collaborative care, including advocates, law enforcement, and other healthcare/social work providers, strengthens the potential for healthy outcomes.

- Legislation exists to support victims of sexual violence, along with numerous national resources.

Sexual violence is one of the most difficult experiences endured by a human being. Victims of sexual violence describe the shame, the pain, the vulnerability, the fear, and the lack of control. Nurses and other healthcare professionals frequently provide care to victims of sexual violence and oftentimes have no awareness of their history of trauma. Sexual assault forensic examiners (SAFEs), also referred to as sexual assault nurse examiners (SANEs), provide medical and forensic care in the initial hours and days following an act of sexual violence, if the victim seeks care (Ledray, Faugno, & Speck, 2001). These nurses are prepared to treat and care for victims of sexual violence, with an understanding of the complexity of emotional, physical, and psychosocial needs that may result.

The purpose of this chapter is to orient the non-forensic nurse to sexual violence and related crimes such as stalking and strangulation. Aspects of perpetration, although not a focus of this chapter, will be discussed to increase the nurse's awareness of how types of perpetration affect victim response and subsequent care that is offered. Current evidence-based nursing responses and interventions will be presented, as well as resources useful to nurses and to victims of sexual violence and their families, friends, and other sources of social support.

OVERVIEW OF SEXUAL VIOLENCE

According to the Centers for Disease Control and Prevention (CDC), "sexual violence (SV) is any sexual act that is perpetrated against someone's will. [Sexual violence] encompasses a range of offenses, including a completed nonconsensual sex act (i.e., rape), an attempted nonconsensual sex act, abusive sexual contact (i.e., unwanted touching), and non-contact sexual abuse (e.g., threatened sexual violence, exhibitionism, verbal sexual harassment)" (CDC, 2014a, p. 1.) The following sections describe in detail these four types of sexual violence, the different levels of consent or non-consent, other key terms that nurses need to know when dealing with victims of sexual violence, and the trend of sexual violence in the United States.

FOUR TYPES OF SEXUAL VIOLENCE

According to the CDC (2014a, p. 1), the four types of sexual violence are:

- A completed sex act is defined as contact between the penis and the vulva or the penis and the anus involving penetration, however slight; contact between the mouth and penis, vulva, or anus; or penetration of the anal or genital opening of another person by a hand, finger, or other object.

- An attempted (but not completed) sex act.

- Abusive sexual contact is defined as intentional touching, either directly or through the clothing, of the genitalia, anus, groin, breast, inner thigh, or buttocks of any person without his or her consent, or of a person who is unable to consent or refuse.

- Non-contact sexual abuse does not include physical contact of a sexual nature between the perpetrator and the victim. It includes acts such as voyeurism; intentional exposure of an individual to exhibitionism; unwanted exposure to pornography; verbal or behavioral sexual harassment; threats of sexual violence to accomplish some other end; or taking nude photographs of a sexual nature of another person without his or her consent or knowledge, or of a person who is unable to consent or refuse.

ESTABLISHING CONSENT

A key factor in establishing that an act of sexual violence has occurred is the inability of someone to consent or to refuse (Basile, Smith, Breiding, Black, & Mahendra, 2014, p. 11):

- **Consent:** Words or overt actions by a person who is legally or functionally competent to give informed approval, indicating a freely given agreement to have sexual intercourse or sexual contact. This definition may be extended to include consent as an affirmative, conscious, and voluntary agreement to engage in sexual activity.

- **Inability to give consent:** A freely given agreement to have sexual intercourse or sexual contact could not occur because of the victim's age, illness, mental or physical disability, being asleep or unconscious, or being too intoxicated (e.g., incapacitation, lack of consciousness, or lack of awareness) through his or her voluntary or involuntary use of alcohol or drugs.

- **Inability to refuse:** Disagreement to engage in a sexual act was precluded because of the use or possession of guns or other non-bodily weapons, or due to physical violence, threats of physical violence, intimidation or pressure, or misuse of authority.

With advances in genetic testing of specimens and the ability to rule out a high percentage of the population being at the scene of a crime, fewer situations occur in which an assailant can confidently deny his or her physical involvement with the victim. DNA is left everywhere and can be collected from endless sources (e.g., cell phone, bedding, car seat, another body, clothing, food). An individual will more often make a claim that the sexual act or contact was consensual. The legal process is then an argument of consent, not whether something occurred.

KEY TERMS SURROUNDING SEXUAL VIOLENCE

The terms, definitions, and key facts of sexual violence are:

- **Chain of custody/evidence:** A continuous succession of persons responsible for the evidence with the purpose to ensure there is neither alteration nor loss of evidence. The documentation of the chain of custody is a record of times, places, and persons who have been responsible for the evidence. Transfers should be kept to a minimum, and when transfers are made, they should be documented carefully.

  All transfers of custody of evidence must be logged with the name of the persons transferring custody, the name of the persons receiving custody, and the date and time of each transfer. The documentation may be attached to the evidence envelope.

Drug facilitated sexual violence: "When drugs or alcohol are used to compromise an individual's ability to consent to sexual activity. In addition, drugs and alcohol are often used in order to minimize the resistance and memory of the victim of a sexual assault" (Rape, Abuse and Incest National Network [RAINN], n.d.).

Hate crime: "The victimization of an individual based on that individual's race, religion, national origin, ethnic identification, gender, or sexual orientation" (RAINN, n.d.).

Rape: "Sexual contact or penetration achieved without consent, with use of physical force, coercion, deception, threat, or when the victim is mentally incapacitated or impaired, physically impaired (due to voluntary or involuntary alcohol or drug consumption), or asleep or unconscious" (Pandora's Project, n.d.).

Acquaintance assault/rape: "When coercive sexual activities that occur against a person's will by means of force, violence, duress, or fear of bodily injury are imposed upon them by someone they know (a friend, date, acquaintance, etc.)" (RAINN, n.d.).

Partner rape: "Sexual acts committed without a person's consent and/or against a person's will when the perpetrator is the individual's current partner (married or not), previous partner, or co-habitator" (RAINN, n.d.).

Stranger rape: Sexual acts committed by a stranger without a person's consent and/or against a person's will. RAINN (n.d.) identified three major categories of stranger rape:

Blitz sexual assault: The perpetrator rapidly and brutally assaults the victim with no prior contact. Blitz assaults usually occur at night in a public place.

Contact sexual assault: The perpetrator contacts the victim and tries to gain her or his trust and confidence before assaulting her or him. Contact perpetrators pick their victims in bars, lure them into their cars, or otherwise try to coerce the victim into a situation of sexual assault.

  ■ *Home invasion sexual assault:* A stranger breaks into the victim's home to commit the assault.

■ **Sexual violence:** "Any sexual act that is perpetrated against someone's will" (Black et al., 2011).

■ **Sexual exploitation by helping professionals:** "Sexual contact of any kind between a helping professional (doctor, therapist, teacher, priest, professor, police officer, lawyer, etc.) and a client/patient" (RAINN, n.d.).

■ **Sexual harassment:** "Unwelcome sexual advances, requests for sexual favors, and other verbal or physical conduct of a sexual nature in which submission to or rejection of such conduct explicitly or implicitly affects an individual's work or school performance or creates an intimidating, hostile, or offensive work or school environment" (RAINN, n.d.).

■ **Sexual homicide:** The combination of lethal violence with a sexual element (Holmes & Holmes, 2001).

■ **Stalking:** "A pattern of unwanted harassing or threatening tactics used by a perpetrator and included tactics related to unwanted contacts, unwanted tracking and following, intrusion, and technology-assisted tactics" (Black et al., 2011).

CERTIFICATION FOR FORENSIC NURSES

There are different terms currently used for nurses who conduct sexual assault forensic examinations, including most commonly, sexual assault nurse examiner (SANE) and forensic nurse examiner (FNE). There are two national certification examinations, one focused on care of children (SANE-P) and the other focused on care of adults and adolescents (SANE-A); there is also board certification (Advanced Forensic Nursing-Board Certified), which requires meeting specific eligibility criteria and a portfolio review, but not an examination.

Sexual Violence Trends in the United States

The National Intimate Partner and Sexual Violence Survey (Black, 2011) was conducted to collect data on sexual violence, stalking, and intimate partner violence from English- and Spanish-speaking adults in the U.S.; interviews were conducted via randomized calls to landline and cell phones. Survey data have yielded valuable insights regarding trends of sexual violence in the U.S., and differences, for example, by gender, ethnicity, and age of first unwanted sexual experience. Key survey results include:

- Nearly 1 in 5 (19.3%, or over 23 million) women reported being raped in their lifetime (compared with 1.7% of men).

- Nearly half (43.7%) of the female respondents and nearly a quarter (23.4%) of the male respondents reported experiencing other forms of sexual assault (other than rape), such as sexual coercion or unwanted sexual contact.

- 15.2% of the female respondents and 5.7% of the men reported being a victim of stalking in their lifetime.

- Among the female respondents who reported experiencing rape, most (78.7%) were first raped before they were 25 years of age.

- Reports of rape vary by ethnicity and sex.

Although one cannot predict who might be a perpetrator of a sexually violent crime such as rape or sexual assault, there are risk factors that could indicate potential for perpetration. Exposure to childhood violence, for example, is a well-known predictor of perpetration of sexual violence. Significant risk factors common in the backgrounds of adolescent perpetrators of sexual violence or aggression include "experiencing intra- or extra-familial sexual abuse, witnessing family violence, frequent use of illegal drugs, anabolic steroid use, daily alcohol use, gang membership, high levels of suicide risk behavior" (Borowsky, Hogan, & Ireland, 1997). Another significant indicator is the absence of key protective factors, such as family connectedness (CDC, 2015).

The study of victims has yielded much information on responses to sexual violence. Little evidence points to a prototype of individuals who are victimized by sexual violence. However, more evidence has been gathered that describes sexual violence offenders. Female victims reported predominantly male perpetrators, whereas for male victims, the sex of the perpetrator varied by the specific form of violence examined. Male rape victims predominantly had male perpetrators, but other forms of sexual violence experienced by men were either perpetrated predominantly by women (e.g., being made to penetrate and sexual coercion) or split more evenly among male and female perpetrators (e.g., unwanted sexual contact and noncontact unwanted sexual experiences) (Breiding et al., 2014).

Criminologists have identified four major typologies of rapists (Groth, Burgess, & Holmstrom, 1977; Hazelwood, 2009):

- **Power reassurance:** The power reassurance rapist, or *gentleman* rapist, is the least violent and most common offender. The purpose of the assault is to reassure himself of his masculinity and bolster his self-esteem.

- **Power assertive:** The power assertive rapist is motivated by an ability to dominate another person. This rapist is sexually selfish and is not concerned about the victim's emotional or physical wellbeing.

- **Angry retaliatory:** The angry retaliatory rapist uses rape to punish women and express rage. These rapes are usually brutal and violent.

- **Anger excitation:** The anger excitation rapist is a sadist who gets sexual gratification from inducing torture and suffering.

These typologies are useful for nurses who provide care for offenders to understand their motivation.

MINNESOTA SEX OFFENDER PROGRAM

Some states have developed programs designed to provide specialized treatment to sex offenders. Minnesota is a national leader in the implementation of a multifaceted treatment approach. As of early January 2015, the Minnesota Sex Offender Program (MSOP) was providing treatment to over 700 individuals. To be in the program, an individual must have completed any prison sentences and then must be court-ordered to civil commitment within MSOP, typically for an unspecified amount of time (Minnesota Department of Human Services, 2014). Legislation introduced in the mid-1990s expanded civil commitment processes beyond the mentally ill and dangerous to include sexually dangerous persons, or sexually psychopathic personalities. The current treatment program has three progressive phases and goals:

- Phase 1: Acclimation to treatment, engagement, self-management
- Phase 2: Disclosure, unpacking offense history, identification of abuse patterns, skills building, increased awareness of self and others
- Phase 3: Deinstitutionalization, advanced skills building, transitions, consistent use of pro-social coping skills

These phases often incorporate the following clinical treatment activities:

- Individual, group, and family therapy
- Psychoeducational modules
- Vocational programming
- Therapeutic recreation
- Education
- Spiritual services
- Volunteer opportunities

Successful progression through these phases can result in advancement to community preparation services (CPS), an intensive reintegration process designed to gradually increase privileges in non-secure environments. Factors that go into the decision to approve a petition for movement toward CPS, provisional discharge, or full discharge back into the community include:

- The client's progress and treatment needs

- The need for security to continue treatment
- The need for continued treatment at a facility
- Whether a transfer can be done with a reasonable degree of public safety

ASSESSING, FINDING, AND DOCUMENTING SEXUAL VIOLENCE

The Sexual Assault Forensic Examination is a unique combination of medical and forensic assessment and care for victims of sexual violence. In the absence of a SANE within the hospital system, an emergency department nurse can provide care to a sexual assault patient and follow the step-by-step processes outlined in an evidence-collection kit in collaboration with other healthcare team members. As with every patient cared for in the emergency department, informed consent is obtained before care is delivered, and throughout the exam process, a distinct consent process for the sexual assault exam is followed and documented.

Because staffing the sexual assault nurse examiner role around the clock at the hospital is not typical, she/he will be called in when a victim of sexual violence presents to the emergency department and consents to or requests a sexual assault exam. Response times vary by geographic area, but in general it is expected that an on-call SANE can respond within 30 to 45 minutes. A victim advocate is also called in if that service is available in that hospital. Emergency department personnel immediately address acute injuries, with sensitivity to the need to preserve possible evidence. Upon stabilization, and in the absence of acute injuries, the SANE will proceed with providing comprehensive medical and forensic care.

Comprehensive care is essential in providing healthcare services to victims of sexual violence (Patel, Panchal, Piotrowski, & Patel, 2008; also see Chapter 6, "Assessment of Wounds and Injury"), including the following:

- Thorough documentation of health history and the incident

- Immediate assessment and treatment of any physical trauma, including strangulation

- Mental health assessment and care

- Prophylactic treatment for risk of sexually transmitted infections, including gonorrhea, chlamydia, trichomoniasis, and HIV (CDC, 2010)

- Counseling and offering emergency contraception

In addition, care for a victim of sexual violence includes specific forensic components:

- Forensic exam (often using a head-to-toe assessment approach)

- Specimen collection and secure storage or transfer to law enforcement

- Photographs of injuries (genital and non-genital) (refer to Chapter 6 for photography tips)

- Fluorescence/alternate light source

- Thorough documentation (Eisert et al., 2010)

When the exam is completed, the patient returns to the emergency department for additional medical care and social work consultation and is admitted for suicidality or discharged to home, a nursing home, a shelter, or another safe place. Collected specimens, clothing, and digital photographs will be securely stored and released through a chain of custody process to law enforcement if a police report has been made regarding the incident. In the absence of a police report, the collected items are locked securely at the hospital for a designated period of time to accommodate the possibility that a police report will be made.

The evidence collection kit, or "rape kit," might contain collected cotton swabs (e.g., swabs for saliva, semen/seminal fluid, blood, skin cells, saliva), blood and urine samples, and pubic hair combings or fingernail clippings/swabbings. If a police report is not made, the evidence will not be analyzed, because it is law enforcement that requests this analysis as part of the investigation process. Collaboration among the SANE and law enforcement increases the likelihood that a rape kit will be submitted for analysis in the investigation process (Patterson & Campbell, 2012).

Protocols for the care of victims of sexual violence continue to vary by healthcare setting across the U.S., and these protocols are adapted as changes evolve in knowledge, technology, and legislation. Certainly, national standards of care inform some protocol decisions (e.g., HIV prophylaxis), but for many, best practices and supportive evidence are not as well developed (e.g., strangulation assessment). Further, the time frame in which a sexual assault exam should be conducted following the incident is not an absolute. In some healthcare settings, for adolescents/adults, the complete exam is generally conducted up to 120 hours after the assault; this time frame is in part informed by studies showing that sperm can be successfully obtained from a vaginal cotton swab days after an assault (Mayntz-Press, Sims, Hall, & Ballantyne, 2008; Taylor, 2010). Ballantyne (2013) recently documented the ability to obtain male donor profiles from swabs collected 9 days post-coital.

RELEVANT LAWS AND STATUTES REGARDING SEXUAL VIOLENCE

Much of the policy framework and funding for care of victims of sexual assault in the U.S. comes from the federal Violence Against Women Act (VAWA). VAWA enacted the federal rape shield law, which ensures that information about a victim's previous sexual history cannot be brought up in court regardless of the state. The Department of Justice Office on Violence Against Women oversees compliance with VAWA statutes. Two very important regulations established by VAWA are that victims do *not* need to cooperate with law enforcement to receive medical care and a sexual assault exam, including evidence collection at the time of the exam, and that victims will not be charged for a sexual assault exam.

While VAWA ensures that victims do not need to cooperate with law enforcement to receive a sexual assault exam, procedures for confidential reporting exist in some states and not in others. California and Maryland have developed statewide systems that allow for anonymous reporting where a victim's name is not tied to evidence provided to law enforcement. Most states do not have such a system in place. A few local areas have implemented third party/anonymous reporting, including St. Louis County in northern Minnesota in 2009.

Laws and specific protocols for care of sexual assault patients can vary also based on the location where the assault took place or other factors. In California, for example, higher education institutions that receive state funds must have an affirmative consent policy. *Affirmative consent* requires both parties' voluntary agreement to engage in sexual activity, which can be revoked at any point. Affirmative consent policies are becoming more common on college campuses, and nurses who care for patients who were assaulted in campus settings should be prepared to explain what the policies mean when caring for patients who frequently are hesitant to label what happened to them as "sexual assault." Over 800 colleges and universities around the country have adopted such policies.

REFERENCES ADDRESSING SEXUAL VIOLENCE

- *Trauma and Recovery*, Judith Herman (book)
- *Not My Life* (film): Documentary about the realities of human trafficking across the world.
- *The Invisible War* (film): An investigative documentary about the epidemic of rape of soldiers within the U.S. military.
- *Frontline: Rape in the Fields* (film): Documentary about the hidden reality of rape on the job for immigrant women.
- *Miss America by Day*, Marilyn Van Derbur (book): A former Miss America tells the story of how she was sexually violated by her prominent, millionaire father from age 5 to age 18. She was 53 years old before she was able to speak the words in public.
- *Shattered: Reclaiming a Life Torn Apart by Violence*, Debra Puglisi Sharp (book): Real-life story of a nurse who is attacked and raped in her home by a stranger after he murders her husband, and her hope, determination, and agonizing journey back to life.
- *Recovering from Rape*, Linda Ledray (book): Practical advice on overcoming the trauma and coping with police, hospitals, and the courts—for the survivors of sexual assault and their families, lovers, and friends.
- *Lucky*, Alice Sebold (book): Describes her experience of rape while in college and details her years of struggle and ultimate recovery.

ASSISTING VICTIMS, FAMILIES, AND SIGNIFICANT OTHERS

Anyone can be a victim of a crime. With over 3.8 million violent crimes occurring in the U.S. in 2010 (Truman, 2011), there is a clear need for the healthcare system to actively engage in violence prevention and intervention initiatives. Because the emergency department of a hospital is the most likely place a victim of violence will turn to, it's imperative that staff, particularly nurses, are educated and are prepared to address the forensic aspects of injuries resulting from violence (Henderson, Harada, & Amar, 2012). With attention toward providing comprehensive, holistic healthcare and forensic care, an effective nurse will meet each victim of sexual violence where she or he is at that moment, for example:

- The adolescent with suspected drug-facilitated sexual assault

- The woman brutally assaulted by her partner, yet unwilling to make a police report

- The gay man reporting assault by a former partner after enduring the abuse for years

- The deaf girl assaulted by an acquaintance on her way to the mall

- The woman involved in prostitution, assaulted by a client and scared of her pimp

- The young adult assaulted in the park by a stranger asking directions

- The immigrant woman raped by her friend's husband

- The college student suspecting assault after waking up in a strange car

Every incident of sexual violence is distinctive and experienced in a unique way by each victim. Care of victims of sexual violence requires thoughtful, thorough assessment and treatment that is offered in a context of belief, support, and non-judgmental care. Compounded by previous life experiences, there can be a significant sense of revictimization that requires careful and emotionally intelligent intervention and support. See Chapter 17, "Trauma-Informed Care," for additional information regarding trauma-informed care, which is critically important for survivors of sexual violence.

Every nurse needs a personal awareness that enables connection to every patient, which encourages trust and disclosure, enhances the patient's capacity to receive information and support, and enhances decision-making about healthcare services. There are core values, characteristics, and skills that can encourage the best healthcare experience for a victim of sexual violence, including:

- Respect

- Empathy

- Honesty

- Trust

- Listening

- Mindfulness

- Emotional intelligence

Advocacy is a key strategy that has demonstrated significant positive effects in the care of patients who have experienced sexual violence (Campbell, 2006). The presence of an advocate minimizes the perception that the forensic nurse is functioning as an advocate (Campbell, Patterson, & Lichty, 2005). Some documented patient outcomes of victim advocate presence during a SANE exam include (Campbell, 2006):

- More patients agreeing to receive STI/HIV prophylaxis

- More likely to receive information about pregnancy prophylaxis

- Better mental health outcomes and fewer feelings of guilt

- Less distress related to legal system involvement

It's also been shown that patients are more likely to continue with care, including medical follow-up and counseling (Preston, 2003), and their chances of becoming a victim a second time and developing post-traumatic stress disorder symptoms are reduced (Campbell, 2008).

TRANS-DISCIPLINARY RESOURCES AND REFERRALS

Regardless of specialty, all nurses will encounter patients who have experienced sexual violence. This section details additional resources that nurses can access to learn more about sexual violence, as well as resources that can be offered to patients who need additional support.

International Association of Forensic Nurses

The International Association of Forensic Nurses (IAFN) is a network of over 3,000 members who practice and support forensic nursing. The IAFN publishes the *Journal of Forensic Nursing*. It also offers multiple CEU-eligible trainings, including a virtual practicum on the forensic and clinical management of sexual assault and a 40-hour sexual assault nurse examiner (SANE) training. SANEs are registered nurses who have completed specialized education and clinical preparation in the medical forensic care of the patient who has experienced sexual assault or abuse, and are an important resource for these patients. The IAFN also offers free webinars and specialized sexual assault forensic examination (SAFE) topics. The Indian Health Service funds the IAFN's Tribal Forensic Healthcare Training Project, which offers trainings for healthcare providers to improve the response to domestic and sexual violence in hospitals, health clinics, and health stations within the Indian health system.

IAFN provides additional resources for nurses, online training, and in-person training that you can find out about at http://www.forensicnurses.org/?page=EducationMainPage.

National Coalition of Anti-Violence Programs

The National Coalition of Anti-Violence Programs (NCAVP) is dedicated to reducing violence and its impacts on lesbian, gay, bisexual, transgender, queer, and HIV-affected (LGBTQH) communities. It takes special knowledge to be culturally competent when it comes to these communities and their experiences around sexual violence; many mainstream organizations that lack appropriate training can be a source of revictimization for LGBTQH clients. The NCAVP publishes a member list including local organizations across the U.S. and in Montreal, Quebec, and Toronto, Canada.

NCAVP provides additional resources for nurses, online training, and in-person training that you can find out about at www.avp.org/about-avp/national-coalition-of-anti-violence-programs.

National Sexual Violence Resource Center

The National Sexual Violence Resource Center (NSVRC) promotes a mission of providing leadership in sexual violence prevention and response through collaboration, resource sharing and creation, and research promotion. The NSVRC publishes a toolkit for *sexual assault response teams* (SART), which are coordinated, multidisciplinary, and victim-centered first response teams for victims of sexual assault. The NSVRC also runs a SART listserv, a forum for discussion among community and professional organizations and agencies that respond to sexual violence. One project includes the Healthcare Initiative, which provides information on the impact of sexual violence on health and how healthcare providers can respond to and prevent sexual violence.

You can find out more about the resources for nurses and patients and online training NSVRC provides at www.nsvrc.org.

Rape, Abuse and Incest National Network

The Rape, Abuse and Incest National Network (RAINN) is the largest anti–sexual violence organization in the United States. RAINN operates the National Sexual Assault Hotline, a free, anonymous telephone and web-based helpline for people who have experienced sexual violence and their loved ones. RAINN also operates the Department of Defense Safe Helpline for sexual assault survivors in the military. RAINN's website has a search feature to find a local crisis center, as well as general information about sexual assault, healing, and prevention.

RAINN also provides an excellent resource for learning about the laws in your state.

RAINN offers a variety of resources for nurses and patients at www.rainn.org.

Safe Dates

Safe Dates is an evidence-based school curriculum for primary prevention of dating violence, including sexual abuse. The curriculum is intended for 8th- and 9th-grade students, and it is an important resource for public health and school nurses. The goals of the program include changing adolescent dating violence and gender-role norms, improving peer help-giving and dating conflict-resolution skills, promoting victim and perpetrator beliefs in the need for help and seeking help through the community resources that provide it, and decreasing dating abuse victimization and perpetration (Foshee, 2004).

You can find resources for nurses and in-person training at www.hazelden.org/web/go/safedates.

CASE STUDY: SEXUAL VIOLENCE

Sarah, a 16-year-old White adolescent, arrived to the emergency department with her mother. She told the triage nurse she thought she had been raped the night before but she wasn't sure. The SANE and advocate were paged and both arrived within 30 minutes of the call. The SANE introduced herself and observed the adolescent, noting her clean clothing and casual conversation with mom. "I am a nurse and I come to the hospital to take care of patients who have been raped or think they might have been. I would like to explain what I can do and you can then tell me what you would like or what you would not like." After explaining the examination process and options for preventing pregnancy, HIV, and other STIs, the SANE obtained consent from the adolescent to receive care. Sarah was not sure what had happened, but as she told the SANE what she could remember, it became clear that signs of possible assault existed. Sarah described drinking a lot of alcohol and going to her friend's bedroom to sleep. She remembered her friends helping her onto the bed and leaving the room. She vaguely remembered a guy being in the room and then leaving. She did not remember removing her clothing, but when she woke up later, she was missing clothing. As part of the exam, the SANE asked questions using trauma-informed interviewing techniques, including a specific question, "What is something you cannot forget about this experience?" Expecting to hear more about not being able to remember, the SANE was surprised when Sarah immediately shared, "I can't forget that some of my friends recorded what had happened and put the recording up on Snapchat. They were worried I was dead because I wasn't responding to them. But now everyone can see what happened. I thought they were my friends but they really aren't. I don't know how I can face these people again." Sarah was worried about what would happen if she made a police report, and although she could understand the importance and value in making the report, she left the hospital without agreeing to have the police called. She and her mother agreed to consider contacting the police after they had taken some time to think it through. Sarah did, however, consent to having a rape kit completed, which was documented and stored following chain of custody protocols. Because Sarah wasn't sure what had happened, swabs were collected from all possible penetration sites, along with samples of blood and urine. Sarah did not report any injuries, and a thorough examination confirmed there was not any bruising or other apparent injury to photograph. Sarah was encouraged to pay attention to any physical changes over the subsequent day or two, because some bruising might not appear immediately. Sarah received medications to prevent STIs and pregnancy. She agreed to receive follow-up calls from the advocacy center and SANE office, which would provide another opportunity to discuss making a police report, as well as address any questions or needs related to counseling and the healing process. Sarah's mother was supportive and repeatedly stated that she was there for Sarah and would stand by any decision Sarah made regarding talking with the police.

The SANE emphasized that Sarah was being strong in coming to the hospital for care and encouraged Sarah to consider making a police report, while acknowledging her fears and concerns related to the social network of friends surrounding her. The SANE respected Sarah's decisions, and as she left the hospital, Sarah was tired but felt she had received good care. She had been heard and her choices had been respected.

SUMMARY

Sexual violence is a pervasive and insidious public health and safety concern. Despite being commonly thought of as a women's issue, evidence supports that men are also sexually victimized. Sexual violence often occurs in conjunction with other perpetrator-initiated crimes and risk behaviors (e.g., burglary, intimate partner violence, substance use, prostitution/trafficking). Sexual violence also affects the physical and mental health and wellbeing of survivors.

Sexual assault nurse examiners (SANEs) fulfill a key role in the care of victims of sexual violence. Care includes health assessment and treatment as well as forensic assessment, specimen collection, and documentation to maintain proper legal chain of custody processes. Collaborative care, including advocates, law enforcement, and other healthcare/social work providers, strengthens potential for healthy outcomes. Legislation and national resources exist to support prevention of and response to sexual violence, including supporting victims and their families.

REFERENCES

Ballantyne, J. (2013). *DNA profiling of the semen donor in extended interval post-coital samples*. Retrieved from https://www.ncjrs.gov/pdffiles1/nij/grants/241299.pdf

Basile, K. C., Smith, S. G., Breiding, M. J., Black, M. C., & Mahendra, R. R. (2014). *Sexual violence surveillance: Uniform definitions and recommended data elements*. Retrieved from http://www.cdc.gov/violenceprevention/pdf/sv_surveillance_definitionsl-2009-a.pdf

Black, M. C., Basile, K. C., Breiding, M. J., Smith, S. G., Walters, M. L., Merrick, M. T., ... Stevens, M. R. (2011). *The National Intimate Partner and Sexual Violence Survey (NISVS): 2010 summary report*. Atlanta, GA: National Center for Injury Prevention and Control, Centers for Disease Control and Prevention.

Borowsky, I. W., Hogan, M., & Ireland, M. (1997). Adolescent sexual aggression: Risk and protective factors. *Pediatrics, 100*(6), E7. Retrieved from http://pediatrics.aappublications.org/content/100/6/e7.full

Breiding, M. J., Smith, S. G., Basile, K. C., Walters, M. L., Chen, J., & Merrick, M. T. (2014). Prevalence and characteristics of sexual violence, stalking, and intimate partner violence victimization—National Intimate Partner and Sexual Violence Survey, United States, 2011. *CDC Surveillance Summaries. MMWR, 63*(SS08), 1–18. Retrieved from http://www.cdc.gov/mmwr/preview/mmwrhtml/ss6308a1.htm

Campbell, R. (2006). Rape survivors' experiences with legal and medical systems: Do rape victim advocates make a difference? *Violence Against Women, 12*(1), 30–45.

Campbell, R. (2008). The psychological impact of rape victims. *American Psychologist, 63*(8), 702–717.

Campbell, R., Patterson, D., & Lichty, L. (2005). The effectiveness of sexual assault nurse examiner (SANE) programs: A review of psychological, medical, legal, and community outcomes. *Trauma, Violence, & Abuse, 6*(4), 313–329.

Centers for Disease Control and Prevention (CDC). (2015). *Sexual violence: Risk and protective factors.* Retrieved from http://www.cdc.gov/ViolencePrevention/sexualviolence/riskprotectivefactors.html

Centers for Disease Control and Prevention (CDC). (2014a). *Sexual violence: Definitions.* Retrieved January 23, 2015, from http://www.cdc.gov/violenceprevention/sexualviolence/definitions.html

Centers for Disease Control and Prevention (CDC). (2014b). *2010 STD treatment guidelines: Sexual assault and STDs.* Retrieved from http://www.cdc.gov/std/treatment/2010/sexual-assault.htm

Eisert, P. J., Eldredge, K., Hartlaub, T., Huggins, E., Keirn, G., O'Brien, P., ... March, K. S. (2010). Development of forensic evidence collection guidelines for the emergency department. *Crit Care Nurs Quarterly, 33*(2), 190–199.

Foshee, V. (2004). Safe Dates: An adolescent dating abuse prevention curriculum. Center City, MN: Hazelden Publishing.

Groth, A. N., Burgess, A. W., & Holmstrom, L. L. (1977). Rape: Power, anger and sexuality. *American Journal of Psychiatry, 134*, 1239–1243.

Hazelwood, R. R. (2009). Analyzing the rape and profiling the offender. In R. R. Hazelwood & A. W. Burgess (Eds.), *Practical aspects of rape investigation: A multidisciplinary approach.* Boca Raton, FL: CRC Press, 4th edition, 97–122.

Henderson, E., Harada, N., & Amar, A. (2012). Caring for the forensic population: Recognizing the educational needs of emergency department nurses and physicians. *Journal of Forensic Nursing, 8*(4), 170–177. doi: 10.1111/j.1939-3938.2012.01144.x

Holmes, R. M., & Holmes, S. T. (2001). *Murder in America* (2nd ed.). Thousand Oaks, CA: Sage.

International Association of Forensic Nurses (IAFN). (n.d.). Retrieved from http://www.forensicnurses.org/?page=EducationMainPage

Ledray, L., Faugno, D., & Speck, P. (2001). SANE: Advocate, forensic technician, nurse? *Journal of Emergency Nursing, 27*(1), 91–93.

Mayntz-Press, K. A., Sims, L. M., Hall, A., & Ballantyne, J. (2008). Y-STR profiling in extended interval (≥3 days) postcoital cervicovaginal samples. *J Forensic Sci, 53*(2), 342–348. doi: 10.1111/j.1556-4029.2008.00672.x

Minnesota Department of Human Services. (2014). *Sex offender treatment*. Retrieved from http://mn.gov/dhs/people-we-serve/adults/services/sex-offender-treatment/

Pandora's Project. (n.d.). *What is rape?* Retrieved from http://www.pandys.org/whatisrape.html

Patel, A., Panchal, H., Piotrowski, Z., & Patel, D. (2008). Comprehensive medical care for victims of sexual violence: A survey of Illinois hospital emergency departments. *Contraception, 77*(6), 426–430.

Patterson, D., & Campbell, R. (2012). The problem of untested sexual assault kits: Why are some kits never submitted to a crime laboratory? *Journal of Interpersonal Violence, 27*(11), 2259–2275.

Preston, L. (2003). The sexual assault nurse examiner and the rape crisis center advocate: A necessary partnership. *Topics in Emergency Medicine, 25*(3), 242–246.

Rape, Abuse and Incest National Network (RAINN). (n.d.). Retrieved from https://www.rainn.org/

Taylor, T. (2010). Extending the time to collect DNA in sexual assault cases. *NIJ Journal, 267*. Retrieved from http://www.nij.gov/journals/267/pages/extending.aspx

Truman, J. S. (2011). National Crime Victimization Survey: Criminal Victimization, 2010. U.S. Department of Justice, Office of Justice Programs, Bureau of Justice Statistics. NCJ, 235508.

11

CHILD MALTREATMENT

Annie Lewis-O'Connor, PhD, NP-BC, MPH, FAAN; and Adine Latimore, MSN, PPCNP-BC, SANE

"It is the responsibility of every adult ... to make sure that children hear what we have learned from the lessons of life and to hear over and over that we love them and that they are not alone."

–Marian Wright Edelman (Edelman, Wright, 1992)

KEY POINTS IN THIS CHAPTER

- Child maltreatment includes physical, sexual, and emotional abuse and neglect of a child under the age of 18 by a parent, caregiver, or another person in a custodial role.

- Child maltreatment adversely affects a child's immediate and long-term physical and psychological health and well-being.

- Nurses are in a prime role to recognize and intervene with children who have experienced child maltreatment and to provide prevention education.

- Knowledge of resources and models of care ensure that children and families get the needed help to cope with child maltreatment and its consequences.

Globally, children are exposed to violence. This chapter provides information to help nurses recognize and intervene with children and families experiencing child maltreatment. An overview of the problem, including scope, prevalence, and laws, is presented to increase the nurse's contextual knowledge of child maltreatment. The discussion includes practical strategies for screening, documentation, and responding to child maltreatment.

OVERVIEW OF CHILD MALTREATMENT

Child maltreatment, sometimes referred to as *child abuse and neglect,* includes all forms of physical and emotional maltreatment, sexual abuse, neglect, and exploitation that results in actual or potential harm to the child's health, development, or dignity (World Health Organization [WHO], 2015).

Sadly, exposure to violence and abuse is a daily occurrence for many children throughout the world. They may experience it directly or indirectly, as the intended targets or as witnesses, in their homes, their schools, their neighborhoods, through the media, or in the context of war. In the past 3 decades, the research and evidence have grown exponentially in understanding the impact of violence on children. Key facts are (WHO, 2015):

- A quarter of all adults report physical abuse during childhood.

- One in 5 women and 1 in 13 men report sexual abuse as a child.

- Consequences of child maltreatment include impaired lifelong physical and mental health and poor social and occupational outcomes, and influence a country's economic and social development.

THE ADVERSE CHILDHOOD EXPERIENCES STUDY

The Adverse Childhood Experiences (ACE) Study is a landmark research study focusing on the role of childhood adversity—in other words, childhood toxic exposures, including violence and abuse, and their relationship to long-term health consequences (Anda et al., 2011). The study identified categories of ACE exposures in children and then followed them longitudinally to determine health outcomes. The researchers found that increases in the number of categories experienced resulted in increases in severity of illness risk factors, psychosocial and behavior problems, and serious disease or other physical health problems, as well as increases in healthcare utilization (Anda, Brown, Felitti, Dube, & Giles, 2008; Anda, Butchart, Felitti, & Brown, 2010; Anda et al., 2011; Brown et al., 2009; Cuijpers et al., 2011). Illness risk factors and psychosocial/behavioral problems include smoking, obesity, physical inactivity, depression, suicide attempts, alcoholism, drug abuse, sexual risk-taking, and sexually transmitted diseases. Serious disease or other physical health problems include heart disease, cancer, stroke, chronic bronchitis, chronic obstructive pulmonary disease (COPD), chronic pain, diabetes, hepatitis, and skeletal fractures.

Typically, children who witness violence in their homes do so during their growth years, during the phase of life when they are learning about themselves, their relationships with others, and the world around them. Childhood is most commonly regarded as a time of innocence and predictability; however, this depiction is by no means the reality for large numbers of children who grow up amid violence. For these young people, the world is experienced as a place where violence is an integral part of everyday life, where danger is commonplace, and where interactions are chaotic and unpredictable. The central developmental task for these children is to find safety in a world that feels unsafe and seek trust from people who have been untrustworthy.

RURAL VS. URBAN CHALLENGES TO CHILD DEVELOPMENT

Is there an increased incidence of in child abuse depending on whether one is in an urban or rural environment? First let's define these areas. An *urban* environment is a densely settled area that meets minimum population requirements of at least 2,500 people, at least 1,500 of which reside outside institutional group quarters. The Census Bureau identifies two types of urban areas—UA's: urbanized areas of 50,000 or more people, and UC's: urban clusters, at least 2,500 people but fewer than 50,000 (U.S. Census Bureau, 2015). *Rural* encompasses all populations, housing, and territory not included within an urban area. Comparisons of urban and rural areas reveal differences in the incidence of documented child abuse and disparity in available resources. According to Sedlak and colleagues (2010), incidents of overall abuse in rural counties were 1.7 times that of the rate in urban counties; sexual abuse in rural counties was twice the rate as urban counties and 1.6 times the rate as major urban areas. The risk of emotional abuse for children in rural counties was 2.6 times that in major urban counties. Child maltreatment and the context in which it occurs bring challenges. It is imperative that nurses gather information on local resources and services that are available to assist victims and their families.

SOCIAL DETERMINANTS OF HEALTH

The complexities of child maltreatment are rooted in the *social determinants of health* (SDOH)—the economic and social conditions, along with their distribution among the population—that influence individual and group differences in health status. According to the Office of Disease Prevention and Health Promotion and its Healthy People 2020 program, health starts in homes, schools, workplaces, neighborhoods, and communities. In part, health is determined by access to social and economic opportunities; the resources and supports available in homes, neighborhoods, and communities; the quality of schooling; and the nature of social interactions and relationships, as shown in Figure 11.1. The conditions in which a child lives explain, in part, why some children are healthier than others and why children more generally are not as healthy as they could be (Office of Disease Prevention and Health Promotion, n.d.).

These factors are interrelated and can affect whether a child experiences violence. Violence occurs more often in areas with economic instability (Sedlak et al., 2010). Poverty, unemployment, food insecurity, and housing instability all create more stress on individuals and families, which can increase the vulnerability of children within families. Neighborhoods and schools can be sites for violence and also contribute to the norms and acceptability of violence. Because violence is also a social determinant of health, the recognition of the factors and the role they play in improving child health can guide nurses in prevention and intervention strategies.

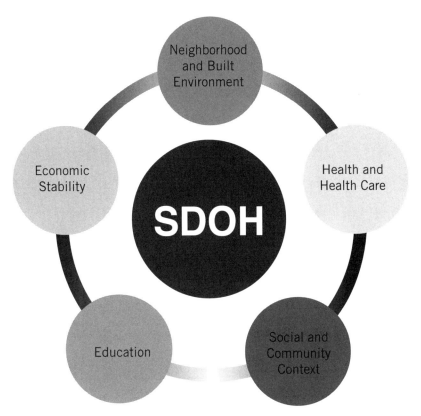

FIGURE 11.1 THE SOCIAL DETERMINANTS OF HEALTH (SDOH).

Addressing these disparities is central to eliminating the child's exposure to violence and abuse.

THE PERPETRATORS OF CHILD ABUSE AND NEGLECT

As unlikely as it might seem, the most common perpetrators of child maltreatment are parents and caregivers. Other perpetrators are the unmarried partner of a child's parent or other relatives. Data from the Administration on Children, Youth, and Families (2014) suggests that most perpetrators are White women between the ages of 18 and 44. The largest three groups of perpetrators are White (49.3%), African American (20.1%), and Hispanic (19.5%). More than half are women (53.9%). In terms of types of abuse, women are more often perpetrators of medical neglect (76%), men of sexual abuse (87.8%), and there's a fairly even split in physical child abuse between men (49.6%) and women (48.2%).

Certain factors put adults at risk for becoming abusers. For example, many abusive and neglectful adults were victims of abuse themselves. Although not everyone with these risk factors is an abuser, every caretaker at risk exhibits one or more of the following characteristics (Miller-Perrin & Perrin, 2006):

- Immaturity, lack of parenting skills, or unrealistic expectations of a child

- Unmet emotional needs, isolation, or poor impulse control

- A significant disruption of normal life, such as divorce, death of a loved one, loss of a job or source of income, or significant illness

- An accumulation of small stressors in combination with other risk factors that result in the parent or caretaker losing control

- Substance abuse

These factors don't necessarily cause abuse but could warrant further investigation and parenting education and support.

PREVENTION STRATEGIES FOR CHILD ABUSE

Healthcare to prevent child abuse falls into three categories:

- *Prevention* is education and prevention regarding developing a disease or from environmental hazards.

    It involves educating young mothers about safety and protecting their young children (anticipatory guidance). Because most children are maltreated by someone they know, young parents must be aware and monitor their children for risk exposures to prevent harm and promote safety.

▪ *Secondary prevention* includes interventions when a diagnosis or condition has occurred with the goal of mitigating the effects and restoring optimal health.

It might involve early detection of exposures to child maltreatment and employing safeguards to protect and mitigate health consequences. This might include early interventions through identification. For example, a young teenager gives birth to a baby. She discloses many stressors in the home and lacks confidence in parenting her new baby. A nurse from a home visitation program could provide ongoing support and assessment and serve as a catalyst for resources. Later in this chapter, we discuss the Nurse-Family Partnership program.

▪ *Tertiary prevention* focuses on optimizing health and wellness for patients with chronic illness and/or significant sequelae from events that affect health.

It might help a young adolescent cope with the physical and mental health consequences experienced through years of abuse as a young child.

A combination of all preventions strategies offers the best opportunity to identify at-risk individuals, improve health, and prevent exposures to violence and abuse.

SCREENING AND EXAMINING FOR CHILD ABUSE

One of the most effective ways to screen for children under age 12 for maltreatment is through a dialogue with the caretaker of the child. An important lesson learned from the intimate partner violence community and advocates is that screening using a checklist format is not effective. Rather, more disclosures are made when patients feel more engaged in a discussion. For example, the nurse could state, "I would like to ask you some questions about how things are going at home, is that okay with you? In your words, how are things going at home? What do you enjoy the most, the least? What kind of supports do you have?"

Such dialogue opens up a conversation and provides an opportunity to build a relationship that promotes trust and a partnership.

When a child is older than 12, often the provider can see the child and caretaker together and then ask to speak with the child alone. This provides an opportunity to build a rapport with the tween/adolescent and the healthcare provider and explore the patient's relationships, strengths, and challenges. If at any time the patient discloses exposures to abuse and or neglect, this is reportable to the child welfare agency in all 50 U.S. states. This is also the case among industrialized nations; however, it is not true in all areas of the globe.

SCREENING INSTRUMENTS

Most screening instruments that are validated for assessing for child maltreatment have been used retrospectively with an adult population for the purposes of research and do not translate well into clinical settings. A good example of this is the ACE Study, which screened adults for their experiences of abuse as a child. Children who present in the healthcare system either have signs and symptoms of abuse and/or neglect, present with a caretaker who has concerns for abuse, or are brought in by law enforcement or child protective services. Most pediatric providers will ask some general questions about safety and caretakers' concerns. As children get older, they are often seen alone with the provider and asked questions about bullying, safety, and relationships.

Although many validated tools aren't used in the pediatric setting, most experienced pediatric providers are aware of concerns for abuse. In the future, healthcare providers may use more targeted screening via computer-based inquiry. There is also talk in the field about screening caretakers and children for ACE categories (see the earlier section "The Adverse Childhood Experiences Study").

EXAMINING CHILDREN

The examination of a child is based on a "do no harm" premise. It's important that you consider the developmental stage of the child, not just the age of the child. A child should never be restrained, and conscious sedation is never encouraged. On few occasions, a child may require evaluation under anesthesia; for example, vaginal bleeding or a significant ano-genital injury.

Approaching the child for an examination requires the healthcare team to work in harmony. Some tips are:

- Work at a pace that works for the child.

- Inform the child that at any point she/he can stop the examination by raising a hand. This gesture allows the child to feel safe and have control.

- Engage the child in play while you assess the child's physical condition.

Your physical assessment begins the moment a child walks into your office. Observe the child's gait. Is it steady? Is there a limp? How is the parent-child interaction? Instances of maltreatment are often hidden, or explanations of injuries are not consistent with the physical examination (Adams, 2011).

More often than not, children are not going to disclose how the injury occurred, especially if the offender is in the room. Your job is to advocate for a child when you have any suspicion or concern that an injury was deliberate, and then to notify the proper authority.

DOCUMENTING INJURIES

Wounds, bruises, and burns are easily visible, but the mechanism that caused the injury may be difficult to name. Document the injury the best way possible; documentation can take these forms:

- Radiography if broken bones are suspected

- Photographs for bruises, burns, bite marks, and/or superficial injuries

- The history as provided by child and/or caretaker

- Objective data—what you see, palpate, smell (e.g., gasoline odor), and hear

Obtain consent from a parent/guardian/caretaker before images are taken. In the event the child discloses that the caretaker who has accompanied the child is the person who has harmed the child, separate the child and caretaker, hold the child, and contact child services for an emergency response. Once consent is obtained, document the type of camera you're using, your name, the date of the photographs, and name of the patient. The initial photograph should be an overview or full picture of the child, the second photograph should be mid-range or specific area involved, and the third photograph should be a closeup. More than three images can be taken; if using a digital camera, check photos for clarity and take more pictures as you need. You should also use a proper tool to measure the injury involved. You can buy the ABFO #2 photo scale at http://www.crime-scene.com/store/A-6200.shtml. If the photo scale is not available, you may use a ruler or anything whose size cannot be challenged; for example, a coin.

Another imperative concept to embrace is that of cultural perspective. The United States is known as a country of diversity and one with many cultures. Cultures bring with them many practices and rituals, some of which may mimic child abuse. In the Afro-Caribbean religion of Santeria, many children are marked with crosses on their body when they become initiated into that religion (Fontes, 2005). There are also many medical practices that leave marks, bruises, or burns. For example, coining, where coins are rubbed on a child's skin; cupping, where hot cups are applied to a child's skin and a vacuum is formed; and moxibustion, where small items are heated up and applied to parts of the body (Fontes, 2005). Many cultures believe that these practices help with healing and the relief of symptoms and are not intended to be an act of abuse or violence. You may still have to report to child protection, but you can also support and advocate for this family and their cultural practices.

RESPONDING TO CHILD VICTIMS AND THEIR FAMILIES

When a child discloses to you or a parent reports to you that his or her child has been a victim of abuse or suspects abuse, what do you do? The initial response should be to stay calm. This may be a shock to you, but it has also been a shock to the family. This is a time when a parent and child may need a calm voice in a world that has now been turned upside down. Anxiety, fear, and thoughts such as, "What do I do now?" have moved to the top of this family's list.

If a child discloses to you, make sure you listen to the child. Praise the child for coming forward and talking about it and also let the child know that you are available to help him or her. That help should be in the form of trauma-informed care (addressed in Chapter 17, "Trauma-Informed Care"). It's important to explain to the non-abusing caretaker that the law requires you to make a report on behalf of the child (note: This report is not against an abuser but is rather filed on behalf of a child). Minimal facts of the incident should be obtained (i.e., who, what, when, where), but you do not want to interview the child. For example, questions such as, "Who did that? What happened? Where did this happen? When did this happen? Is anything hurting you?" can help you understand what happened to the child, but ask only the questions necessary to guide the medical evaluation of the child. Details of the incident are better left to the authorities or a forensic interviewer who specializes in talking to children that have been abused. You also must remember that most children do not disclose everything at one time; it may be a more gradual process. Forensic interviewers are trained to help children with their disclosures.

If a parent reports to you, be supportive and nonjudgmental. Ask the parents what information they have, how they found out, or what the child has told them about the incident. This information will be used to notify the child services organization in your area. Does the parent have support? Are mental health services/crisis intervention needed for the parent at this time? The child should also be referred to a medical provider, preferably one who specializes in the examination of children that have been abused, for an examination. A medical examination may be necessary to collect physical/biological evidence, depending on when the last incident happened, and to also screen for infections if genital contact was disclosed.

CHILD ABUSE REPORTING LAWS

Media coverage of child abuse or child maltreatment is very common; some of the most horrific cases are reported and capture our attention. The attention suggests that child maltreatment is new. However, that is not the case. In fact, in 1874, the case of 10-year-old Mary Ellen McCormack was brought to light. She was a foster child in New York who was treated horrifically by her foster mother. Mary Ellen testified in court of being whipped and beaten almost every day (Watkins, 1990). She was removed from that foster home and her foster mother was convicted and received jail time. Mary Ellen's case put a face to child abuse, as documented by the American Humane Society. In 1875, a year later, the world's first organization devoted entirely to child protection, due largely in part to McCormack's case, came into existence. The New York Society for the Prevention of Cruelty to Children was formed (Myers, 2008).

Many states followed with their own laws and statutes that are based on the standard set by the Federal Child Abuse Prevention and Treatment Act (CAPTA). This federal law defines child abuse and neglect as any recent act or failure to act on the part of a parent or caretaker that results in death, serious physical or emotional harm, sexual abuse or exploitation, or that presents an imminent risk of serious harm (Child Abuse Prevention and Treatment Act, 2010).

Today, all states have child abuse laws. There may be variations of course, but in general, the laws are in place to protect children:

- **State Child Abuse Laws** lists each state and its respective laws: http://statelaws. findlaw.com/family-laws/child-abuse.html

- **The Child Welfare Information Gateway** is an excellent resource for information on state statutes regarding child welfare and maltreatment: https://www.childwelfare.gov/topics/systemwide/laws-policies/state

These state laws contain guidelines for reporting child abuse. A nurse is not responsible for determining whether abuse has occurred; rather, the nurse is responsible for filing a report to the appropriate agency in the state when concerns for the safety and wellbeing of a child are present. The investigation will explore if abuse occurred resulting in harm to the child. For example, under Massachusetts law, the Department of Children and Families (DCF) is the state agency that receives all reports of suspected abuse and/or neglect of children under the age of 18 (Massachusetts DCF, 2015). The nurse should file a report if he or she suspects abuse; the role of the state agency is to conduct the investigation.

Another variation on child reporting is that of Native American children. A different law applies to these children: the Indian Child Welfare Act (ICWA) of 1978 (National Indian Child Welfare Association, 2015). (Native American and Indian are used interchangeably to identify the same group of people.) This federal law was enacted in 1978 because Native American children were being removed from their homes and placed with non–Native American foster homes, adoptive homes, etc., when there were concerns of abuse. This law seeks to keep Native American children with Native American families. More information on this law is at http://www.nicwa.org/indian_child_welfare_act. Globally, the United Nations enacted laws to protect children internationally. "The Convention on the Rights of the Child" (United Nations Office of the High Commissioner for Human Rights, crc 1989 & 1990) is the most comprehensive document on the rights of children (a child is defined as below the age of 18). This law includes children's rights to protect their identity, cultural protections, and protections for the disabled and refugees, parental guidance, and laws regarding separation from parents. This document has a multitude of rights including 54 articles. Of the nine human rights treaties in effect today, this is the longest and most comprehensive one documented.

Providers of Care

The health delivery system has evolved over the past few decades. Recognizing the prevalence of child maltreatment and the need for informed evidence-based care, a number of specialists were added to the healthcare team. Some of those experts include:

- **Sexual assault nurse examiners** (SANEs) can be one of the first providers to see a child after the child has disclosed abuse. These nurses provide expert, developmentally appropriate care; and forensic examinations that include photo documentation, the collection of evidence, and emotional support to children. Nurses, nurse practitioners, and midwives work in these roles.

- **Pediatricians, board certified in child maltreatment,** are responsible for the diagnosis and treatment of children and adolescents who are suspected victims of any form of child maltreatment. Usually these pediatricians serve on child protection teams.

- **School nurses** have a unique opportunity to provide care to these children. A school nurse is with these children most of the day and may be the first person to whom a child discloses. The National Association of School Nurses (NASN) stands in support of early recognition and treatment for children who are victims of child maltreatment. School nurses have the ability to recognize early signs of abuse and assist these children by assessing, reporting, and referring to appropriate agencies for intervention and treatment (NASN, 2014).

- **General practitioners** have a unique role in that they see children for various illnesses throughout the year and have an opportunity to assess at each visit for indicators of maltreatment.

MODELS OF CARE AND INTERVENTIONS

There are also many resources you can turn to for advice on how to treat and prevent child abuse:

- **Family Justice Center Alliance (FJCA)** (http://familyjusticecenter.com): The FJCA serves as a distinct group of partners and agencies within the community who work together for the purposes of providing a welcoming and safe environment for survivors of child maltreatment and domestic violence.

- **National Children's Alliance** (http://www.nationalchildrensalliance.org): Formed in 1988, National Children's Alliance provides support, technical assistance, and quality assurance for Children's Advocacy Centers (CAC), along with serving as a voice for abused children for more than 25 years.

- **National Children's Advocacy Center (NCAC)** (http://www.nationalcac.org): This unique agency brings together a multidisciplinary response to severe physical and sexual child abuse by enabling law enforcement, prosecutors, child protective services, and medical and mental health professionals to work together as a collaborative team to investigate, prosecute cases, provide medical care, and support victims of child abuse. A CAC provides outreach and education in the community and serves as a resource for the community. CAC programs work to minimize trauma, break the cycle of abuse, and provide communities with an added bonus—increased prosecution rates for perpetrators.

- **Child Protection Teams:** This is a team of experts in many fields that care for victims of child abuse. Team members may include pediatricians, nurse practitioners, social workers, clergy, and mental health providers who work together to assess victims of abuse in a hospital setting.

- **Child Fatality Review Board:** These boards work in some states to review the deaths of children and make recommendations for public policy to enhance prevention strategies. Child abuse deaths are preventable, and child fatality review boards can help by continuing to inform and educate regarding prevention strategies. In 2012, the Child Welfare Information Gateway reported that 1,640 children died as a result of child abuse, and more than 70% of those children were 2 years old or younger (Child Welfare Information Gateway, n.d.).

- **Forensic Child Interviewers:** These are trained experts in interviewing children in a non-leading, objective manner. The information gained during these interviews can be used in court and can help inform the medical and psychological evaluation.

- **Nurse-Family Partnership** (http://www.nursefamilypartnership.org): One of the strongest evidence-based interventions, Nurse-Family Partnership has shown effective outcomes over 3 decades.

Randomized controlled trials were conducted with three diverse populations beginning in Elmira, New York, in 1977; in Memphis, Tennessee, in 1990; and in Denver, Colorado, in 1994 (Eckenrode et al., 2000; Olds, Henderson, Chamberlin, & Tatelbaum, 1986). All three trials targeted first-time, low-income mothers. The long-term outcomes for mothers and children in these three trials were significantly improved when home visitation was used as an intervention. In fact, in medical and scientific journals, Nurse-Family Partnership is most often cited as the most effective intervention to prevent child abuse and neglect, which contributes to childhood injury. Injury, in turn, is the leading cause of death for children from age 1 to early adulthood.

Follow-up research continues today, and the Nurse-Family Partnership is being implemented in Canada, The Netherlands, England, Scotland, Northern Ireland, and Australia.

See more at http://www.nursefamilypartnership.org/proven-results/published-research.

CASE STUDY: CHILD ABUSE

You are a pediatric nurse working in a primary care setting. A mother arrives with her two small children for their annual physical. She appears anxious and unable to focus on questions as she cares for her children. You ask: "You seem upset, is there anything you would like to talk about?" and she begins to cry. What steps would you take next?

Intervention:

Ask a colleague to supervise the children and take the mother into a quiet place. Request that while you meet with the mother you are not interrupted. Inform the mother that you are there to support her and that you would like to ask her some questions. Start with general questions moving toward more specific. "How are you? Are you working outside the home? What kind of supports do you have?" Then move to specific questions: "In your relationship, do you ever feel afraid or scared? Does your partner ever push, shove, or physically hurt you? If you could change two things about your partner, what would you like to change?" This dialogue can open a conversation. In the event it doesn't, the mother may simply not be ready to discuss. Let her know that she can call at any time. If the mother discloses fear and feeling unsafe, then a natural course of inquiry would be to ask: "How do you feel this is affecting your children?" It's important for the mother to be aware that if she raises concerns that the children are not safe or are at risk for abuse, a report will need to be made to the child welfare agency on behalf of the children. This process should be done with kindness and support. It is highly recommended to employ the assistance of a social worker or experienced colleague on the healthcare team.

Summary

Child maltreatment occurs all too frequently in families. Nurses routinely encounter children and their families in their jobs across practice settings. It's important that nurses recognize the effects of violence across the life span and can describe the role of the health provider in the recognition, response, and prevention of violence. An understanding of child maltreatment helps nurses to identify child maltreatment, implement targeted care, and refer children and families to appropriate resources.

References

Adams, J. (2011). Medical evaluation of suspected child sexual abuse: 2011 update. *Journal of Child Sexual Abuse, 20*(5), 588–605.

Anda, R. F., Brown, D. W., Felitti, V. J., Dube, S. R., & Giles, W. H. (2008). Adverse childhood experiences and prescription drug use in a cohort study of adult HMO patients. *BMC Public Health, 8,* 198. doi: 10.1186/1471-2458-8-198

Anda, R. F., Butchart, A., Felitti, V. J., & Brown, D. W. (2010). Building a framework for global surveillance of the public health implications of adverse childhood experiences. *Am J Prev Med, 39*(1), 93–98.

Anda, R. F., Felitti, V. J., Bremner, J. D., Walker, J. D., Whitfield, C., Perry, B. D., ... Giles, W. H. (2011). The enduring effects of abuse and related adverse experiences in childhood: A convergence of evidence from neurobiology and epidemiology. *Eur Arch Psychiatry Clin Neurosci., 256*(3), 174–186.

Brown, D. W., Anda, R. F., Tiemeier, H., Felitti, V. J., Croft, J. B., & Giles, W. H. (2009). Adverse childhood experiences and the risk of premature mortality. *Am J Prev Med, 37,* 389–396. doi: 10.1016/j.amepre.2009.06.021

Child Abuse Prevention Treatment Act (CAPTA). (1974 & 2010). Retrieved 03/25/2015 from http://www.acf.hhs.gov/sites/default/files/cb/capta2010.pdf

Child Welfare Information Gateway. (n.d.). *Definitions of child abuse and neglect in federal law.* Washington, DC: U.S. Department of Health and Human Services, Children's Bureau. Retrieved from https://www.childwelfare.gov/can/defining/federal.cfm

Cuijpers, P., Smit, F., Unger, F., Stikkelbroek, Y., Ten Have, M., & de Graaf, R. (2011). The disease burden of childhood adversities in adults: A population-based study. *Child Abuse and Neglect, 35,* 937–945. doi: 10.1016/j.chiabu.2011.06.005

Eckenrode, J., Ganzel, B., Henderson, C. R., Smith, E., Olds, D. L., Powers, J., … Sidora, K. (2000). Preventing child abuse and neglect with a program of nurse home visitation: The limiting effects of domestic violence. *JAMA, 284,* 1385–1391.

Edelman, M. W. (1992). *The measure of our success: A letter to my children and yours.* Boston, MA: Beacon Press.

Fontes, L. A. (2005). *Child abuse and culture: Working with diverse families.* New York, NY: The Guilford Press.

Massachusetts Department of Children and Families (DCF). (2015). Retrieved from www.mass. gov?eohhs/docs/dcf/can-mandated-reporters-guide.pdf

Miller-Perrin, C. L., and Perrin, R. D. (2006). *Child maltreatment: An introduction.* Thousand Oaks, CA: Sage Publications.

Myers, J. B. (2008). A short history of child protection in America. Hein Online 42 Fam. L.Q. 449, 2008–2009.

National Association of School Nurses (NASN). (2014). *NASN Position statement-Child maltreatment, care of victims of: The school nurses role.* Retrieved from http://www.nasn.org/ PolicyAdvocacy/PositionPapersandReports/NASNPositionStatementsFullView/tabid/462/ smid/824/ArticleID/639/Default.aspx

National Indian Child Welfare Association (NICWA). (2015). *Indian Child Welfare Act of 1978.* Retrieved from http://www.nicwa.org/indian_child_welfare_act/

Office of Disease Prevention and Health Promotion. (n.d.). *Social determinants of health.* Retrieved from https://www.healthypeople.gov/2020/topics-objectives/topic/social-determinants-health

Olds, D., Henderson, C., Chamberlin, R., & Tatelbaum. R. (1986). Preventing child abuse and neglect: A randomized trial of nurse home visitation. *Pediatrics, 78,* 65–78.

Secretary's Advisory Committee on Health Promotion and Disease Prevention Objectives for 2020. (2010). *Healthy People 2020: An opportunity to address the societal determinants of health in the United States.* Retrieved from http://www.healthypeople.gov/2020/topics-objectives/topic/social-determinants-health

Sedlak, A. J., Mettenburg, J., Basena, M., Petta, I., McPherson, K., Greene, A., & Li, S. (2010). *Fourth National Incidence Study of Child Abuse and Neglect (NIS–4): Report to Congress, executive summary.* Washington, DC: DHHS, Administration for Children and Families. Retrieved from http://www.law.harvard.edu/programs/about/cap/cap-conferences/ rd-conference/rd-conference-papers/sedlaknis.pdf

United Nations Office of the High Commissioner for Human Rights. (crc 1989 & 1990). *Convention on the Rights of the Child.* Retrieved from www.ohchr.org/en/professionalinterest/pages/crc.aspx

United States Census Bureau. (2015). Retrieved from https://www.census.gov/geo/reference/urban-rural.html

United States Department of Health and Human Services, Administration for Children and Families, Administration on Children, Youth and Families, Children's Bureau. (2015). Child maltreatment 2013. Retrieved from http://www.acf.hhs.gov/programs/cb/research-data-technology/statistics-research/child-maltreatment

Watkins, S. A. (1990). The Mary Ellen myth: Connecting child welfare history. *Social Work,* 35(6), 500–503.

World Health Organization (WHO). (2015). *Child maltreatment.* Retrieved from http://www.who.int/topics/child_abuse/en/

12

ELDER ABUSE

Andrea M. Yevchak, PhD, RN

KEY POINTS IN THIS CHAPTER

- Elder abuse is pervasive, yet often goes undetected.

- Multiples types of elder abuse exist with varying definitions and laws based on individual states.

- Elder abuse may go undetected due to the mistaken association with age-associated changes.

- Intervening in elder abuse begins with careful assessment and documentation, followed by appropriate referral and ongoing management.

The global aging population is increasing exponentially. Aging brings about physical and cognitive changes, as well as psychosocial changes such as living arrangement, that can increase the risk of neglect, maltreatment, abuse, and exploitation of older adults (Homeier, 2014). It's imperative that healthcare professionals be able to recognize and manage elder mistreatment and abuse, especially with the increasing numbers of older adults living across settings of care. The purpose of this chapter is to present information on the problem of elder abuse; define different types of elder abuse; identify ways to detect and manage abuse across settings of care; describe different populations at higher risk for elder abuse; and provide healthcare providers with a clinical example and resources for elder abuse.

DEFINING ELDER ABUSE

Elder abuse occurs independent of gender, ethnicity, cultural background, or socioeconomic status (Burnett, Achenbaum, & Murphy, 2014); however, the true breadth of elder abuse is unknown because it remains undetected and underreported (Acierno et al., 2010). Yearly, about 10% of older adults report emotional, physical, or sexual abuse or potential neglect (Acierno et al., 2010). Financial forms of elder abuse are the most reported (Burnett et al., 2014). Adult Protective Services (APS) data also demonstrate increasing prevalence of elder abuse (National Center on Elder Abuse [NCEA], 2015).

In 1987, elder abuse was added in amendments to the Older Americans Act, but it is defined according to state guidelines and regulations that may vary dramatically, making detection and reporting difficult for healthcare professionals. However, some standards do exist. The National Center on Elder Abuse (NCEA, 2015) lists three basic categories of elder abuse:

- **Domestic elder abuse:** When someone who has a special relationship with the older adult commits the abuse or maltreatment, it's considered *domestic abuse.* Special relationships can be spousal or familial, friends, or caregivers.

- **Institutional elder abuse:** *Institutional abuse* refers to maltreatment within a residential facility, such as a long-term care facility, and is usually committed by someone who has an obligation or duty to provide for the older adult.

- **Self-neglect or self-abuse:** *Self-neglect or self-abuse* is defined as behaviors of the older adult that affect his/her own health and/or safety. Inherent in this definition is that the older adult has the mental capacity to understand his/her actions.

Elder abuse has significant personal and economic consequences. Older adults who experience abuse, regardless of underlying physical and cognitive function, are at a higher risk of dying earlier than their peers (Burnett et al., 2014). It's also associated with a higher rate of healthcare utilization and institutional placement (LoFaso & Rosen, 2014). Economic implications, beyond those of financial abuse, are also significant (LoFaso & Rosen, 2014). This includes emergency department visits, hospital admissions, and additional medical testing and treatments.

Older adults at higher risk of experiencing maltreatment and abuse include those who are female, of an advanced age, frail, have cognitive or mental health impairments (e.g., dementia, delirium, depression, etc.), living with others, experiencing social isolation, and those who abuse substances (Acierno et al., 2010; Burnett et al., 2014; NCEA, 2015). Those who abuse older adults tend to be those individuals closest, such as a spouse, child, family member, or friend. Additional characteristics of offenders are that they may have a history of personal or family abuse; have cognitive impairment, mental illness, or be mentally challenged; have financial issues; or have dependency on drugs or alcohol (Burnett et al., 2014). There are no known definitive demographic characteristics of those who abuse older adults (NCEA, 2015).

One of the first steps in prevention, detection, and management of elder abuse is education. Elder abuse may go undetected because of the underlying ageism within current society (Capezuti, 2011). Because of these biases, both older adults and others may view elder abuse as an expected consequence of aging. In addition, many of the physiological changes associated with aging may make it difficult to distinguish age-associated changes from elder abuse (Burnett et al., 2014).

DETECTING ELDER ABUSE

Elder abuse is not easily detected. The aging process and multiple presentations of abuse can complicate detection (Burnett et al., 2014). Each broad category of elder abuse listed by the NCEA includes seven types. Table 12.1 outlines the definitions along with the physical and psychological signs and symptoms according to the NCEA (2015) and others (Burnett et al., 2014; Vognar & Gibbs, 2014). All categories include the older adult's reporting or stating of abuse.

TABLE 12.1 TYPES OF ABUSE

Type of Abuse	Definition	Signs and Symptoms
Physical abuse	Use of bodily force that may result in injury, pain, or long-term consequences; can also include medications used as restraints, force-feeding, and other forms of physical punishment	Bruises, black eyes, welts, cuts, bite marks Fractures Various internal injuries Repeated falls Torn clothes or broken assistive devices such as eyeglasses or hearing aids Laboratory data suggesting overuse of medications Sudden change in behavior Frequent emergency department visits
Sexual abuse	Any nonconsensual sexual act with an older adult; includes those who are not able to provide consent	Bruising around the breasts or genital area Unexplained sexually transmitted diseases Unexplained vaginal or rectal bleeding Torn, stained, or bloody clothing Difficulty walking or sitting
Emotional or psychological abuse	Includes verbal or nonverbal acts, such as isolation, threats, intimidation, etc. that cause anguish, pain, or distress	Emotional volatility Becoming withdrawn or unresponsive Change in behavior or personality Depression Suicidal ideation Hypervigilance

Neglect	Refusal or failure to fulfill agreed upon responsibilities to an older adult; usually involving essential items for survival like shelter, food, water, clothing, etc.	Dehydration or malnutrition Poor hygiene Untreated medical condition Unsafe living conditions Decubitus ulcers Unexplained deterioration in health Failure to thrive Lack of preventative healthcare and maintenance Repeated emergency department visits or hospital admissions
Abandonment	Leaving an older adult for whom there is responsibility for providing care	Can occur across settings of care, including public locations such as a mall or grocery store
Financial or material exploitation	Illegal or unintended use of an older adult's money, property, or other assets	Sudden change in financial status or routines Adding additional names to bank signature cards or credit cards Unpaid bills Forged signatures Provision of services that are not needed for the older adult
Self-abuse or self-neglect	Behaviors or actions taken by the older adult that threaten his or her health and/or safety	Change in appearance Depression Sudden withdrawal or isolation Unexplained change in health status Dehydration Malnutrition

In addition to these signs and symptoms, certain medical conditions are often seen in cases of elder abuse. These may include, but are not limited to (LoFaso & Rosen, 2014):

- Hyperthermia or hypothermia

- Muscle wasting

- Infections, such as recurrent urinary tract infections, aspiration pneumonia, and infection wounds

Multiple normal physiological changes come naturally with aging. Therefore, it's important for healthcare professionals to be able to distinguish age-related changes from elder abuse. As an example, physiological changes in an older adult's skin make it more likely to be damaged from daily activities. Many injuries that could be caused by elder abuse, such as bruising or lacerations, may be attributed to a normal consequence of aging and thin, fragile skin if not fully assessed (Gibbs, 2014; LoFaso & Rosen, 2014).

Forensic nursing knowledge that you bring to the situation can help to distinguish age-related changes from those of elder abuse. For example, bruising occurs frequently in older adults due to age-related thinning of the skin and/or medications that increase the likelihood of experiencing bruising even with very mild trauma, such as anticoagulants or systemic steroids (Gibbs, 2014). It's important to note with bruises both the location and stage of the bruise to distinguish between age-related bruises and abuse:

- Typically, age-related bruising occurs on areas that are accidentally damaged during daily activities, such as the upper and lower extremities (Gibbs, 2014; Ziminski, Phillips, & Woods, 2012). These body parts may be easily hit against a surface while reaching for a dish to prepare a meal or while taking a bath. Non-accidental bruising is likely to occur on concealed areas such as the neck, ears, buttocks, or perineal areas. Also, patterns of bruising that may indicate abuse include those showing multiples stages of healing.

- Older adults, for the most part, should be able to recall the event that caused the bruise (Gibbs, 2014). Similar distinctions should be present in additional skin injuries such as lacerations and burns that are frequently associated with physical abuse. Ulcerations, including pressure ulcers, are associated with neglect and self-neglect, because this type of injury is often preventable (Gibbs, 2014).

In a case of suspected maltreatment or abuse, functional and cognitive capacity should be evaluated to understand an individual's baseline. For example, an older adult presents with a moderate to severe burn. The individual explains that the burn was received while conducting meal preparation, yet you are aware that physical and cognitive limitations make this individual dependent upon others for all meal preparation. This scenario is not explainable, and an underlying factor for consideration may be abuse or neglect. This is important in understanding and explaining accidental injuries from those associated with abuse (Gibbs, 2014). Repeated accidental injuries should be investigated, especially if the explanation does not consistently match the injury.

Techniques for Detecting Abuse

Interdisciplinary assessment for elder abuse begins by establishing rapport. This can be done differently based on the setting, whether it's through a long-standing relationship with an individual in the community or in a crisis situation in the emergency department. Older adults and their caregivers should be interviewed in a safe, private environment if abuse is suspected. General open-ended questions are an appropriate way to start the interview and to begin to establish rapport. Examples include:

- "Tell me about your current living situation."

- "Have there been any changes at home recently?"

- "Is there anything going on at home that you would like to tell me more about?"

- "Can you explain to me what assistance you need at home?"

- "Tell me more about those who help you at home."

- "Can you describe a typical day for me?"

Continue questioning into specific areas where you might suspect abuse; for example, following up with questioning about their current living situation to focus on safety or time spent alone in the house. You can tailor the focused questions to the suspected type of abuse as well.

While interviewing the older adult, look for these signs:

- They may be withdrawn or use silence as an answer.

- They may appear fearful or apprehensive. Take notice of eye contact, or lack thereof.

- Older adults may be hesitant to share information in cases of abuse as a protective mechanism for themselves, and also for protection of the perpetrator (Vognar & Gibbs, 2014).

- Take note if the suspected perpetrator of the abuse doesn't allow the older adult to be interviewed alone for fear of what the older adult may say when alone.

Interviewing those surrounding the suspected abuse can also begin with open-ended questions. Look for these signs (Burnett et al., 2014):

- It's important to understand how the suspected abuser views the older adult's physical and cognitive abilities, as well as his or her responsibilities.

- Note whether any threatening statements are made during the interview.

- Take notice if the suspected abuser is defensive or places blame in other directions.

- By contrast, the suspected abuser may also become overprotective of the older adult.

After the interviews have been conducted, document any inconsistencies and describe nonverbal responses and behaviors (for example, a person stating that he or she is fine but refusing to make eye contact). Identify any patterns within the history, such as cancellations of routine preventative or health maintenance appointments or frequent visits to the emergency department.

Potentially the best mechanism for assessing elder abuse is the incorporation of a standardized, routine screening into comprehensive, interdisciplinary care for older adults (Burnett et al., 2014). This includes screening older adults for any significant physical or cognitive changes, as well as for psychosocial issues like depression. Standardized assessment should also address social support and financial issues (Burnett et al., 2014). The following tools can be used for this purpose, each having its own strengths and weaknesses. None of these "diagnose" elder abuse, but they can help establish a baseline and identify individuals in need of more comprehensive, interdisciplinary assessment. Screening tools include:

- Elder Assessment Instrument (EAI) (Fulmer, Paveza, Abraham, & Fairchild, 2000)

- Brief Abuse Screen for the Elderly (BASE) (Fulmer, Guadagno, Bitondo dyer, & Connolly, 2004)

- Elder Abuse Suspicion Index (EASI) (Yaffe, Weiss, Wolfson, & Lithwick, 2007)

- Vulnerability to Abuse Screening Scale (VASS) (Schofield & Mishra, 2003)

- Geriatric Mistreatment Scale (GMS) (Giraldo-Rodriguez & Rosas-Carrasco, 2013)

- Hwalek-Sengstock Elder Abuse Screening Test (HS-EAST) (Neale, Hwalek, Scott, Sengstock, & Stahl, 1991)

- Indicators of Abuse (IOA) (Reis & Nahmiash, 1998)

DOCUMENTING ELDER ABUSE

Different standards depend on the setting, but in general the record should be clearly written and as detailed as possible (Gibbs, 2014). Include all interview data gathered from the older adult and the caregiver(s), as well as facts regarding the interview circumstances. Always record pertinent history regarding suspected or actual abuse as well as objective, standardized measures of physical and cognitive functioning.

In cases of physical abuse, include with your documentation any photographic evidence (Gibbs, 2014). Measurement of injuries such as bruises or ulcers is important. Photographs should be taken at various angles and distances and with adequate lighting. If you can, document evidence over a period of time to show progression of the abuse (Gibbs, 2014).

ELDER ABUSE INTERVENTION AND MANAGEMENT STRATEGIES

Interventions and management strategies regarding elder abuse focus on the safety of the older adult. A multifaceted approach has been identified to ensure early recognition of elder abuse and includes the following (Capezuti, 2011):

- Detection of potential or actual abuse

- Referral as the first step in intervention

- Continued monitoring

After careful assessment for and documentation of signs and symptoms related to elder abuse, referral to an appropriate source for intervention is critical. Referrals depend on the level of abuse:

- If abuse is suspected but not substantiated, an ideal agency for referral is Adult Protective Services (APS), which is typically composed of social workers or caseworkers (Twomey & Weber, 2014).

- Where there is immediate danger of elder abuse, referral should include:

    - Emergency and police services (Burnett et al., 2014)

    - Long-term care nursing facilities may act as a shelter for older adults if they are unable to return to their former residence (Vognar & Gibbs, 2014).

    - An interdisciplinary team including a forensic nurse and/or pathologist is recommended as available to address all aspects of elder abuse, including personal and legal, to provide a plan of care moving forward for the older adult (Twomey & Weber, 2014).

■ Where self-abuse or self-neglect is suspected, the healthcare proxy or durable power of attorney, if applicable, is an ideal person to seek help from (Burnett et al., 2014). If the older adult does not have family or friends available, APS can be used as a referral.

RELEVANT LAWS AND STATUTES REGARDING ELDER ABUSE

Elder abuse laws and regulations are typically held under the umbrella of Adult Protective Services (APS). These laws and regulations vary by state, as does the agency within that state that is responsible for upholding them. In general, states have a responsibility to protect older adults who have experienced abuse or those who are at-risk for abuse. This includes older adults living in the community, as well as in institutional and long-term care settings.

Within the community, laws and regulations typically exist to provide penalties against those who conduct criminal offenses toward an older adult. Within institutional and long-term care settings, federal regulations protect the rights of older adults. States may also enact additional penalties on top of the existing federal regulations. In these settings, most states have mandatory reporting requirements for registered nurses, additional healthcare employees, as well as employees of the facility.

As explained within this chapter, types and definitions of abuse can also vary by state, including at what age an adult becomes an "older adult." Additional information and details for each state can be found on the National Center on Elder Abuse (NCEA) website at http://www.ncea.aoa.gov.

When reporting a case of suspected abuse, you need to have all available details, such as the older adult's name, address, contact information, the rationale for concern, the nature of the incident, nature and need for protective services, and the physical and cognitive functioning of the older adult involved. After initial screening, reports are assigned to a caseworker who conducts an investigation and intervenes using additional services as necessary. Reports may also be categorized according to level of potential severity, which can vary by state. APS has a duty to address all emergency cases immediately. Less severe cases can be investigated anywhere from 1 to 14 days after the initial report (Vognar & Gibbs, 2014).

Mandated reporting varies and is dependent upon state statutes. Refer to the NCEA website (http://www.ncea.aoa.gov/) for additional information related to your specific state. In general, most states afford protection from retaliation, liability, intimidation, and penalty to those who report suspected cases of abuse in good faith or reasonable suspicion. In some cases, the reporter can even remain anonymous. It is an ethical concern for healthcare providers to report suspected cases of abuse according to federal laws: the Older Americans Act (OAA) of 2006 and the Elder Justice Act (EJA) of 2010 (Hess, 2011).

RESOURCES TO HELP WITH ELDER ABUSE

Resources for elder maltreatment and abuse differ by state, but Adult Protective Services (APS) also refers to categories of social services, typically in the community, that are responsible for looking into reported cases of elder maltreatment or abuse (NCEA, 2015). They are generally considered the first line of defense in protection and prevention of elder abuse. In some cases, states overlap resources. The Area Agency on Aging (AOA) or County Department of Social Services may be responsible for the investigation of alleged cases of elder abuse.

Law enforcement is involved in certain situations, which can vary by state, but typically include the courts, victim services, a district attorney or civil attorney, and law enforcement officers (Twomey & Weber, 2014). The police officer can be an employee of the state, city, borough, town, township, or county. In states whose statutes make elder abuse a crime, there is a requirement to report suspected abuse. These cases traditionally involve physical and/or sexual abuse.

In institutional settings, such as a nursing home, the Long-Term Care Ombudsman can help with reports of elder abuse (NCEA, 2015). The National Center on Elder Abuse website lists additional information on state-by-state resources for reporting abuse. In addition, the Eldercare Locator website can be helpful in identifying the APS reporting number for each state. Table 12.2 lists additional resources.

TABLE 12.2 ONLINE RESOURCES FOR ELDER ABUSE

Resource Name	Website Address
National Center on Elder Abuse	http://www.ncea.aoa.gov/
Center for Elders and the Courts	http://www.eldersandcourts.org/
National Council on Aging	http://www.ncoa.org/public-policy-action/elder-justice/
Center of Excellence on Elder Abuse and Neglect at the University of California at Irvine School of Medicine	http://www.centeronelderabuse.org/
American Bar Association	http://www.americanbar.org/groups/law_aging/resources/elder_abuse.html
Eldercare Locator	http://www.eldercare.gov/eldercare.net/public/resources/topic/Elder_Abuse.aspx
National Committee for the Prevention of Elder Abuse	http://www.preventelderabuse.org/
American Psychological Association	http://www.apa.org/pi/aging/resources/guides/elder-abuse.aspx
Centers for Disease Control and Prevention	http://www.cdc.gov/violenceprevention/elderabuse/
National Resource Center on LGBT Aging	http://www.lgbtagingcenter.org/resources/resources.cfm?s=5

According to the National Center on Elder Abuse, interdisciplinary teams may specialize in certain aspects of elder abuse. Financial Abuse Specialist Teams (FAST) include public and/or private agencies, such as those within law, real estate, banking, etc. Another type of team is the Elder Death Review Team (EDRT), which typically includes a medical examiner, coroner, district attorney, or other public official. Geriatric specialists and forensic experts may also consult on these cases of elder abuse. Certain communities may have Elder Abuse Forensic Centers (NCEA, 2015).

CASE STUDY: ELDER ABUSE

The emergency department is crowded. Mary is an 82-year-old woman presenting for shoulder pain after a fall. She ambulates with supervision assistance and is accompanied by her daughter. Mary states that she lives alone, but with daily assistance from her daughter. She cannot tell you her medications or chronic conditions. Regarding her physical appearance, she appears frail. Her clothes are not clean and you notice dirt under her fingernails; however, she did have a fall at home this evening.

During the physical assessment, Mary remains relatively quiet, not making eye contact or conversation. She does answer questions appropriately and follows directions. It is noted that she has some areas of redness and bruises distributed over her upper extremities and torso. When asked about the bruising, Mary's daughter chimes in, stating that her mother is a bit unsteady and has a tendency to fall; Mary agrees. No additional assessments were completed on Mary's lower extremities to note redness or bruising or to objectively assess her physical and cognitive limitations. The daughter continues to talk about her mother's physical limitations within the home and explains the amount of care she provides around the clock. She also takes care of her family, which includes three children, and works full-time as a teacher.

It is noted that the daughter does not leave Mary's room at all during the emergency department visit. She also appears to be attentive to her mother, retrieving drinks as needed and assisting her mother to use the toilet. The nursing staff is relieved and thankful for the additional help on such a busy evening.

This scenario depicts a potential case of abuse. Although Mary's appearance may be considered expected after a fall at home and a rushed visit to the emergency department, there is no additional follow-up or questioning. Objective assessments of physical or cognitive abilities are not completed, nor are assessments for bruising on her lower extremities that may be consistent with multiple falls. The daughter in this case appears to be caring for her mother, and staff note nothing out of the ordinary. It is a busy clinical scenario, and elder abuse is not suspected. Mary is frail, perhaps contributing to her falls, but it may also be related to long-term neglect resulting in malnutrition and dehydration.

With regards to what you have learned in this chapter, what are some forensic principles you might apply in a case such as this?

■ Are there any indications that a further assessment should be conducted?

■ What potential signs of abuse are present in this case?

■ What can the nurse in this situation do if s/he suspects abuse?

■ What protocols are in place in your hospital regarding such cases?

SUMMARY

Elder abuse is pervasive, yet often goes undetected. Nurses need to understand that multiple types of elder abuse exist with varying definitions, and the laws that cover elder abuse can vary from state to state. It's often easy to misdiagnose elder abuse as injuries associated with age.

Nurses should always carefully assess and document any suspected abuse and follow up with the appropriate referrals and managed care.

REFERENCES

Acierno, R., Hernandez, M. A., Amstadter, A. B., Resnick, H. S., Steve, K., Muzzy, W., & Kilpatrick, D. G. (2010). Prevalence and correlates of emotional, physical, sexual, and financial abuse and potential neglect in the United States: The National Elder Mistreatment Study. *Am J Public Health, 100*(2), 292–297. doi: 10.2105/ajph.2009.163089

Burnett, J., Achenbaum, W. A., & Murphy, K. P. (2014). Prevention and early identification of elder abuse. *Clinics in Geriatric Medicine, 30*(4), 743–759. doi: http://dx.doi.org/10.1016/j.cger.2014.08.013

Capezuti, E. (2011). Recognizing and referring suspected elder mistreatment. *Geriatric Nursing, 32*(3), 209–211. doi: http://dx.doi.org/10.1016/j.gerinurse.2011.04.005

Fulmer, T., Guadagno, L., Bitondo dyer, C., & Connolly, M. T. (2004). Progress in elder abuse screening and assessment instruments. *Journal of the American Geriatrics Society, 52*(2), 297–304. doi: 10.1111/j.1532-5415.2004.52074.x

Fulmer, T., Paveza, G., Abraham, I., & Fairchild, S. (2000). Elder neglect assessment in the emergency department. *Journal of Emergency Nursing, 26*(5), 436–443. doi: http://dx.doi.org/10.1067/men.2000.110621

Gibbs, L. M. (2014). Understanding the medical markers of elder abuse and neglect: Physical examination findings. *Clinics in Geriatric Medicine, 30*(4), 687–712. doi: http://dx.doi.org/10.1016/j.cger.2014.08.002

Giraldo-Rodriguez, L., & Rosas-Carrasco, O. (2013). Development and psychometric properties of the Geriatric Mistreatment Scale. *Geriatr Gerontol Int, 13*(2), 466–474. doi: 10.1111/j.1447-0594.2012.00894.x

Hess, S. (2011). The role of health care providers in recognizing and reporting elder abuse. *J Gerontol Nurs, 37*(11), 28–34; quiz 36–27. doi: 10.3928/00989134-20110831-02

Homeier, D. (2014). Aging: Physiology, disease, and abuse. *Clinics in Geriatric Medicine, 30*(4), 671–686. doi: http://dx.doi.org/10.1016/j.cger.2014.08.001

LoFaso, V. M., & Rosen, T. (2014). Medical and laboratory indicators of elder abuse and neglect. *Clinics in Geriatric Medicine, 30*(4), 713–728. doi: http://dx.doi.org/10.1016/j.cger.2014.08.003

National Center on Elder Abuse (NCEA). (2015). *Elder abuse information.* Retrieved from http://www.ncea.aoa.gov/

Neale, A. V., Hwalek, M. A., Scott, R. O., Sengstock, M. C., & Stahl, C. (1991). Validation of the Hwalek-Sengstock Elder Abuse Screening Test. *Journal of Applied Gerontology, 10*(4), 406–418. doi: 10.1177/073346489101000403

Reis, M., & Nahmiash, D. (1998). Validation of the Indicators of Abuse (IOA) Screen. *The Gerontologist, 38*(4), 471–480. doi: 10.1093/geront/38.4.471

Schofield, M. J., & Mishra, G. D. (2003). Validity of self-report screening scale for elder abuse: Women's Health Australia Study. *Gerontologist, 43*(1), 110–120.

Twomey, M. S., & Weber, C. (2014). Health professionals' roles and relationships with other agencies. *Clinics in Geriatric Medicine, 30*(4), 881–895. doi: http://dx.doi.org/10.1016/j.cger.2014.08.014

Vognar, L., & Gibbs, L. M. (2014). Care of the victim. *Clinics in Geriatric Medicine, 30*(4), 869–880. doi: http://dx.doi.org/10.1016/j.cger.2014.08.012

Yaffe, M. J., Weiss, D., Wolfson, C., & Lithwick, M. (2007). Detection and prevalence of abuse of older males: Perspectives from family practice. *Journal of Elder Abuse & Neglect, 19*(1–2), 47–60. doi: 10.1300/J084v19n01_04

Ziminski, C. E., Phillips, L. R., & Woods, D. L. (2012). Raising the index of suspicion for elder abuse: Cognitive impairment, falls, and injury patterns in the emergency department. *Geriatric Nursing, 33*(2), 105–112. doi: http://dx.doi.org/10.1016/j.gerinurse.2011.12.003

13

FORENSIC MENTAL HEALTH NURSING

L. Kathleen Sekula, PhD, PMHCNS, FAAN; and
Angela F. Amar, PhD, RN, FAAN

KEY POINTS IN THIS CHAPTER

- Nurses working with patients with mental disorders and co-existing forensic issues outside of forensic settings must consider the medicolegal aspects of patient care.

- Documentation has the added element of potential impact on legal outcomes and the ability of the victim or the perpetrator to receive proper care.

- Knowledge of the mental health dynamics of these patients can keep the healthcare staff, patients, and others safe.

Forensic mental health nursing is the intersection of mental health and the legal system. Forensic psychiatric nurses work with offenders who have been deemed mentally disordered and need additional attention separate from the judicial/penitentiary system. Forensic psychiatric nurses work with mentally disordered offenders in secure psychiatric services where they assess the patient (victim or perpetrator) and gather evidence that may influence conviction, sentencing, recidivism, treatment, and prevention (Lyons, 2009). Forensic psychiatric nurses use their training to aid in the rehabilitation of criminal offenders, assess the wellbeing of crime victims, and serve as expert consultants for criminal proceedings. They most commonly work for law enforcement agencies and at facilities such as prisons, mental hospitals, and juvenile detention centers.

Nurses often interface with patients who exhibit mental health issues in many practice settings: hospitals, clinics, physician and nurse practitioner offices, corrections settings, etc. The patient may present as a psychiatric emergency or may present for other healthcare problems, during which time the patient may exhibit long-standing mental disorders. Many of these patients may have forensic issues related to their care. They may have entered the clinical setting with a weapon, been injured during an altercation with law enforcement or directly with a victim, been a victim of a crime, or been involved in one of many other scenarios in which a person with mental disorders requires medical attention while also having legal problems. Frequently, the healthcare team must deal with the personality disorders common in offenders, concerns regarding violence and safety, and those with factitious disorders trying to feign mental illness to avoid jail or legal consequences.

The nurse who understands the impact of mental disorders in patients throughout the healthcare system can make a difference in the way clinicians perceive and treat these patients as well how the patient may progress to a healthy outcome within the system. What is documented in forensic psychiatric cases may be used at a later date and under different circumstances in a court case to either support the patient regarding a legal issue or help to support a victim in a case related to a particular patient. This chapter provides basic information on mental health and psychiatric nursing in patients with concurrent legal issues.

THE ROLE OF THE FORENSIC NURSE

Forensic psychiatric or mental health nurses deal with mental health issues of victims and offenders. The forensic psychiatric nurse (Sekula & Colbert, 2013):

- Assesses:

    - Perpetrator's ability to formulate intent

    - Risk for violence and for committing additional crimes

    - Competency to proceed in trial

- Writes and submits formal reports to the court

- Serves as expert and fact witness

- Consults with attorneys and law enforcement personnel

- Provides therapy

Nurses in non-forensic mental health settings can use knowledge of these roles and functions in providing care to offenders.

Forensic mental health interfaces in many ways with patients who present in non-mental health settings. How you respond to these patients can make a difference in outcomes. The majority of mentally disordered patients do not have forensic issues. Some do. For the purposes of this chapter, issues related to patients with co-existing mental disorders and forensic issues in non-forensic settings will be addressed. People who do not have mental health problems commit the majority of violent crimes. In fact, adults with serious mental illness are more likely to become victims of crimes at higher rates than individuals in the general population (Crisanti, Frueh, Archambeau, Steffen, & Wolff, 2014). It's important for the non-forensic nurse to be aware of how his or her practice has the potential to impact care of forensic patients. Excellent documentation, collection of evidence, and positive interactions with forensic psychiatric patients is paramount to good practice.

ANTISOCIAL PERSONALITY DISORDER PATIENTS

Antisocial personality disorder (APD) is a common psychiatric diagnosis associated with criminal behavior. Persons with antisocial personality disorder display consistent disregard for others through exploitation and repeated unlawful actions. Hallmark features include lack of remorse for their actions, repeated neglect of responsibilities, and destructive or illegal acts. This disorder often manifests in childhood as conduct disorder. Often, they are court ordered for evaluation or treatment. They may also seek healthcare for injuries sustained during the commission of a crime or during an incarceration.

Patients with APD can be challenging to nurses. These clients also tell lies, manipulate and exploit others, and show little insight about their behavior or empathy for those injured or affected. Developing a therapeutic relationship is difficult. Acts of kindness are seen as weakness from the staff. These patients may attempt to manipulate the nursing staff through flattery, seduction, and guilt. Nurses must establish and maintain clear boundaries by explaining exactly which behaviors are inappropriate. Do not assume patients already know what's appropriate. For example, "I am your nurse, taking you to get an X-ray is not a date." Frequent team meetings to discuss care are important. Everyone must remember that these patients use flattery and seduction for secondary gain. Any signs of manipulation should be documented with dates, times, and circumstances. Everyone on the team must communicate the same expectations of behavior and consequences for breaches. Once the patient has been informed of consequences, they must be enforced.

MALINGERING PATIENT

Another patient challenge is the malingering patient. A *malingering patient* intentionally produces false or exaggerated physical or psychological symptoms to obtain incentives such as avoiding military duty, avoiding work, gaining financial compensation, evading criminal prosecution, or obtaining drugs (American Psychological Association [APA], 2013). The intentional and deliberate behavior differentiates malingering from conversion and somatoform disorders, in which the production of physical symptoms is unconsciously motivated.

Strongly suspect malingering when there is a medicolegal presentation. For example, an attorney refers a patient or a patient is seeking compensation for injury. Other clues include a marked discrepancy between the claimed distress and the objective findings, lack of cooperation during evaluation and in complying with prescribed treatment, and presence of an antisocial personality disorder (Bienenfeld, Talavera, Harsch, & Ahmed, 2015). The person who is malingering often has superficial knowledge of the feigned disorder. For example, a patient faking a musculoskeletal problem of the lower arm would not be able to predict the range of movements affected by the disorder in occupational therapy.

Malingering can be difficult to identify. Many of the exaggerations about illness can be common with individuals diagnosed with mental illness. A determination of malingering typically requires the identification of a motivating factor, multiple sources of converging evidence, and the systematic ruling out of probable alternative explanations (Mason, Cardell, & Armstrong, 2014). Observation can be helpful. Patients sometimes demonstrate "sicker" behaviors when the doctor visits. Nurses then are aware of behaviors that are not indicative of the feigned disorder. For example, the nurse observes the patient conversing intelligently and playing board games with other patients. However, whenever the doctor is on the unit, the patient only stares in space, acts in a bizarre manner, and speaks in gibberish. Persons demonstrating malingering psychotic disorders often exaggerate hallucinations and delusions but cannot mimic formal thought disorders. They usually cannot feign blunted affect, concrete thinking, or impaired interpersonal relatedness (Bienenfeld et al., 2015). Direct confrontation and accusations of malingering are seldom met with success. However, discussions can include inconsistencies in symptoms and patterns of disease reported and actual presentations. Supportive confrontation should involve at least two members of staff, with an emphasis on the patient being a person who needs help, with the assurance that care will continue (Mason et al., 2014). Carefully document behavior, especially including inconsistencies in behavior. These patients rarely accept recommendations for psychiatric consultation.

FORENSIC PSYCHIATRIC ISSUES

In this section, we focus on incidences where psychiatric mental health issues intersect with the law. When a patient enters the healthcare setting, assessment and documentation, safety and security, and determining treatment options are the clinician's main focus.

ASSESSING MENTAL HEALTH

When the patient presents in the healthcare setting and the nurse suspects that there may be mental dysfunction (either acute or chronic symptomatology), there are steps to take that will establish the path on which the case will progress. Assessment should begin as with any patient entering the setting. How does the patient present? How does the patient look (dress, hygiene, eye contact, posture, communication)? From that point one moves on to why the patient is presenting at this time. What is the patient's mood state and affect? Does the patient feel safe? Is the patient paranoid? Just as one would assess for any patient, one would assess:

- Medical history

- Educational background

- Occupational history

- Psychiatric history

- Substance abuse history

- Noting any mention of legal issues in the past or present

An issue at hand in these circumstances may often be that the nurse is working in a clinical area where psychiatric expertise is not easily available, and it may be in an emergency setting where the priority is on the physical health concerns of the patient. Once again, it is important for the nurse to be aware of his/her intuition. Does something seem *off*? If so, then it is paramount that the clinician document what he or she *observes*. Negative attitudes about psychiatric patients can affect the nurse's ability to properly evaluate and treat this vulnerable population and may even have adverse effects on the care of the patient. These are often not easy cases. And so, education regarding the complexities of care (including difficulties with diagnoses) is key to enhancing positive outcomes and doing no harm to the patient. If the clinician can determine the patient's needs, even though perhaps he or she is demonstrating vague and non-specific symptoms, then the clinician may indeed be able to determine if the psychiatric symptoms are being exacerbated by a physical illness. Is the patient under the influence of drugs or alcohol? What is the next step when it is determined that the patient is intoxicated? Is the patient suicidal or homicidal?

It is also helpful to have an understanding of how the *Diagnostic and Statistical Manual of Mental Disorders* (DSM-5) interfaces with forensics (APA, 2013). The DSM-5 diagnostic criteria and text are primarily designed to assist psychiatric clinicians in clinical assessments, case formulation, and treatment planning; the courts and attorneys also use it as a reference when attempting to determine the forensic consequences of mental disorders. While someone with psychiatric experience and expertise will serve as the clinician for diagnoses of the patient with psychiatric disorders, the DSM-5 is a good source of information for the generalist when exploring the symptoms that contribute to the various diagnoses.

DOCUMENTING MENTAL HEALTH

Forensic medical interviewing is essentially the same as general medical interviewing/history taking (O'Brien, 2001). However, the most significant difference between forensic and general interviewing/history taking is the attention to documentation that is necessary. The observation and interview process must be as objective and detailed as possible. Observations of the patient and conversations with the patient should be carefully documented, and any impressions or conclusions should be based only on the data available. Legal conclusions should be avoided. The role of the nurse is not to judge the forensic aspects of a case but to provide objective data. Clinicians can draw clinical conclusions and express an opinion as to how these conclusions are consistent with a particular cause without stating it as a factual conclusion (O'Brien, 2001). Legal conclusions will occur within the legal system once all of the facts are collected.

When documenting, use plain language, do not paraphrase, use the patient's own words, and give patients time to answer. Meet with them in a quiet setting where they feel safe and secure and have privacy. Explain everything that you are doing. Do not touch them without permission. Let them know when a procedure is going to be conducted or if laboratory samples are going to be taken. Patients with psychiatric symptoms may have special needs regarding security and safety.

SAFETY

Violence or aggressive behaviors are important concerns for working with forensic psychiatric patients. Factors that influence an individual's proclivity for violence include the client's diagnosis, history of violent behavior, young age, neurobiology, and genetic predisposition. Previous diagnoses of psychosis, substance abuse, organic brain disorders, dementia, mental retardation, or personality disorder are highly correlated risk factors for assault (Quintal, 2002). The strongest predictor of future violence is past violence. Patients with histories of violence must be monitored closely. The use of violence is often an attempt to gain control in a system where control seems lost. Patients resort to aggression when they are unable to manipulate the staff or do not get what they want. It's important for staff to remain neutral and avoid engaging in power struggles with the patient. Staff should also avoid becoming defensive when patients make disparaging remarks. Self-awareness of the nurse's past history with violence or manipulation as well as attitudes and beliefs regarding violence and victimization are important. A nurse who has been assaulted by a patient before may have difficulty caring for patients with violent pasts. It's easy to feel fear in the face of aggression. Fear can cause the nurse to avoid the patient or bend the rules. Careful and consistent team approaches to these patients helps to ensure a therapeutic approach that does not compromise safety or patient care.

When a patient enters a clinical setting and is acting out, the clinician is responsible to handle the situation in the best way possible. The first step is to recognize the problem. Violence can occur anywhere in the healthcare setting and can involve patient-patient, patient-staff, staff-staff, or any combination of these interactions, with families often also involved. Early behaviors that are indicative of aggression include pacing, restlessness, tense facial expression and body language, shouting, use of obscenities, and overreacting to stimuli. In addition, each patient has triggers to aggression and specific behaviors that are manifested in response to those triggers. Triggers can include things like hearing *no* to a request or loud noises on the unit. Keeping the unit safe involves a proactive approach to early identification of aggression and reduction of risk (Delaney & Johnson, 2006).

De-escalation is verbally talking the patient down. The goal is to work with patients to find solutions, approaching them calmly and avoiding a power struggle (Johnson & Hauser, 2001). Practice guidelines established by Richmond and colleagues (2012) suggest that staff be trained in verbal de-escalation, milieu therapy and safety, and principles of de-escalation. Try these techniques for de-escalation:

- Respect personal space

- Do not be provocative

- Establish verbal contact

- Be concise

- Identify wants and feelings

- Listen closely to what the patient is saying

- Agree or agree to disagree

- Lay down the law and set clear limits

- Offer choices and optimism

- Debrief the patient and staff

Personal space is critical. For most individuals, personal space is arm's length. If an individual's personal space is invaded, the individual may perceive that he has been physically touched, which could escalate the situation. Maintaining safe distance from the agitated patient and being aware of potential weapons in the space can help the nurse to avoid injury. Keeping the person talking can prevent aggression. The goal of therapy is to get patients to talk about, rather than act on, their feelings. Most patients act out because of unmet needs or concerns. The nurse must identify these needs and concerns in order to be able to determine other methods of meeting the patient's needs without resorting to aggression. Offer choices when possible and try to present the positive options first followed by negative options. Medications can be offered as a way to calm the patient so that further discussion can occur. This is in contrast to medication being offered to sedate the patient. If medication is used to sedate the patient, it is important to have additional conversations with the patient to process the incident and to discuss alternative ways of managing angry feelings in the future. In dealing with an agitated patient, only one staff member should speak. This approach avoids confusion and decreases stimulation. Debriefing is important so that staff can process the incident, learn from any unintended consequences, and prevent future aggression.

If the situation gets out of hand and physical aggression is imminent or has already occurred, follow the established protocol. The nurse must know of the available resources and the limits of those resources, in addition to knowing where to find additional help when needed. Use good communication skills combined with a respectful approach when meeting the patient. If security is needed, be clear when calling for assistance regarding exactly what is happening with the patient. Use the least restrictive measures necessary when restraining the patient. The use of violence or physical restraint reinforces the patient's belief that violence is necessary to solve problems. Therapeutic communication skills should be the first line of assistance. The clinician conveys caring, develops trust, and establishes rapport by listening to the patient.

Sometimes the patient is not communicative and is unable to convey his problems/concerns to the staff. When this happens, other resources can be sought.

Sometimes the family, friends, co-workers, or someone else in the patient's life may be present to assist with information. It's paramount that the nurse documents each source with the information given. When it's unclear why the patient is not communicative, a mental status examination or cognitive capacity screening examination should be conducted in an attempt to determine the reason for the patient's non-communication (O'Brien, 2001).

One must always determine the safety of both the patient and the staff with all patient interactions, especially with patients who have psychiatric disorders. Many times, the patient presents in an agitated state. Although agitation measurement scales are available, they are rarely used (Zun, 2012). The clinician uses more subjective measures based on what she believes the level of agitation is. In this case, it is more difficult to determine the proper use of restraints without using some reliable measure that helps determine the patient's level of anxiety. Issues related to agitation have the potential to affect both the patient and the clinician. When physical or pharmacological use of restraints for agitated patients is being considered, one must clearly assess and document the rationale for those restraints. The Joint Commission for Accreditation of Healthcare Organization and the Centers for Medicare and Medicaid Services (CMS) now have clear restrictions on the use of restraints in hospitals across the country. These restrictions came about in direct response to deaths reported as resulting from restraints (Berzlanovich, Schopfer, & Keil, 2012). Forensic consequences can arise when restraints are not applied properly.

If a patient enters the healthcare setting with a weapon, security must be called immediately. Know what the procedures for such incidences entail and know them before a critical incident arises. In many cases such as this, outside law enforcement is called. Again, the nurse should document what occurred from the time the patient entered until the patient left. Psychiatric issues should also be documented objectively and thoroughly. While this documentation may lead to charges being filed or not filed, an important implication is that if psychiatric symptoms affected how the patient was behaving, that documentation can help get the forensic psychiatric patient the services he or she needs.

COMPETENCY/INSANITY

Court cases with forensic mental health patients often include discussions of competency and insanity. The legal system allows that individuals must be determined competent to stand trial so that they can make a well-reasoned defense. Defendants who are not deemed competent to stand trial based on mental, physical, or cognitive impairment may receive postponement of criminal proceedings. Therefore, it's necessary to conduct a careful assessment of an individual's relevant functional abilities and clinical conditions. The assessment, usually conducted by an experienced forensic clinician, would include a determination of the patient's knowledge that society would see the act as wrong, perception of consequences, any organic conditions, stressful events before the crime was committed, and use of drugs or alcohol.

Insanity is a legal term that refers to a person's ability to know right from wrong at the time of a criminal offense. Not guilty by reason of insanity is a legal argument that a person should not be held liable for a crime if the act is attributable to mental illness that interferes with rationality or excusing condition (not knowing right from wrong). Insanity refers to the mental state at the time of the crime. It may exist with or without the presence of a psychiatric disorder. An experienced forensic clinician conducts insanity determinations.

A nurse in the general clinical setting may not understand the importance of the role he or she may play in determining the competence of a particular patient. However, a nurse's documentation may have direct impact on final determination of competence of that patient. While the advanced practice forensic psychiatric nurse is prepared to serve on the legal team when conducting a competency evaluation, the documentation by the nurse in any setting where the patient presented may be pertinent to that patient's legal case and can then be used as documentation by the team. For this reason, a nurse should always attend to the importance of documenting in an objective manner. It's not the responsibility of the nurse to make a judgment as to whether the patient is a victim or a perpetrator. He or she should simply document what is observed and what happens during the time he or she is involved with each patient. The clinician prepared to determine competence relies on the clinical data, along with an in-depth interview and all other relevant information, in order to make a sound decision regarding competence.

The purpose of the evaluation is to determine competency to stand trial, assess the individual's relevant functional abilities and clinical conditions that may affect psychiatric status, and to evaluate criminal responsibility. Risk of violence, need for civil commitment, workplace disability, harassment and discrimination claims, and determination of damages in civil cases are among the many reasons for forensic evaluations. Forensic mental health screening and evaluation is defined as the process conducted by mental health personnel, at the direction of criminal justice authorities, for the purposes of delineating, acquiring, and providing information about the mental condition of client-offenders that is useful in decision-making in the criminal justice system. Evaluators are retained by third parties. Goals are not clinical but legal or financial.

Legal tests of sanity may include the McNaughton rules, irresistible impulse, and guilty but mentally ill. The *McNaughton rules* derive from a trial in 1843 in which Daniel McNaughton was tried for the murder of a public official. McNaughton believed there was a conspiracy among the Tories of England to destroy him. In an attempt to assassinate the Prime Minister, who was the Tory leader, McNaughton mistakenly shot and killed the Prime Minister's secretary. McNaughton was judged to be criminally insane and acquitted of the murder (but institutionalized for the remainder of his life). There was a public outcry over the leniency of this verdict. The House of Lords convened a special session of the judges to give an advisory opinion regarding the law of England governing the insanity defense. The judges advised that to be considered legally insane, the accused person with a mental disorder either must not know the nature and quality of the act or must not know whether the act is right or wrong. Whether or not the individual is responsible for his or her action is the underlying issue in the McNaughton rules. *Irresistible impulse* was added to the McNaughton rules in 1929. This addition stipulates that even if the defendant knew the criminal act was wrong but could not control his or her behavior because of a psychiatric illness or a mental defect, the defendant is not guilty (Sekula & Colbert, 2013, p. 602).

The advanced practice forensic psychiatric nurse is prepared with both psychiatric and forensic expertise and is therefore prepared to assess the patient for psychiatric symptoms as well as legal implications in his or her care. However, the nurse caring for the patient in the healthcare system may be the one whose documentation is most pertinent to outcomes for the patient, because he or she may have presented in the healthcare setting at this critical time point. The nurse may have assessed for drug and alcohol use, state of agitation, or verbalization of suicidality or homicidality; any utterances by the patient can be documented in the patient's own words in the clinical notes.

What is important in this focus area for nurse generalists caring for the forensic psychiatric patient is that they observe and document accurately, remain objective and nonjudgmental, and remain focused on the needs of the patients.

CASE STUDY: MENTAL HEALTH

For nurses working in the generalist setting, it's important to know that their documentation regarding any patient who may have mental health disorders along with forensic issues may be the most important documentation when making determinations regarding the patient's care and outcomes in the legal system.

You are a nurse in the emergency department at a large metropolitan hospital. Charles, a 46 year-old unemployed carpenter, is admitted from the county jail for severe abdominal pain and headaches. He is argumentative with the triage nurse, saying that he is being treated differently from other patients. When the attending nurse begins her assessment of the patient, he tells her that he has "unbearable" pain and that it had gone untreated for several days while in jail. He tells the nurse that he feels that he "must be admitted" to the hospital because he feels he may have a serious illness, which the county jail is ignoring.

The nurse conducts a physical assessment because of the reported severity of the pain. Lab tests are requested, and then a physical and mental health history is conducted. He reports that the corrections department for several years has victimized him and that he was wrongly accused of theft from the company for which he worked as a carpenter. He has been divorced for 5 years and has three children who he states will have nothing to do with him because his ex-wife "turned them against me." He reports minimal use of drugs and ETOH but acknowledges that many of the problems between him and his ex-wife occurred because of his drug and ETOH use. As the nurse continues questioning and documenting, Charles tells her that she is the first person who seemed to "even care about my problems. You are really a good nurse! I know you can help me."

Taking what you have learned in this chapter, consider the following:

- What are some observations that you might make given what Charles has stated?

- How do you plan to talk with him about his statements regarding the corrections system, his court case, his family, and his statement that you are a really good nurse?

- What are the most important considerations as you work with Charles?

- How can you be both supportive and yet set proper limits?

As the nurse in charge of this case, consider the importance of letting Charles know that you are here to assist him with his problems for which he was admitted to the emergency department. You are not here to address his problems with the corrections system, his employer, or his family. A thorough physical assessment should focus on the validity of his self-reported symptoms, being fully supportive of the fact that they may be "real" symptoms but also taking into consideration that he may be malingering in order to be admitted to the hospital. How do you respond to his flattering remarks? What is the basis for your response knowing what you have learned from this chapter? What is your most important role in this case?

SUMMARY

This chapter provided a review of the main points regarding the interface between psychiatric mental illness and the healthcare system when legal implications are involved. A major point that was stressed is the importance of accurate and objective documentation by all who interface with patients in the healthcare setting. The nurse must remain objective in all documentation because interjecting his or her subjective feelings regarding a victim or a perpetrator may impact legal outcomes and may affect the ability of the victim or the perpetrator to receive proper care. It is not a nurse's job to judge but to document correctly and objectively. The role that all nurses can play when caring for the forensic mental health patient was also highlighted.

REFERENCES

American Psychological Association (APA). (2013). *Diagnostic and statistical manual of mental disorders* (5th ed.). Washington, DC: Author.

Berzlanovich, A. M., Schopfer, J., & Keil, W. (2012). Deaths due to physical restraint. *Deutsches Ärzteblatt International, 109*(3), 27–32. doi: 10.3238/arztebl.2012.0027

Bienenfeld, D., Talavera, F., Harsch, H. H., & Ahmed, I. (2015). *Malingering clinical presentations*. Retrieved from Emedicine.Medscape.com/article/293206-clinical

Crisanti, A. S., Frueh, B. C., Archambeau, O., Steffen, J. J., & Wolff, N. (2014). Prevalence and correlates of criminal victimization among new admissions to outpatient mental health services in Hawaii. *Community Mental Health Journal, 50*(3), 296–304. doi: 10.1007/s10597-013-9688-1

Delaney, K. R., & Johnson, M. E. (2006). Keeping the unit safe: Mapping psychiatric nursing skills. *Journal of the American Psychiatric Nurses Association, 12*(4), 198–207.

Johnson, M. E., & Hauser, P. M. (2001). The practices of expert psychiatric nurses: Accompanying the patient to a calmer personal space. *Issues in Mental Health Nursing, 22*(7), 651–668.

Lyons, T. (2009). Role of the forensic psychiatric nurse. *Journal of Forensic Nursing, 5*(1), 53–57. doi: 10.1111/j.1939-3938.2009.01033.x

Mason, A. M., Cardell, R., & Armstrong, M. (2014). Malingering psychosis: Guidelines for assessment and management. *Perspectives in Psychiatric Care, 50*(1), 51–55.

O'Brien, J. S. (2001). Interviewing techniques. In J. S. Olshaker, M. C. Jackson, & W. S. Smock (Eds.), *Forensic emergency medicine* (pp. 55–62). Philadelphia, PA: Lippincott Williams & Wilkins.

Quintal, S. A. (2002). Violence against psychiatric nurses: An untreated epidemic? *Journal of Psychosocial Nursing & Mental Health Services, 40*(1), 46–55.

Richmond, J. S., Berlin, J. S., Fishkind, A. B., Holloman, G. H., Zeller, S. L., Wilson, M. P., ... Ng, A. T. (2012). Verbal de-escalation of the agitated patient: Consensus statement of the American Association for Emergency Psychiatry Project BETA De-escalation Workgroup. *Western Journal of Emergency Medicine, 13*(1), 17–25.

Sekula, L. K., & Colbert, A. M. (2013). Forensic psychiatric nursing. In E. M. Varcarolis & M. J. Halter (Eds.), *Foundations of psychiatric mental health nursing* (7th ed., Vol. 1), (pp. 598–610). St. Louis, MO: Elsevier.

Zun, L. S. (2012). Pitfalls in the care of the psychiatric patient in the emergency department. *Journal of Emergency Medicine, 43*(5), 829–835.

CHAPTER 14

DEATH INVESTIGATION

Stacey A. Mitchell, DNP, MBA, RN, SANE-A, SANE-P; and
Stacy A. Drake, PhD, MPH, RN, AFN-BC, D-ABMDI

KEY POINTS IN THIS CHAPTER

- Deaths that are sudden and unexpected or deaths that result from complications of injuries, drug toxicity, or chemical exposure must be reported to the medicolegal authority.

- Clothing should accompany the body to the medicolegal death investigation agency.

- There are exceptions under HIPAA that allow for the release of information after death.

- Be cautious of how you interpret postmortem changes; describe what you observe and palpitate using descriptive terms.

- If a patient with a remote history of trauma dies, the death should be reported to the medicolegal death investigation agency.

According to the Centers for Disease Control and Prevention (CDC, 2014a), the leading cause of death for adolescents and young adults is unintentional injury. This includes car crashes, drug overdoses that are not suicidal in nature, and drowning. Homicide and suicide rank high in this age group also (CDC, 2014a). In older adults, death is usually caused by a disease process such as heart disease, cancer, stroke, or Alzheimer's disease (CDC, 2014a). However, falls are the leading cause of elderly traumatic deaths.

On a daily basis, nurses provide care to patients who die. The cause may be the result of traumatic injuries or a natural disease process. In addition to caring for families who experience the death of a loved one, legal responsibilities must be considered after someone dies. Depending on jurisdiction, nurses may be required to report the death to the medical examiner or coroner. Nurses should be familiar with the laws and the types of deaths that require medical examiner or coroner notification.

Death investigation is a subspecialty of forensic nursing. Although there are few forensic nurse death investigators, they fulfill an important role. The death investigation process gathers health and other medical information to determine the circumstances surrounding the death. Many agencies use information about death as part of their daily duties. For example, the prosecutor's office uses injuries and medical treatment documented in murder trials and other types of court cases. The health department uses stats to track and trend death and how it occurs, such as from overdoses. Product improvement comes from studying deaths or injuries related to consumer products. Forensic nurse death investigators gather information, assess scenes, and assist the medical examiner or coroner with determining the cause and manner of death. Although it may seem tedious to gather the information needed to report a death, this information serves of vital importance for family and communities. The purpose of this chapter is to describe the field of death investigation and the roles of healthcare workers.

DEATH INVESTIGATION SYSTEMS

The first thing nurses must determine is the type of death investigation system that operates in their area. The United States has three types of death investigation systems:

- The **coroner system** is the oldest and traces back over 600 years to England (DiMaio & DiMaio, 2001). During this time, by the order of the king, the coroner would collect taxes and document information about those who had died in towns and villages (Constantino, Crane, & Young, 2013). Inquests were conducted to determine whether the death was intentional or unintentional. If evidence showed the death to be intentional, the coroner would arrest the accused and present the information at trial (Constantino et al., 2013). The colonists brought this system with them to the New World. Over time, this became the structure for investigating deaths in America.

  Today, the coroner is an elected position where, depending on the state, the qualifications are minimal. In some states, the coroner doesn't have to be a physician or possess any experience in investigating death (DiMaio & DiMaio, 2001). A funeral director, sheriff, layperson, or nurse may be elected into this position. Regardless of who is in this role, additional training and continuing education is a requirement for anyone working as a coroner (Garbacz Bader & Gabriel, 2010).

- The **medical examiner** system was first identified in Massachusetts in 1877. The state was divided into sectors and had a designated physician who was called the "medical examiner" (DiMaio & DiMaio, 2001). This system evolved over the years. It was not until 1918 that the medical examiner system became what it is known as today (DiMaio & DiMaio, 2001). *Medical examiners* are licensed physicians with expertise in pathology or forensic pathology. The governing body of the jurisdiction in which they function appoints them. The medical examiner investigates deaths as designated by the legislature as being suspicious, violent, unexpected, and unexplained. Responsible for all aspects of the investigation, the medical examiner oversees or performs the autopsy examination, scene investigation, and any laboratory testing (Constantino et al.,

2013)

- The **mixed** death investigation system is a hybrid of both a coroner and medical examiner system. Nurses work in the medical examiner's office doing investigations.

The following sections discuss both the coroner and medical examiner roles in depth as well as other positions that investigate deaths that nurses may interact with.

CORONER AND MEDICAL EXAMINER

The principal role of either the coroner or medical examiner is to determine the cause and manner of death:

- The **cause of death** is the reason why a person died, such as from an injury or disease process (DiMaio & DiMaio, 2001; Constantino et al, 2013). For example, if a person was shot in the head, the cause of death would be listed on the death certificate as "Gunshot wound of the head." Cancer and heart disease are other examples of causes of death.

- The **manner of death** is the category in which the death falls (DiMaio & DiMaio, 2001). The manners of death include natural, homicide, suicide, accident, and undetermined. The medical examiner or coroner uses information obtained during the autopsy examination, scene investigation documents and photographs, police reports, and results from any postmortem laboratory studies to determine the cause and manner of death.

Both the medical examiner and the coroner collaborate with law enforcement and the criminal justice system. Injury information such as bullet trajectory, type of injury, and cause of death are discussed with detectives. Expert witness testimony is presented to judges and juries regarding autopsy and forensic laboratory findings. During testimony, attorneys for either side may explore with the medical examiner or coroner alternative scenarios about how the death may have occurred (Constantino et al., 2013).

Forensic Pathologist

A *forensic pathologist* is a licensed physician who has specific training in anatomic and/or clinical pathology in addition to a subspecialty certification in forensic pathology (Constantino et al., 2013; Garbacz Bader & Gabriel, 2010). Medical examiners are forensic pathologists (Garbacz Bader & Gabriel, 2010). Coroners, on the other hand, may not be trained as forensic pathologists. When a coroner is not a licensed physician, a forensic pathologist is contracted to conduct the autopsy examination, review scene investigation materials (photographs, statements, police reports, etc.), and order any laboratory studies (Garbacz Bader & Gabriel, 2010). Depending on the jurisdiction, the forensic pathologist may make a recommendation to the coroner as to the cause and manner of death.

Medicolegal Death Investigator

A *medicolegal death investigator* (MDI) is a professional who investigates deaths that fall under the jurisdiction of the medical examiner or coroner. There are no degree requirements to become a medicolegal death investigator (American Board of Medicolegal Death Investigators [ABMDI], 2015). A background in healthcare, forensic science, or anthropology is useful, because the MDI must possess the most knowledge of anatomy, physiology, and pharmacology at a death scene (ABMDI, 2015). The MDI examines death reports to determine whether the death falls under medical examiner or coroner jurisdiction. Duties include responding to the death scene, documenting the condition of the body, photographing or videoing the scene, and identifying wounds and medications. More importantly, the MDI makes death notifications and works with grieving families.

When hospitals or law enforcement contacts the medical examiner or coroner, the person who obtains the necessary information is most likely the MDI. As a healthcare provider calling in a death report, the nurse is asked to provide all information about the patient, circumstances of any injuries, and any medical treatment that was rendered.

FORENSIC NURSE DEATH INVESTIGATORS

A *forensic nurse death investigator* (FNDI) is a registered nurse who has received specialized education and clinical preparation in conducting a death investigation (International Association of Forensic Nurses [IAFN], 2013). While nursing education is the foundation, a medicolegal death investigation course provides the FNDI with the knowledge, skills, and abilities to conduct a competent death investigation. The nursing process is interwoven throughout the death investigation. The FNDI assesses the scene and the decedent, plans for evidence collection or family notification of death, implements referrals for family members, and evaluates all actions taken (IAFN, 2013).

The FNDI also obtains death reports. Nurses may encounter an FNDI when calling to see whether a death falls under the medical examiner's or coroner's jurisdiction. The FNDI may respond to the hospital when there is a death that is considered high profile or for the death of an infant or child. These deaths require special attention.

LEGAL REQUIREMENTS SURROUNDING DEATH INVESTIGATION

On a macro level, nurses utilize information from death investigations—commonly referred to as *mortality data* (CDC, 2014b; Hanzlick, 2006)—to identify and monitor the health of a population within a region. Nurses, along with other healthcare providers, also use this data to set priorities for research endeavors and to allocate funds for research investment. Mortality data includes causes and manners of death (CDC, 2014b). The cause and manner of death come from death certificates (CDC, 2014b; Godwin, 2005; Hanzlick, 2006). It's at the micro level where small details can make a big difference for aggregated death certificate data.

A death certificate is necessary for every person who dies. Professionals who are responsible for signing death certificates include primary physicians, nurse practitioners, medical examiners, coroners, or justices of the peace. Although death investigation laws vary from jurisdiction to jurisdiction, only medical examiners or coroners can sign death certificates for decedents who died from non-natural causes, i.e., accident, suicide, homicide, or undetermined. When a person dies from sudden, unexpected, or traumatic causes, the law mandates that the death be reported to a statutorily established medicolegal death investigation agency. The death investigation process typically starts with the nurse or another healthcare provider recognizing or identifying that a patient's death requires reporting to the medicolegal death investigator who is designated, by law, to sign the death certificate.

The nurse's role in identifying and reporting a death to the medicolegal death investigation agency should not be minimized. The majority of deaths occur in the presence of a healthcare provider (Lynch, 2002). Frequently, the nurse has the responsibility of recognizing whether or not the death should be reported to the local medical examiner or coroner. The intent of this chapter is not to transform you into a death investigator but rather to demonstrate how your role contributes to medicolegal death investigation at a micro level (e.g., classification of death certificate) and how that information is later used at a macro level (e.g., aggregated mortality data for program planning or funding priorities) (Godwin, 2005; Hanzlick, 2006).

RELEVANT LAWS AND STATUTES

Every medicolegal death investigation agency has authority or jurisdiction to:

- Investigate circumstances surrounding a person's death through state, county, or city statutes. These statutes provide the authority to investigate the circumstances surrounding a death in an effort to determine the cause and manner of death.

- Ensure people are appropriately identified (Dolinak, Matshes, & Lew, 2005). For example, if a patient in the hospital dies without being identified, the death is reportable to the local agency, and scientific identification will occur either via fingerprints, dental, DNA, or other testing.

■ Collect appropriate physical and biological evidence during the course of their examinations (Dolinak et al., 2005; Spitz, 1993).

The statutes provide guidance on the types of deaths that are reportable to the medicolegal death investigation agency. Most healthcare organizations work with their local medical examiner or coroner office to establish policies and procedures that adhere to the statutory requirements. These policies and procedures provide guidance in identifying a patient whose circumstances of death may require medicolegal death investigation. These policies may also include procedures for handling the body. For example, if the body is transferred to the medicolegal death investigation agency, all therapeutic devices should remain in place, e.g., intravenous lines, endotracheal tubes. It's also important to know that the Health Insurance Portability and Accountability Act (HIPAA) has exceptions that allow for the release of information after death.

Nurses should report these types of deaths to the medical examiner or coroner (Texas Code of Criminal Procedure, Chapter 49.25, n.d.), although jurisdictions do vary; all nurses should know the laws and statutes of their specific states:

■ Deaths of individuals in the custody of law enforcement, including jail or prison inmates

■ Deaths within 24 hours of admission to a hospital may or may not be reportable

■ Deaths from any unnatural cause (except legal execution):

  ■ Drowning, suffocation, smothering, burns, electrocution, lightning, radiation, chemical or thermal injury, starvation, environmental exposure, neglect

  ■ Unexpected death during, associated with, or as a result of diagnostic or therapeutic medical or surgical procedures

- Deaths from narcotics or other addictions, other drugs, including toxic agents, or toxic exposure. By convention, deaths from acute toxicity are considered non-natural, while deaths from chronic complications of toxic exposures are typically considered natural. Acute alcohol toxicity, for example, is non-natural, while death from alcoholic cirrhosis is considered natural.

- Death thought to be associated with, or resulting from, occupational injury

- Abortions are typically non-reportable, but fetal deaths from maternal trauma are.

- Deaths occurring from apparent natural causes during the course of a criminal act, e.g., victim collapses during a robbery

- Death following injury-producing accidents (e.g., falls, motor vehicle crash), if recovery was considered incomplete or if the accident is thought to have contributed to the cause of death (regardless of the interval between accident and death)

- Legal executions may or may not be included (or specifically excluded) from the list of reportable deaths.

- When a body is found and the circumstances of death are unknown

- When circumstances raise the suspicion that a death was from unlawful means:

  - Death from apparent homicide

  - Death from firearms, stabs, strangulation

  - Death while in custody of law enforcement

- Suicides, or suspicion thereof

- Deaths unattended by a physician; deaths in which the physician is unsure of cause of death:

  - Sudden death occurring in a person without a known natural cause

  - Deaths from acute or unexplained rapidly fatal illness, for which a reasonable natural cause has not been established

  - Deaths of persons in nursing homes or other institutions where medical treatment is not provided by licensed medical personnel

  - Deaths where no physician can certify that death is due solely to natural causes

  - Deaths that occurred within 24 hours of care but where the underlying cause of death is unknown

- Child deaths (less than 6 years of age), including fetal deaths where gestational age is equal to or greater than 20 weeks and/or weight is equal to or greater than 350 grams

- Death of an unknown person

AUTOPSIES, ORGAN DONATION, AND CHAIN OF CUSTODY

When jurisdiction is retained—i.e., the death falls within the statuary authority of a medical examiner or coroner—consent from the next of kin to proceed with an investigation is not required. The authority to conduct an investigation, including an autopsy, comes from the statutory mandate. If jurisdiction is not retained—i.e., the death doesn't require medicolegal death investigation and next of kin requests an autopsy—the nurse should contact the pathology department to arrange for in-hospital autopsy services. If the hospital cannot provide this service, private pathologists can be contacted to perform an autopsy for a fee. In either case, autopsies performed outside the jurisdiction of the medicolegal death system are only performed under consent from the next of kin (Hanzlick, 2007). For example, if a patient dies as a result of cardiovascular disease, the nurse understands that this death is natural and not reportable to the medicolegal authority. If the treating physician or the family wants an autopsy performed, consent from the family must be obtained.

Federal law dictates that hospitals report all inpatient deaths to organ and tissue agencies (Uniform Law Commission, 2015). In most healthcare agencies, nurses have the responsibility of notifying the organ and tissue procurement agencies. The procurement agencies will determine eligibility and approach next of kin for consent. So what happens when the death requires a medicolegal death investigation and is also eligible for organ/tissue donation? Most medicolegal death investigation agencies have a working relationship with procurement agencies, and it's typically the responsibility of the procurement agencies to contact the medical examiner or coroner to obtain permission to recover organs and tissues according to family consent.

When a person dies and the body is within the jurisdiction of the medical examiner or coroner, the body, the property, and clothing the person was wearing should be released to either the death investigation agency or law enforcement. This is especially true for clothing, regardless if bloody or torn, because clothing provides invaluable evidence, e.g., gunshot residue patterns (Dolinak et al., 2005; Spitz, 1993). Additionally, body parts, which may have been removed during surgery (e.g., skull flaps) may need to accompany the body to the medicolegal death investigation agency, or be subsequently transferred. For example, if part of the skull was removed during craniotomy for treatment of a gunshot wound, the reconstruction of that part of the skull may aid the forensic pathologist with determination of direction, number of shots, or even range of fire. Lastly, it is important to understand that the body as a whole is viewed as evidence; therefore, accounting for the location of the body and who had contact or possession of the body and any property (i.e., chain of custody) is important for legal proceedings. For example, most agencies have a chain of custody form that needs to be signed by the person transporting the decedent to the morgue and requires another signature for the person who accepts the transfer. A separate chain of custody will generally be required for clothing or other personal effects.

ASSESSMENT FINDINGS, TECHNIQUES, AND DOCUMENTATION

The nurse's clinical assessment and documentation may be one of the most important and significant pieces of evidence detailing the circumstances surrounding a death or detailing injuries. It is very common that the records for the death admission will accompany the body to the medical examiner's or coroner's office and subsequently appear in court. It is also very common that medical records from prior admissions or specific documents (e.g., radiographic findings or medication administration records) will be requested. These documents are essential for any medicolegal death investigation. The investigators, pathologists, or nurse case managers will typically review the records in an effort to summarize the decedent's health history and chain of events leading to death. The nurse's documentation is obviously an important part of the medicolegal death investigation. When a death is reported in which the decedent has a history of remote trauma and a subsequent sequence of complications preceding death, a record review is essential. Documentation of the initial admission circumstances, along with any injuries (i.e., location, type, statements as to how injury occurred), are all critical in establishing cause and manner of death. Thus, it is important to document as accurately and objectively as possible at all times.

When a patient dies, certain pathophysiologic changes occur, called *postmortem changes*. For the most part, a hospital patient will be in a relatively controlled temperature, free from insects and sun exposure. Thus, the degree to which postmortem changes will be observed in a healthcare setting is generally limited. The individual changes are discussed separately but occur simultaneously and are dependent upon many factors.

When assessing postmortem changes in a deceased patient, the techniques used include inspection and palpation. The following postmortem changes can be assessed:

- **Algor mortis:** Cooling of the body after death. The body typically assumes the ambient temperature (Dolinak et al., 2005). Algor mortis is assessed through palpation. A febrile patient takes longer to equalize to ambient temperature than an afebrile patient.

- **Livor mortis (lividity):** A purple-red discoloration of the skin from settling of blood within the vascular tree (Dolinak et al., 2005). Although this can be seen in living patients, it's prevalent postmortem. Lividity patterns develop in gravity-dependent areas of the body over time. Typically, hospital patients develop lividity on the posterior aspect. Portions of the body exposed to pressure (e.g., the buttocks and shoulders in a supine decedent) are devoid of lividity. The lividity can change if a body is moved; however, after approximately 8 to 12 hours the settled blood leaks from the capillaries into the subcutaneous tissues. After this occurs, the lividity is "fixed." At that point, lividity develops in a newly dependent part of the body if the position is changed but won't blanch from the previously dependent portions. Lividity is clearly visible, and whether or not it is fixed is assessed by palpation. If lividity blanches under firm pressure of an examiner's thumb, for example, it is not yet fixed. Blood also settles to dependent parts of internal organs as well, although this phenomenon is not generally referred to as livor mortis (Dolinak et al., 2005).

- **Rigor mortis:** Stiffening of muscles due to chemical changes in the myoplasm (Dolinak et al., 2005). This begins after death; however, it's not readily assessed until hours later. The muscles stiffen in the position in which the person died. Elevated temperature or exercise just before death may accelerate development of rigor mortis. Rigor mortis is assessed through inspection and palpation.

- **Drying of tissues:** A red or gray discoloration occurs in the sclera in areas exposed to air (also known as *tache noir*). A red or purple discoloration may occur in the other mucus membranes, lips, mouth, and genitals (Dolinak et al., 2005), but generally takes longer. Regardless, these changes are all postmortem artifacts and should not be interpreted as trauma. Drying of tissues is assessed through inspection.

- **Putrefaction:** Occurs from bacterial proliferation with accompanying gas formation (Dolinak et al., 2005). Putrefaction begins immediately after death and is eventually manifested by "bloating" that becomes progressively more noticeable over time. It's assessed through inspection. Skin slippage can occur as the bacteria digest the superficial subcutaneous connective tissues holding the epidermis in place. The proliferation of bacteria in the bloodstream also causes the tissues to appear green or brown because of chemical changes to the hemoglobin.

Although putrefactive changes are not typically seen in decedents within a hospital setting, especially if the body is placed quickly in a refrigerated environment, there is one important exception. In septic patients, circulating bacteria are already throughout the bloodstream tissues at the time of death, and putrefaction may proceed at a surprisingly rapid pace, even if the body is immediately transferred to a cool ambient temperature (such as a cooled morgue or holding area) (Dolinak et al., 2005).

■ **Dilated anus:** The anus becomes dilated, particularly in children, after death. This is an artifactual change that can be noted via inspection and should not be interpreted as an indicator of sexual assault.

As the postmortem interval increases, additional changes occur; however, in the healthcare setting these changes are rarely, if ever, observed. The changes include mummification or leathering/browning of the skin; *adipocere,* or conversion of adipose tissue to a waxy substance (usually in wet or moist environments); and skeletonization. An example of documenting postmortem changes could be as follows: body is cool to the touch, blanching lividity in posterior aspects of body; rigor is palpable in small muscles (e.g., fingers and jaw) but not in large muscle groups (hips or knees).

Documentation is fundamental for the nursing profession. A nurse documenting an assessment of a patient that will require a medicolegal death investigation must realize that many people will review the records, and in fact, the records are a legal document. Obviously, the documentation should be thorough, factual, and objective.

STRATEGIES TO ASSIST FAMILIES

Death can cause many emotions. Deaths that are sudden, unexpected, or traumatic cause additional stress, and if these stresses are not considered and recognized, they can have lifelong impacts. This section includes strategies you can implement when interacting with families experiencing the loss of a loved one from sudden and unexpected circumstances.

It's best to direct communication to the legal next of kin. Every state has laws outlining the legal next of kin. In most states it follows as such: spouse (common law spouse is recognized); adult children; parents; adult siblings. For a minor the sequence includes parents; adult siblings; grandparents. A legal written document may also specify next of kin for healthcare decisions. All healthcare organizations have a policy regarding legal next of kin for the purpose of consent for treatment or disposition of the body.

Communication both verbal and written is key. When communicating with the legal next of kin, it's critical to provide concise and simple information, avoiding medical jargon and technical terms. Communication with a family must be done in a professional and honest manner. When a family asks questions regarding medicolegal death investigation processes or any other topic and you don't know the answer, the response should simply be, "I don't know," but qualified with an offer to inquire and subsequently provide the accurate information. Informing family of something that may or may not be true creates conflict between agencies and family. Common inquiries include information about funeral arrangements or the time frame in which the medical examiner or coroner will hold the body. Another question regarding medicolegal investigation involves whether or not an autopsy will be performed and the time frame in which the final autopsy report will be ready. These questions should be deferred to the appropriate death investigation authority. In fact, depending on the circumstances of death and local statutes, the availability of the report to next of kin or others varies.

Regarding written communication, the family should be provided with the contact information for the medical legal death investigator, case number, and other referral information depending upon the circumstances of the death. Grief service resources should be provided, including information for coping with suicide, homicide, child deaths, and accidental deaths. Some resources you can refer families to are:

- Centers for Disease Control and Prevention (CDC): www.cdc.gov

- National Association of Medical Examiners (NAME): www.thename.org

- American Board of Medicolegal Death Investigators (ABMDI): www.abmdi.org

- American Academy of Forensic Sciences (AAFS): www.aafs.org

- International Association of Forensic Nurses (IAFN): www.iafn.org

- Child Protective Services

- Adult Protective Services

- Your local health department

- Your local funeral home(s)

CASE STUDIES: DEATH INVESTIGATIONS

Two short case studies are provided to portray differences in types and circumstances of death.

CASE STUDY 1

You are the nurse working the evening shift at a nursing home when one of your patients dies. The patient is an 82-year-old woman who was admitted to the nursing home initially for rehabilitation following a fall that resulted in a right intertrochanteric hip fracture. Additional health history includes diabetes, congestive heart failure, and hypothyroidism. Her mobility status before the fall included walking with the aid of a cane with the ability to ascend and descend 5 to 10 steps. At the time of death she was status post-surgery by 1 month and only able to sit in a chair. Two days ago, she had started antibiotics for a new diagnosis of bronchopneumonia. Her primary care physician states that she is willing to sign the death certificate.

Questions:

1. Is this death reportable to the medical examiner or coroner?

2. Is the primary physician able to sign the death certificate?

Discussion:

The death is reportable to the medical examiner or coroner because the initiating factor leading to the death included trauma, specifically a fall. Because trauma played a role in causing the death, the manner of death is accidental. Because the death is not due to natural causes, the primary care physician cannot sign the death certificate.

CASE STUDY 2

You are the nurse working in the emergency department (ED) when emergency services arrive with cardiopulmonary resuscitation in progress of a patient who sustained a gunshot wound. Providers cut the clothing off in an attempt to perform a thoracotomy. The patient was pronounced dead 10 minutes after arrival.

Questions:

1. Is the death reportable to the medical examiner or coroner?

2. What do you do with the patient's clothing that was cut off?

Discussion:

The death is reportable because it's due to trauma, the gunshot wound. The manner of death could be either homicide or suicide. The nursing documentation, along with the physician's chart, will be critical to determining the correct manner of death. The clothing that is removed must be sent with the body to the medical examiner or coroner for examination. It should not be balled up, but folded with any defects facing upward. All clothing should be placed in paper bags and signed over to either the medical examiner/coroner or law enforcement.

Summary

Nurses often interact with those who conduct death investigations. It's imperative that the nurse is aware of the local death investigation law to ensure that deaths are reported appropriately and potential evidence is not discarded. Communication between death investigation and healthcare agencies is critical in establishing policies and procedures addressing jurisdiction and preparation of the deceased patient in the event the death falls under medical examiner or coroner law. Nurses should have a basic understanding of the role those involved in the death investigation play to facilitate the best outcomes for the decedent, families, and society. It's in using this knowledge that the nurse alleviates stress and confusion family members may experience after the sudden, unexpected, or traumatic death of a loved one. Lastly, the decedent is provided an independent investigation and examination to better establish the cause and manner of death.

References

American Board of Medicolegal Death Investigators (ABMDI). (2015). *FAQ*. Retrieved from http://www.abmdi.org/faq

Centers for Disease Control and Prevention (CDC). (2014a). *10 leading causes of death by age group, United States-2012*. Retrieved from http://www.cdc.gov/injury/wisqars/pdf/leading_causes_of_death_by_age_group_2012-a.pdf

Centers for Disease Control and Prevention (CDC). (2014b). *Mortality data*. Retrieved from http://www.cdc.gov/nchs/deaths.htm

Constantino, R. E., Crane, P. A., & Young, S. E. (2013). *Forensic nursing: Evidence-based principles and practice*. Philadelphia, PA: F. A. Davis Company.

DiMaio, V. J., & DiMaio, D. (2001). *Forensic pathology* (2nd ed.). Boca Raton, FL: CRC Press.

Dolinak, D., Matshes, E., & Lew, E. (2005). *Forensic pathology: Principles and practice*. Burlington, MA: Elsevier, Inc.

Garbacz Bader, D. M., & Gabriel, S. (2010). *Forensic nursing: A concise manual*. Boca Raton, FL: CRC Press.

Godwin, T. A. (2005). End of life: Natural or unnatural death investigation and certification. *Disease a Month, 51*, 218–277.

Hanzlick, R. (2006). Medical examiners, coroners, and public health. *Arch Pathol Lab Med, 130*, 1274–1282.

Hanzlick, R. (2007). *Death investigation systems and procedures*. Boca Raton, FL: CRC Press.

International Association of Forensic Nurses (IAFN). (2013). *Forensic nurse death investigator education guidelines*. Retrieved from https://c.ymcdn.com/sites/iafn.site-ym.com/resource/resmgr/Education/Nurse_Death_Investigator_Edu.pdf

Lynch, M. J. (2002). The autopsy: Legal and ethical principles. *Pathology, 34,* 67–70.

Spitz, W. U. (1993). *Medicolegal investigation of death: Guidelines for the application of pathology to crime investigation* (3rd ed.). Farmington Hills, MI: Gale Group.

Texas Code of Criminal Procedures 49.25 (n.d.). Retrieved from http://www.statutes.legis.state.tx.us/Docs/CR/htm/CR.49.htm

Uniform Law Commission. (2015). *Anatomical Gift Act (2006)*. Retrieved from http://uniformlaws.org/Act.aspx?title=Anatomical%20Gift%20Act%20%282006%29

15

CORRECTIONAL CARE CONCEPTS FOR NURSING PRACTICE

Anita G. Hufft, PhD, RN; and
Cindy Peternelj-Taylor, RN, MSc, DF-IAFN

"The mood and temper of the public with regard to the treatment of crime and criminals is one of the most unfailing tests of the civilization of any country."

–Sir Winston Churchill

KEY POINTS IN THIS CHAPTER

- Jails, prisons, and correctional institutions as an integral component of the community represent a public health opportunity.

- More than 10 million men and women are imprisoned around the globe; most will return to the community.

- Nurses practicing in penal institutions recognize that in their professional roles, prisoners (and ex-offenders) are viewed and treated as patients.

- Nurses are faced with challenges unique to their roles, the patient population for whom they provide care, the correctional environments in which they practice, and the laws that govern their administration.

- In order to provide competent nursing care, it is imperative that nurses understand the healthcare needs that prisoners experience while incarcerated and bring to the community upon their release.

Jails, correctional facilities, and prisons are often thought of as being separate from the community when, in fact, these penal institutions are an integral part of the community. Distinct in their own culture and providing a unique healthcare environment, secure settings nevertheless are reflective of the broader community and cultures from which they receive prisoners. An understanding of the experience of incarceration and its impact on the health of individuals and populations is critical to the assessment and delivery of population-based healthcare, and it is a critical component of successful integration of offenders back into the community. This chapter defines the offender population and explores the factors affecting health and healthcare during incarceration and upon re-entry, providing a framework for the assessment and care of offenders in community settings.

From a public health perspective, the health of the incarcerated population is a direct reflection of the state of health of the community at large. In his remarks to the National Conference of the National Commission on Correctional Health Care (NCCHC) in 2003, Vice Admiral Carmona, the United States Surgeon General, remarked: "Correctional health is a key to public health...tremendously important, not just to the individuals [served], but to the health of the families and communities they come from and to which they will return" (Carmona, 2003, para. 10–12). Increasingly, secure penal institutions are identified as a public health opportunity (Correctional Service Canada, 2003; Herbert, Plugge, Foster, & Doll, 2012; Williams, 2007).

THE ROLE OF NURSES IN A CORRECTIONAL SETTING

Nurses practicing at the interface of the health and criminal justice systems, regardless of where they are located in the world, are faced with daily challenges unique to their roles, the individuals for whom they provide care, the secure environments in which they practice (including prisons, jails, correctional facilities, and a variety of community-based environments), and the laws that govern their administration. The American Nurses Association (ANA, 2013) states that nurses who practice with imprisoned populations are involved with "the protection, promotion, and optimization of health and abilities; prevention of illness and injury; alleviation of suffering through the diagnosis and treatment of human response; advocacy for and delivery of healthcare to individuals, families, communities, and populations under the jurisdiction of the criminal justice system" (p. 1).

As the largest group of healthcare professionals working with those who are imprisoned, nurses have a significant role to play. Through their professional roles and responsibilities, they not only contribute to the health and wellbeing of prisoners (from both an individual and population-based perspective) but also are instrumental in contributing to the health and safety of facility staff and the community at large. From an international perspective, Fraser (2014) concludes that "all staff in prisons should recognize the importance of balancing the need for safe custody and control on the one hand, and care and rehabilitation on the other" (p. 185).

Overview of Offender Populations

The latest available data from the International Centre for Prison Studies indicates that when remanded prisoners (those charged and detained but not yet sentenced) and sentenced prisoners are considered, more than 10.2 million people are incarcerated throughout the world, which equates to a world prison population rate of 144 people per 100,000 population (Walmsley, 2014b). However, prison rates vary greatly between different countries and regions of the world. Table 15.1 shows the incarceration rate for a few countries, with the United States leading the way.

And while incarceration rates vary considerably across different regions, one thing that is consistent is the marked growth of prison populations throughout the world (Walmsley, 2014b). With more than 10 million men and women in custody around the globe, and the fact that most of these individuals will eventually return to the community, it's imperative that all nurses understand the healthcare needs these individuals experience while incarcerated and bring to the community upon release, and how they can use that understanding to not only provide quality care to offenders but moreover to decrease the burden of disease and ultimately improve the healthcare of their communities (Gatherer, Enggist, & Møller, 2014; van den Bergh, Gatherer, Fraser, & Møller, 2011; Wilper et al., 2009).

TABLE 15.1 INCARCERATION RATES BY COUNTRY

Country	Incarceration Rate (per 100,000)
United States	716
Belize	476
Poland	217
Mexico	210
England/Wales	148
Australia	130
Canada	118
Italy	106
Finland	58
Japan	51

Source: Walmsley, 2014b

OFFENDER POPULATION IN THE UNITED STATES

Over 2.2 million people resided in prisons and jails in the United States in 2012. The U.S. leads developed nations in the rate of incarcerations:

- There's been a 500% increase over the past 40 years.

- It has over 5 million ex-offenders on parole or probation and under some form of community-based supervision at any one time (James, 2014).

- Over 93% of inmates in the United States will be released back into the community, presenting healthcare needs that may be compounded by their incarceration (James, 2014).

▒ Of the almost 600,000 inmates released each year, their reintegration will be determined, in part, by the healthcare they receive.

HEALTHCARE NEEDS FOR PRISON POPULATIONS

Because the ability of a community to provide healthcare to all of its members contributes to a safer environment for all its citizens and improves quality of life, it's therefore incumbent upon nurses to understand the needs of this population and to consider strategies for providing healthcare consistent with those needs.

Correctional inmates experience physical and mental illness at a rate higher than the general public and present unique challenges to healthcare providers. Research has affirmed for 20 years that mental illness, substance abuse, chronic disease, and sexually transmitted diseases are concentrated in correctional facilities (Conklin, Lincoln, & Flanigan, 1998). Current evidence suggests that healthcare programming aimed at addressing the specific health challenges that offenders experience while imprisoned, particularly in areas of drug and mental health treatment, may be effective in facilitating the transition to community integration and successful re-entry. Significant numbers of offenders have problems with mental illness, often experiencing co-morbidity associated with substance abuse or physical illnesses and presenting unique challenges to dealing with emerging crises and long-term management, particularly upon release from incarceration (Duncan & Zwemstra, 2014; Office of the Correctional Investigator, 2014).

In a study published by the RAND Corporation, Davis et al. (2009) sought to better understand the public health implications of prisoner re-entry. As a population, prisoners are sicker than the general population, and they suffer from higher rates of infectious diseases, serious mental illnesses, drug abuse, and dependence disorders than the general population. As the country's prison population has risen over the past 2 decades, the number of parolees returning to the community has risen as well. This implies a great demand on community services for both primary care and serious, chronic physical and mental health problems. Parolees have high rates of chronic illnesses such as asthma and hypertension, as well as infectious diseases like hepatitis and tuberculosis that require regular medical help. In addition, significant numbers of HIV-infected patients are represented in the prison population.

The National Institute on Drug Abuse (2014) estimates that about 70% of state and 64% of federal prisoners regularly used drugs prior to incarceration. The study also showed that one in four violent offenders in state prisons committed their offenses under the influence of drugs. In *Understanding the Public Health Implications of Prisoner Reentry in California*, Davis et al. (2009) reported that:

- Two-thirds of California inmates reported having a drug abuse or dependence problem, yet only 22% said they had received treatment since being sent to prison.

- Approximately 50% of prisoners reported having a mental health problem, yet only half of that number indicated they received treatment while incarcerated— about the same rate reported for state prisoners nationally.

- Over 49% of all inmates under the jurisdiction of the Federal Bureau of Prisons (2015) are imprisoned in relation to drug offenses.

In Europe, drug use is disproportionately high among prisoners in comparison to the general population, and health problems including co-morbid communicable diseases (especially blood-borne diseases) and psychiatric disorders are especially prevalent. For drug users, the mortality risk in the first few weeks following release is of particular concern (Montanari et al., 2014). Once released, these individuals bring their unresolved substance abuse and mental health problems back into the community. When these illnesses are not adequately treated, the risks to physical health and re-entry attempts among parolees rise, increasing the likelihood of health decline, failure to integrate into society, re-offending, and re-incarceration.

Understanding Correctional Healthcare

The Eighth Amendment of the U.S. Constitution guarantees healthcare as a right to prisoners and, as such, is the basis for the development of models of correctional healthcare and standards of practice and accreditation of those facilities (Rold, 2006). In Canada, as per the Correctional and Conditional Release Act, individuals who are imprisoned are entitled to both physical and mental healthcare in accordance with professional and community standards (Canadian Public Health Association, 2004). In the World Health Organization's report *Prisons and Health*, Gatherer et al. (2014) identify three factors pertaining to offenders that healthcare personnel must abide by:

- To assume duty of care (to meet their basic needs)

- To understand and view the offenders as vulnerable (due to their dependence on the staff and prison system for all aspects of their lives including protection, safety, and healthcare)

- To recognize that offenders retain their human rights while incarcerated (other than their freedom)

However, the right to care does not mean that prisoners have consistently accessible quality care. Many correctional facilities are overcrowded and understaffed, and the demand for providing appropriate security in a healthcare setting adds stressors for both the patient and the healthcare provider. Most correctional healthcare facilities have very structured procedures for requesting, accessing, and receiving healthcare that demand strict adherence to limited times and settings for the provision of care. Prisoner oversight by correctional officers for some, if not all, procedures limits privacy. Restricted budgets, correctional policies, concerns for safety, and the general culture of many correctional settings in which punishment, rather than rehabilitation, is the focus also limit medications and health intervention options provided to prisoners.

Most primary healthcare services are provided within the correctional setting, but few jails and prisons have resources to care for critically ill patients or patients needing specialized services such as surgery, delivery of a baby, or diagnostic tests. Prisoners are often transported to local or regional community facilities for such care and are often subjected to security measures such as shackling, which are both humiliating and uncomfortable.

U.S. prisons and jails have access to accreditation standards and professional certification set by the National Commission on Correctional Health Care (NCCHC) and the American Correctional Association (ACA), which ensure comparable services to that of the community. These organizations also provide standards publications, peer reviewed journals on correctional healthcare, training, and other services, which promote quality correctional healthcare. U.S. nurses have the opportunity to join these organizations and receive specialized training, attend workshops and conferences, and become certified as a correctional nurse. Most nurses working in U.S. prisons and jails, however, are not certified. Although cited as a benefit to nurses and a factor affecting quality evidence-based practice, certification is not required in most correctional settings (Almost et al., 2013; Schoenly & Knox, 2012). In the United Kingdom, the Royal College of Nurses (RCN) provides guidance for nursing staff regarding health and nursing care in the criminal justice service through its criminal justice forum, publications, toolkits, and newsletters (RCN, 2009).

Correctional nurses provide care for patients who generally have higher rates of many acute and chronic conditions while in an environment with a primary objective of detention, security, and punishment, rather than healthcare. This context for care differentiates correctional nursing from nursing in other settings. Correctional nurses report more overtime hours and limited control over practice due to staffing issues (Almost et al., 2013). Lack of time to discuss inmate care with other healthcare providers may be a critical factor affecting the quality of care provided in correctional settings. Other factors include characteristics of the patients and their experiences in custody.

POPULATION CHARACTERISTICS AND COMMON CONDITIONS

Demographic characteristics among jail and prison inmates are major determinants of healthcare concerns. The majority of prisoners, regardless of where they are in the world, generally come from lower socioeconomic and socially disadvantaged groups and have lower literacy rates in comparison to the general population. Prior to incarceration, many experienced high-risk lifestyles that included poor health habits and irregular or nonexistent healthcare. Prisoners experience higher rates of drug and alcohol abuse and carry a higher burden of both communicable and non-communicable diseases, exposure to violence and abuse, injuries, and mental health problems than the general population. Correctional healthcare often focuses heavily on the treatment of infectious and sexually transmitted diseases, a number of chronic conditions, alcohol-related problems such as withdrawal and cirrhosis, and mental illness. Significant numbers of individuals released from incarceration bring deficits in academic skills, vocational skills, interpersonal skills, and cognitive abilities. Additionally, the maladaptation to environmental stressors, deprivation, and threats to personal safety carry over into the community experience of ex-offenders, increasing the likelihood of self-neglect. Concern for self-injury and suicide is also ever-present (Gaes & Kendig, 2002; Gatherer et al., 2014; Hammett, Roberts, & Kennedy, 2001; Lansing et al., 2014; Mallik-Kane & Visher, 2008; Wilson & Tully, 2009).

SPECIAL NEEDS OF WOMEN

For an ever-increasing number of women in all the continents, imprisonment has become a harsh reality. More than 625,000 women and girls are incarcerated throughout the world (Walmsley, 2014a). The number of parents in prison has multiplied over the past 2 decades (Youth.Gov, n.d.). Over 53% of current prisoners are parents, and an estimated 1,706,600 children in the United States, 20% of whom are children of color, have at least one parent in prison. The rate of incarceration among women has been increasing at a rate 50% higher than men since 1980 (Glaze & Maruschak, 2008).

Most of these women are convicted of non-violent drug-related crimes, and they often have significant histories of physical and sexual abuse, high rates of HIV, and substance abuse problems. Many mothers in jails and prisons serve as the only providers for their families. When they are incarcerated, the entire family suffers, family integrity is threatened, and children are put at risk. Childcare of dependents of incarcerated mothers often falls to relatives, particularly grandparents, who may experience a disproportionate burden due to age and financial status, further creating stress in the family and the community. Almost one out of every nine incarcerated women have children placed in foster care in the U.S. Parents convicted of drug offenses or serving more than 22 months in prison are especially vulnerable to losing custody due to sanctions imposed post-release that prohibit access to cash assistance, food stamps, public housing, and employment training (Schirmer, Nellis, & Mauer, 2009).

In comparison to their male counterparts, women enter correctional facilities with greater rates of sexually transmitted diseases; substance abuse and related sequelae; mental health problems (including post-traumatic stress disorder and self-harming behaviors); communicable diseases such as HIV, AIDS, and hepatitis B and C; and sexually transmitted infections. Over half of female prisoners have dependents for whom they provided exclusive care prior to incarceration (Fisher & Hatton, 2009; Power, Brown, & Usher, 2012; van den Bergh et al., 2011). Also, incarcerated women have special needs that require skilled attention during care delivery. Providing safe nursing care to women who are incarcerated requires gender sensitivity.

INMATE GOALS NOT RELATED TO HEALTH PROBLEMS

Correctional healthcare is complicated by the nature of the patient, in terms of motivation for seeking healthcare and origins of healthcare needs. Prisoners often seek healthcare as a form of manipulation or behavioral adaptation to incarceration (Hufft, 2013; Schoenly, n.d.) in order to establish power, obtain privileges or rewards to which they are not entitled, or just amuse themselves and pass the time. Goals for accessing healthcare services may include environmental comforts or work reduction, removal from an unsafe environment or perceived danger, or access to drugs or other items for barter. Correctional nurses are obliged to assess every patient as objectively as possible and treat each individual according to identified needs, but exposure to manipulative and coercive interactions on a daily basis presents real threats to the delivery of consistent, professional, and quality care to those who truly require such services.

PRISONER ADAPTATION TO THE CORRECTIONAL SETTING

The adaptations required to adjust to a correctional setting are numerous and can have a tremendous impact on an individual inmate's health. The loss of freedom on numerous levels includes everything from movement, clothing, and scheduling of daily life to affiliations. Family and community connections have been severed or severely altered and may include loss of custody of children or loss of a spouse or significant other. The structure of physical facilities and the corrections hierarchy involves formal and informal sources of power, which must be learned and negotiated, and they are all characterized by fear, restrictiveness, and threat of violence. At the very heart of the adaptation to corrections is self-concept, which involves varying degrees of loss, depending on the roles the individual occupied before incarceration. Correctional healthcare includes the assessment of the degree and effectiveness of the prisoner's adaptation and how this affects health status and needs. This carries over to the assessment of the ex-offender, because these same adaptations occur upon release.

EX-OFFENDER POPULATION OVERVIEW

Individuals returning to the community after incarceration have often been exposed to infectious diseases, environments of violence and overcrowding, deprivation from family, and even maltreatment from correctional staff and other inmates. Providers specifically trained to care for their special needs provide these patients care. Only 22 primary care residency programs in the U.S. train physicians in how to care for prisoners or people who have been through the correctional system, and most nurses working in correctional settings receive on-the-job training only, rather than formal preparation for the role. Universally, professional isolation is a real concern for all healthcare professionals working with prisoners. To combat this, Fraser (2014) stresses the importance of healthcare professionals maintaining active and meaningful links to professional organizations within their own countries. Nevertheless, for many inmates, the healthcare received while imprisoned may be the first and possibly the best healthcare they have received. First-time diagnosis of mental health problems and chronic illnesses, along with infectious diseases, often occurs upon presentation for initial assessment during incarceration. However, if a correctional setting adopts the option for "individual health assessment when clinically indicated," as sanctioned by the NCCHC (2008, para. 4), some individuals may be released without ever having received a health assessment. The experience inmates have with the correctional healthcare system is a significant factor affecting future attitudes and health-seeking behaviors.

Lack of knowledge about this special population among healthcare providers working in correctional settings, and those who care for these individuals upon their release from correctional settings, increases the risk of fragmented care, inadequate care, and missed diagnoses. The mentally ill are a particularly vulnerable population who are overrepresented in the prison population. Upon release, it is essential that they access needed treatment and obtain assistance in managing their medications.

What healthcare providers don't know can result in ineffective care strategies. The fact of the matter is that most nurses will care for ex-offenders and won't know it. One in 31 Americans is or has been incarcerated (Pew Center on the States, 2009). Healthcare clinicians may not understand that being released from a correctional facility puts a person at risk for hospitalization and negatively impacts morbidity and mortality rates (Wang, Wang, & Krumholz, 2013). Working with ex-offenders in the community setting is often challenging due to their apathy or reluctance to engage in shared decision-making regarding their health. During incarceration, inmates aren't allowed to assume responsibility for their own healthcare. With few exceptions, they do not make their own healthcare appointments, they do not purchase or administer their own medications, and often they must receive permission from a correctional officer to seek healthcare.

An understanding of the correctional healthcare system alerts correctional healthcare providers to the unique health risks of prison and how they might help patients prevent future incarcerations. Extending this knowledge to nurses working outside the correctional system bridges the gaps in care and increases the likelihood that timely and appropriate care is initiated during re-entry.

Knowledge that someone has a criminal record can sometimes create fear and stereotypes of ex-offenders. Nurses who are unfamiliar with correctional healthcare often base their perceptions on media portrayals of prison life and of those who commit crimes.

Ex-offenders face many challenges upon their return to the community, including gaining access to education and training, and they need immediate assistance with food and shelter, long-term housing, finding employment, and healthcare. Major barriers to successful ex-offender re-entry include a lack of available support services, or ignorance of them when support services are available.

HEALTH NEEDS OF EX-OFFENDERS

In a survey of ex-offenders in New Jersey (Dougherty, 2013), over 30% of the respondents reported healthcare as one of their top three concerns. Ten percent reported life-threatening or emergency medical care needs, and almost all of the respondents were concerned about access to health insurance. The experience of discrimination often deters patients from seeking primary care and leads to the overuse of emergency departments, perceived as sites where patients cannot be turned away. Ex-offenders need links to a medical home and support in appropriate use of healthcare resources, particularly in the area of primary care. With a risk of death after incarceration 3.5 times higher than the general population, ex-offenders are most likely to succumb to drug overdose, cardiovascular disease, homicide, and suicide. It is therefore clear that, upon release from jail or prison, early assessment of risk and referral to appropriate care is an important intervention (Binswanger et al., 2007).

Juvenile offenders often present with developmental disorders, cognitive disorders, and behavioral issues; in particular, they often experience additional, related issues of grief and psychological trauma. There are significant differences in trauma exposure between detained and never-detained youth and subsequent differences in rates of observed aggression and diagnoses of conduct disorders and other mental health disorders (Griel & Loeb, 2009; Wilson & Tully, 2009). All juveniles leaving a correctional setting should receive a high-quality mental health screen. Upon presentation for any health-related service, mental health screening should be implemented. In addition to mental health needs, juvenile needs include physical health and social health and wellbeing.

Poorer physical health among juvenile offenders is reflected in higher rates of substance abuse, head injury, exposure to gunshot wounds and stab wounds, hepatitis C infection and liver disease, and exposure to sexually transmitted communicable diseases, as compared to those never detained. Higher rates of adolescent pregnancy and disordered eating have been observed in female juvenile offenders, indicating a need for focused assessment upon release. Additionally, juvenile offenders' poorer health is affected by the high-risk behaviors in which they engage, which could increase their tendency to resist referrals for healthcare. Their ability to access care is also complicated by lack of education and peer and family support, and these factors need to be assessed and included in any plan of care (Perry & Morris, 2014; Wilson & Tully, 2009).

LAW AND POLICY AFFECTING HEALTHCARE OF EX-OFFENDERS

Sentencing laws are the primary contributors for the incarceration growth trend in the United States and have resulted in overcrowding and accompanying exacerbation of health risks already experienced at a higher rate by the prison population. Seventy five percent of offenders are incarcerated for non-violent, non-sexual offenses, and most of these individuals could be successfully managed in community settings (Dougherty, 2013).

Lack of health insurance coverage has always been a major concern for most ex-offenders in the United States. The National Commission on Correctional Health Care (2014) "believes that optimizing health insurance coverage and continuity represents a vital means for improving healthcare for correctional populations" (para 6). With the passage of the Patient Protection and Affordable Care Act (2010), most inmates will be eligible for coverage through the expansion of Medicaid coverage. Many states terminate Medicaid coverage upon arrest rather than suspending coverage. This causes a delay in reinstatement upon release from incarceration. Suspension of Medicaid, rather than termination, allows for continuity of care through rapid reinstatement after release (Coalition of Correctional Health Authorities and the American Correctional Association, 2012). The deadline for expanding Medicaid to the uninsured, including inmates and those being paroled or placed on probation, was January 1, 2014; yet at the time of this publication, 22 states have not moved to expand Medicaid (State Reforum, 2015).

STRATEGIES FOR MEETING THE HEALTH NEEDS OF EX-OFFENDERS

Providers are responsible for facilitating healthcare access to ex-offenders. In the United States, this would include referring such individuals to social services to determine their eligibility for health insurance under the expansion of Medicaid through the Patient Protection and Affordable Care Act (2010). Nurses should be included in efforts to ensure appropriate referrals in efforts to establish communications and coordination of services with regional correctional facilities as part of ongoing planning for sustained, community-based care following release from incarceration (Patel, Boutwell, Brockmann, & Rich, 2014). In the U.S., ex-offenders represent a considerable proportion of Medicaid eligible individuals, and any efforts to streamline transition to Medicaid, to improve coordination of care, and to access electronic health records across institutions will not only facilitate better care but also decrease the cost of care.

Assessment of health needs is a priority for all patients, and the ex-offender population is no exception. Training about the health risks of incarceration and techniques for asking about a patient's health history during incarceration are essential to an accurate and meaningful assessment. It is important to emphasize a nonjudgmental, objective approach in any patient encounter, but it is imperative to do so in the care of those who have been incarcerated. Putting patients at ease about discussing their experiences while in prison or jail, and helping them to identify their health concerns, some of which may be the consequence of incarceration (as in the case of sexual assault or other forms of violence that are prevalent in jails and prisons), requires that the nurse understand the nature of correctional healthcare, the risks associated with incarceration, and the common responses to those experiences. Teaching ex-offenders how to talk about their incarceration and to learn how to inform others that they've been in prison without disclosing specifics of why are learned responses on the part of the nurse, and an important part of establishing an effective nurse-patient relationship.

When caring for an ex-offender, the nurse must provide a safe environment in which the patient can be honest in revealing relevant health history and experiences, without sacrificing appropriate boundaries and revealing details (such as the reason for incarceration), which may not be relevant to their care and may prejudice the provider.

Although offenders released from prisons have a high need for drug treatment, healthcare, and mental health services, they often face barriers to accessing healthcare. Lack of knowledge to engage the healthcare system, limitations in the availability of services in the communities to which inmates are released, and inability to obtain health insurance, along with a heightened distrust or fear of healthcare providers as authority figures, are among the challenges faced by offenders engaged in re-entry. Those healthcare providers who serve this population may often be unaware of their incarceration and, if they are aware, often do not have access to health records, further exacerbating the ability to provide appropriate continuity of care. The process by which parolees navigate multiple types of health services can be complicated and frustrating, particularly when parolees are not used to having to take responsibility for their own care. In the prison or jail setting, healthcare is provided as a matter of routine, within the context of regimented activities over which the inmate has no control. Once released, the parolee is faced with many tasks; engaging and meeting the demands of the parole system, finding housing, and obtaining employment are some of the priorities for most individuals that overshadow what can be serious health issues. The need for specialized programs such as drug rehabilitation may be a require-ment of parole and an essential component of re-entry. To address this challenge, policy-makers, healthcare providers, and families of offenders need to better understand the healthcare needs of those returning from prison, which communi-ties are dis-proportionately affected by re-entry, and strategies for responding to their needs.

Adoption of the public health model for understanding and facilitating the delivery of healthcare in correctional settings and for those released from corrections provides a context that promotes health agency collaboration, expansion of training opportunities for primary care, cost-effective distribution of scarce healthcare resources, and increased accessibility of health services to underserved and high-risk populations. Public health is about population health:

- Identifying healthcare problems (i.e., surveillance)

- Looking for causes (i.e., through the assessment of risk and protective factors)

- Determining what works and for whom (i.e., developing and evaluating interventions)

- Implementing healthcare plans through effective policy and programming

Through the implementation of primary, secondary, and tertiary prevention interventions, healthcare professionals are able to achieve maximum benefit for the largest number of people. The importance of correctional institutions collaborating with community partners such as health, education, social services, and vocational institutions to best meet the needs of offenders upon release, as well as the communities in which they will return, is fundamental to a public health model (Conklin et al., 1998; Patel et al., 2014; Restum, 2005; Rogers & Seigenthaler, 2001).

Case Study: Correctional Care

A 72-year-old male, with a history of sexual offending against pre-pubescent girls, is currently wheelchair-bound after suffering a stroke. He has limited mobility but has some use of one arm. The prison where he is incarcerated is unable to provide the care that he requires due to limited healthcare resources. His parole officer has applied for a medical parole on his behalf (also referred to as *compassionate release*), and arrangements are being made for his transfer to a local long-term care facility in the community.

Discussion questions:

- What are your thoughts and feelings about his pending transfer to a community-based long-term care facility?

- What are the perceived advantages of such a transfer?

- What barriers might he encounter?

- What information should be included in the nurse-to-nurse referral?

Summary

In therapeutic encounters with prisoners and ex-offenders, it is critical that nurses see the person as a person, and not the crime that was committed. Adopting a nonjudgmental, objective approach facilitates the creation of a safe and trusting relationship necessary for the assessment and implementation of effective interventions, both during incarceration and upon release into the community.

Individuals whose lives are enmeshed with the criminal justice system typically present with a myriad of long-neglected physical and mental healthcare challenges, traumatic life experiences, and communicable diseases often complicated by significant substance abuse problems. Helping ex-offenders to successfully transition to the community, facilitating relapse prevention plans, and assisting with their healthcare challenges are important roles for forensic nurses. Collaborative approaches that bring together policy-makers, healthcare providers, social services, community leaders, and family members are required to address the multitude of stressors and health challenges experienced during incarceration and upon release. Forensic nurses are uniquely situated to assume leadership roles in caring for this underserved population.

References

Almost, J., Doran, D., Ogilvie, L., Miller, C., Kennedy, S., Timmings, C., ... Brookey-Bassett, S. (2013). Exploring work-life issues in provincial correctional settings. *Journal of Forensic Nursing, 9*(1), 3–13.

American Nurses Association (ANA). (2013). *Correctional nursing: Scope and standards of practice* (2nd ed.). Silver Spring, MD: nursesbooks.org.

Binswanger, I. A., Stern, M. F., Deyo, R. A., Heagery, P. J., Cheadle, A., Elmore, J. G., & Koepsell, T. D. (2007). Release from prison: A high risk of death for former inmates. *New England Journal of Medicine, 356*(2), 157–165.

Canadian Public Health Association. (2004). A health care needs assessment of federal inmates. *Canadian Journal of Public Health, 95*(supplement 1), S1–S63.

Carmona, R. H. (2003). *Public safety is public health; Public health is public safety.* National Conference on Correctional Health Care, Austin, TX. Retrieved from http://www.surgeongeneral.gov/news/speeches/correctional10062003.html

Coalition of Correctional Health Authorities and the American Correctional Association. (2012). *Key Elements of the Affordable Care Act: Interface with correctional settings and inmate health care.* Retrieved from http://www.nga.org/files/live/sites/NGA/files/pdf/ACACCHAAffordableCareActMonograph.pdf

Conklin, R. J., Lincoln, R., & Flanigan, T. P. (1998). Notes from the field: A public health model to connect correctional health care with communities. *American Journal of Public Health, 88*(8), 1249–1250.

Correctional Service Canada. (2003). *Infectious diseases prevention and control in Canadian federal penitentiaries 2000–01* (Cat. No. 0-662-67144-9). Ottawa, ON: Author.

Davis, L. M., Nicosia, N., Overton, A., Miyashiro, L., Derose, K. P., Fain, T., ... Williams, E. (2009). *Understanding the public health implications of prisoner reentry in California: Phase I report.* Santa Monica, CA: RAND Corporation. Retrieved from http://www.rand.org/pubs/technical_reports/TR687

Dougherty, J. (2013). *Survey reveals barriers to successful ex-offender re-entry.* Retrieved from https://www.rit.edu/cla/criminaljustice/sites/rit.edu.cla.criminaljustice/files/docs/WorkingPapers/2013/Survey%20Reveals%20Barriers%20to%20Successful%20Ex-Offender%20Re-Entry.pdf

Duncan, G., & Zwemstra, J. C. (2014). Mental health in prison. In S. Enggist, L. Møller, G. Galea, & C. Udesen (Eds.), *Prisons and health* (pp. 87–95). Copenhagen, Denmark: World Health Organization. Retrieved from http://www.euro.who.int/__data/assets/pdf_file/0005/249188/Prisons-and-Health.pdf

Federal Bureau of Prisons. (2015, June 27). *Inmate statistics: Offenses.* Retrieved from http://www.bop.gov/about/statistics/statistics_inmate_offenses.jsp

Fisher, A. A., & Hatton, D. C. (2009). Women prisoners: Health issues and nursing implications. *Nursing Clinics of North America, 44*(3), 365–373. doi: 10.1016/j.cnur.2009.06.010

Fraser, A. (2014). Staff health and well-being in prisons: Leadership and training. In S. Enggist, L. Møller, G. Galea, & C. Udesen (Eds.), *Prisons and health* (pp. 185–189). Copenhagen, Denmark: World Health Organization. Retrieved from http://www.euro.who.int/__data/assets/pdf_file/0005/249188/Prisons-and-Health.pdf

Gaes, G. G., & Kendig, N. (2002). *The skill sets and health care needs of released offenders.* Federal Bureau of Prisons. Retrieved from http://aspe.hhs.gov/hsp/prison2home02/gaes.htm

Gatherer, A., Enggist, S., & Møller, L. (2014). The essentials about prisons. In S. Enggist, L. Møller, G. Galea, & C. Udesen (Eds.), *Prisons and health* (pp. 1–5). Copenhagen, Denmark: World Health Organization. Retrieved from http://www.euro.who.int/__data/assets/pdf_file/0005/249188/Prisons-and-Health.pdf

Glaze, L. E., & Maruschak, L. M. (2008). Parents in prison and their minor children. *Bureau of Justice Studies Special Report*. Retrieved from http://www.bjs.gov/content/pub/pdf/pptmc.pdf

Griel, L. C., & Loeb, S. J. (2009). Health issues faced by adolescents incarcerated in the juvenile justice system. *Journal of Forensic Nursing, 5*, 162–179.

Hammett, T. M., Roberts, C., & Kennedy, S. (2001). Health-related issues in prisoner re-entry. *Crime & Delinquency, 47*(3), 390–490.

Herbert, K., Plugge, E., Foster, C., & Doll, H. (2012). Prevalence of risk factors for non-communicable diseases in prison populations worldwide: A systematic review. *The Lancet, 379*, 1975–1982.

Hufft, A. G. (2013). Theoretical foundations for advanced practice nursing. In R. M. Hammer, B. Moynihan, & E. M. Pagliaro (Eds.), *Forensic nursing: A handbook for practice* (2nd ed.) (pp. 17–29). Burlington, MA: Jones & Bartlett.

James, N. (2014). Offender re-entry: Correctional statistics, reintegration into the community, and recidivism. *Congressional Research Service*. Report 7-5700 RL34287.

Lansing, A. E., Washburn, J. J., Abram, K. M., Thomas, U. C., Welty, L. J., & Teplin, L. A. (2014). Cognitive and academic functioning of juvenile detainees: Implications for correctional populations and public health. *Journal of Correctional Health Care, 20*(1), 18–30.

Mallik-Kane, K., & Visher, C.A. (2008). *Health and prisoner reentry: How physical, mental and substance abuse conditions shape the process of reintegration*. Washington, DC: Urban Institute Justice Policy Center. Retrieved from http://www.urban.org/sites/default/files/alfresco/publication-pdfs/411617-Health-and-Prisoner-Reentry.PDF

Montanari, L., Royuela, L., Pasinetti, M., Giraudon, I., Wiessing, L., & Vicente, J. (2014). Drug use and selected consequences among prison populations in European countries. In S. Enggist, L. Møller, G. Galea, & C. Udesen (Eds.), *Prisons and health* (pp. 107–112). Copenhagen, Denmark: World Health Organization. Retrieved from http://www.euro.who.int/__data/assets/pdf_file/0005/249188/Prisons-and-Health.pdf

National Commission on Correctional Health Care (NCCHC). (2008). *New option for initial health assessment. Spotlight on the Standards*. Retrieved from http://www.ncchc.org/spotlight-on-the-standards-22-2

National Institute on Drug Abuse. (2014). *Drug use, crime, and incarceration*. Retrieved from http://www.drugabuse.gov/related-topics/criminal-justice/drug-addiction-treatment-in-criminal-justice-system

Office of the Correctional Investigator. (2014). *Annual report of the Office of the Correctional*

Investigator 2013-2014. (No. PS100-2014E-PDF). Ottawa, ON: Her Majesty the Queen in Right of Canada. Retrieved from http://www.oci-bec.gc.ca/cnt/rpt/pdf/annrpt/annrpt20132014-eng.pdf

Patel, K., Boutwell, A., Brockmann, B. W., & Rich, J. D. (2014). Integrating correctional and community health care for formerly incarcerated people who are eligible for Medicaid. *Health Affairs, 33*(3), 468–473.

Patient Protection and Affordable Care Act. (2010). Retrieved from http://www.dpc.senate.gov/healthreformbill/healthbill04.pdf

Perry, R. C. W., & Morris, R. E. (2014). Healthcare for youth involved with the correctional system. *Primary Care: Clinics in Office Practice, 41*, 691–705.

Pew Center on the States. (2009). *One in 31: The long reach of American corrections*. Washington, DC: The Pew Charitable Trusts. Retrieved from http://www.convictcriminology.org/pdf/pew/onein31.pdf

Power, J., Brown, S. L., & Usher, A. M. (2013). Non-suicidal self-injury in women offenders: Motivations, emotions, and precipitating events. *International Journal of Forensic Mental Health, 12*, 192–204.

Restum, Z. G. (2005). Public health implications of substandard correctional health care. *American Journal of Public Health, 95*(10), 1689–1691.

Rogers, W. B., & Seigenthaler, C. P. (2001). Correctional health care as a vital part of community health. *Journal of Ambulatory Care Management, 24*(3), 45–50.

Rold, W. J. (2006). *Legal considerations in the delivery of health care services in prisons and jails*. In M. Puisis (Ed.), *Clinical practice in correctional medicine* (2nd ed.) (pp. 520–528). Philadelphia, PA: Mosby-Elsevier.

Royal College of Nursing (RCN). (2009). *Health and nursing care in the criminal justice service*. Retrieved from http://www.rcn.org.uk/development/nursing_communities/rcn_forums/prison_nurses

Schirmer, S., Nellis, A., & Mauer, M. (2009). *Incarcerated parents and their children: Trends 1991–2007*. Washington, DC: The Sentencing Project. Retrieved from http://www.sentencingproject.org/doc/publications/publications/inc_incarceratedparents.pdf

Schoenly, L. (Producer). (n.d.). Manipulation: A significant stressor for correctional nurses [audio podcast]. Retrieved from http://correctionalnurse.net/manipulation-a-significant-stressor/

Schoenly, L., & Knox, C. M. (2012). *Essentials of correctional nursing*. New York, NY: Springer Publishing.

State Reforum. (March 13, 2015). *Map: Where states stand on Medicaid expansion decisions*. Retrieved from https://www.statereforum.org/Medicaid-Expansion-Decisions-Map?gclid=CPiOyJn0qsQCFWQV7AodtH4AbQ van den Bergh, B., Gatherer, A., Fraser, A., & Møller, L. (2011). Imprisonment and women's health: Concerns about gender sensitivity, human rights and public health. *Bulletin of the World Health Organization, 89,* 689–694.

Walmsley, R. (2014a). *World female imprisonment list* (2nd ed.). Retrieved from International Centre for Prison Studies website: http://www.prisonstudies.org/sites/default/files/resources/downloads/wfil_2nd_edition.pdf

Walmsley, R. (2014b). *World prison population list* (10th ed.). Retrieved from International Centre for Prison Studies website: http://www.prisonstudies.org/sites/default/files/resources/downloads/wppl_10.pdf

Wang, E. A., Wang, Y., & Krumholz, H. M. (2013). A high risk of hospitalization following release from correctional facilities in Medicare beneficiaries: A retrospective matched cohort study, 2002 to 2010. *JAMA Internal Medicine, 173*(17), 1621–1628.

Williams, N. H. (2007). Prison health and the health of the public: Ties that bind. *Journal of Correctional Health Care, 13,* 80–92.

Wilper, A. P., Woolhandler, S., Boyd, J. W., Lasser, K. E., McCormick, D., Bor, D. H., & Himmelstein, D. U. (2009). The health and health care of US prisoners: Results of a nation-wide survey. *American Journal of Public Health, 99*(4), 666–672.

Wilson, A., & Tully, P. (2009). Reintegrating young offenders into the community through discharge planning: A review of interventions and needs of youth in secure care. *Australian Journal of Primary Health, 15,* 166–172.

Youth.Gov. (n.d.). *Children of incarcerated parents.* Retrieved from http://youth.gov/youth-topics/children-of-incarcerated-parents

FORENSIC DOCUMENTATION AND TESTIMONY

L. Kathleen Sekula, PhD, PMHCNS, FAAN

KEY POINTS IN THIS CHAPTER

- The first step in proper forensic documentation is assessing the patient and documenting observations.

- Maintaining a chain of custody is key to establishing the validity of evidence.

- Nurses must obtain consent from the victim for collection of evidence and photographs whenever possible.

- Nurses can also contribute to evidence collection without compromising patient care.

- The nurse may be called as a witness regarding any forensic case in which he or she is involved.

Nursing practice interfaces with law in many diverse settings. Proper assessment is a major responsibility of every nurse and is the very basis for all documentation. A systematic assessment includes objective observations and physical findings, and subjective data based on patient perceptions/input. A nurse's intuition may also play a part in the assessment and subsequent documentation of findings. A perceptive nurse may note problems that might otherwise be missed (Lynch, 2011). In addition, all data has to be documented objectively, clearly, and appropriately.

Much has been written about the importance of healthcare professionals helping the legal system by having a basic understanding of guidelines for evidence collection. Due to the type of patients who present in emergency departments as well as other areas in the healthcare setting, clinical nurses often care for victims of violence (McCracken, 1999; Randall, Colman, & Rowe, 2011). Regarding assessment for victimization, a multitude of instruments are available to measure self-harm, interpersonal violence, and child abuse. However, even though many valid and reliable tools and resources are available, this does not mean they are used in practice (Bond & French, 2010). For this reason, it's important that nurses take a leadership role in establishing guidelines for practice in which well-established tools are used in all areas of healthcare to screen for violence (Basile, Hertz, & Back, 2007b).

It's the position of the Emergency Nurses Association that the emergency nurse (Ferrell, 2007):

- Provides physical and emotional care to patients, and also helps preserve the evidentiary material collected in the emergency department

- Collaborates with emergency physicians, social service, and law enforcement personnel to develop guidelines for forensic evidence collection, preservation, and documentation in the emergency care setting

- Stays familiar with the concepts and skills of evidence collection, written and photographic documentation, as well as testifying in legal proceedings

This book provides many suggestions for how the nurse generalist can improve practice by learning some of the techniques of forensic science. This chapter explores the importance of collecting various types of evidence. In addition, the proper documentation of evidence and how the nurse may then be called upon to provide testimony in a case will be discussed.

Outlining the Types of Evidence

Evidence, both testimonial and physical, involves data presented to a court or jury to prove or disprove a claim. It includes any item or information that may be submitted and accepted by a competent court in order to determine the truth of any matter under investigation and can be informational or physical (Sullivan, 2011). Therefore, documentation, including written documentation or what is drawn on a body map by a nurse during the care of a patient, as well as physical evidence (photo documentation, DNA swabs, collection of clothing, etc.) collected by the nurse, can be used in a court proceeding to prove or disprove the merits of a case put forth on behalf of a client by a lawyer.

Testimonial Evidence

Testimonial evidence includes statements made under oath, what is said in court by a witness, and direct evidence. This includes eyewitness accounts, which are what someone saw or heard. A nurse may be called as a witness regarding what happened in the clinical setting while caring for a patient and to describe what he or she saw when the patient entered the hospital and any documentation related to the case.

Physical Evidence Collection

All nurses must learn the similarities and differences in evidence collection at times when a crime is suspected or in any case where a patient's condition warrants suspicion of the patient being a victim or a perpetrator of violence. Locard's principle of exchange sets the stage for understanding how and why evidence collection is so important in conducting scientific investigations. Dr. Edmond Locard (1877–1966), who was a pathologist in Lyon, France, conducted scientific investigations and researched the application of analytical methods to criminal investigations. His theory, that whenever there is contact between two surfaces there is an exchange of materials, was the basis for early evidence collection. Using this theory, the collection of such evidence can lead to the conviction of offenders. The advances that have taken place in processing DNA evidence provide the backdrop for the importance of understanding how every nurse can and should be cognizant of his or her potential role in collecting valuable evidence. We often forget that in addition to caring for the immediate physical problems of patients, we can also contribute to good evidence collection without compromising good care.

Physical evidence includes tangible evidence that can be touched; some of it may be recognized by sight, such as a gun, a knife, a document, or clothing. Types of physical evidence include the following (Lee & Harris, 2011):

- **Pattern evidence:** This evidence is seen in bloodstains, gunshot patterns, and other types of evidence that show a pattern. For example, when a patient who has suffered a gunshot wound enters the healthcare setting, clinicians must be careful to document what they see. Preserve the clothing and note injury patterns and blood patterns on the patient. Chapter 6, "Assessment of Wounds and Injury," provides a comprehensive review of injuries and how to document them appropriately.

- **Conditional evidence:** This evidence is observed at the scene, such as the condition of the room, whether lights are on or off, doors are open or shut, the position of the body, or the surrounding furniture. This information has to be recorded meticulously at the crime scene because the condition can change or be moved over time.

- **Transfer evidence:** This evidence comes under Locard's principle: evidence that results from two surfaces coming in contact with each other, including blood from one person being left behind on another person, fibers from one person's clothing or the person's hair fibers being left behind on a victim.

It can also include *trace* evidence, evidence that's found in small quantities and sometimes cannot be seen by the naked eye. It may include splinters of glass; skin cells; remnants of soil on a piece of clothing; a minute fiber particle; accelerant materials from a fire; and seminal fluid, traces of blood, or hair or fibers on a victim of sexual assault. It sometimes can be seen by microscope or with an alternate light source. In many cases of rape, DNA evidence is collected using cotton swabs on an area where the victim says the perpetrator touched her. While cells containing DNA may not be visible to the naked eye, nurses should try to collect the trace evidence wherever possible.

- **Transient evidence:** This evidence is physical evidence that is temporary in nature and can be easily changed or lost. It's evidence that can degrade or disappear, such as an odor, moisture, temperature, or imprints. It's imperative that such evidence be observed and recorded immediately.

Understanding Basic Principles of Forensic Documentation

While the crime scene is not usually the healthcare setting, the victim or perpetrator may present at the healthcare setting immediately after the crime has occurred. When properly recognized, documented, and preserved, a nurse may be an important link to appropriate outcomes in the legal system when patient cases are linked to legal implications. It's the astute and questioning nurse who will "see" things that others may not pick up on. When that happens, it is of utmost importance that a nurse follows that intuition and assesses and collects evidence whenever possible. In addition to collecting the evidence, the nurse must understand the importance of documenting properly.

Assessing and Documenting Evidence

The first step in evidence collection is the documentation of how and when the patient arrived, and the condition in which the patient arrived. When possible, take photographs of the patient and specific injuries before the patient receives medical treatment (Saferstein, 2011). One should record exactly what is observed and as objectively as possible.

In order to document properly, one must first be able to assess properly. Assessment has always been a key to the nursing process, which includes a head-to-toe assessment, past history of medical issues, and any previous information from other sources that are available. In recent years, nurses have been mandated to assess all incoming patients for current abuse. A routine screening about safety is required to be asked of all patients upon admission to any federally funded healthcare setting. There are several tools that can be used for this purpose, but the tools are only as good as the person who is asking the questions. Every nurse must become comfortable asking the questions in a gentle, non-threatening way. Find out what works best for you when asking a patient if she is in an abusive situation. The nurse's demeanor and the way she asks the questions can affect whether a patient is comfortable revealing abuse. For example, if a nurse states, "We have to ask this question of all persons coming into the hospital. Are you a victim of abuse?" and she asks the question without looking at the patient but looking at her notes, she is not as likely to elicit information. In contrast, by saying, "In this health service, we are concerned about your health and safety, so we ask all women the same questions about violence at home. This is because violence is very common and we want to try to help anyone experiencing violence. Is there anyone in your life you are afraid of hurting you?" This opens up the conversation for the patient to discuss anyone who might be threatening or harming her. There are many ways to ask the questions; becoming comfortable asking the questions is a key factor in the process of questioning.

Many tools and instruments that aid in forensic data collection are well-designed and have been researched in order to establish validity and reliability (Basile, Hertz, & Back, 2007a). Table 16.1 lists just a few of the tools available for intimate partner violence (IPV) and sexual violence.

TABLE 16.1 INTIMATE PARTNER VIOLENCE AND SEXUAL VIOLENCE VICTIMIZATION ASSESSMENT INSTRUMENTS

Scale/Assessment *Developer	Characteristics	Administration
Abuse Assessment Screen (AAS) *McFarlane, Parker, Soeken, & Bullock, 1992	5 items assess frequency and perpetrator of physical, sexual, and emotional abuse by anyone; body map to document area of injury	Clinician administered
American Medical Association Screening Questions *American Medical Association, 1992	10 sample items inquire about physical, sexual, and emotional IPV to be asked in physician's own words	Physician or clinician administered
Danger Assessment *Campbell, 1986	15 items assess a woman's potential danger of homicide by an intimate male partner; available in English and Spanish	Self report
Domestic Violence Initiative Screening Questions *Queensland Government, 1998	6 items assess physical and emotional IPV and desire for professional assistance	Clinician administered
Emergency Department Domestic Violence Screening Questions *Morrison, Allan, & Grunfeld, 2000	5 items assess violence in the home	Self report
Minnesota Tool *md4peace@earthlink.net	13 items and color-coded stickers assess physical, emotional, and sexual IPV	Self report
Ongoing Violence Assessment Tool (OVAT) *Weiss, Ernst, Cham, & Nick, 2003	4 items assess ongoing physical and emotional IPV	Self report
Partner Violence Screen (PVS) *Feldhaus, Koziol-McLain, Amsbury, Norton, Lowenstein, & Abbott, 1997	3 items assess physical IPV in the last year and current safety	Clinician administered

Basile et al.'s excellent compilation of tools (2007a) provides current psychometric properties of established tools and provides information for clinicians to make informed decisions regarding which instruments are most appropriate for use in a given population. The tools are meant to assist in providing better care for all patients entering the healthcare system and to provide tools to improve and facilitate practice. Once completed, the tools can be included in the chart/medical record as part of documentation.

Other tools are available as well:

- **Child abuse:** Several resources are available that identify outstanding tools for screening for abuse of children. Chapter 11, "Child Maltreatment," covers these tools.

- **Military service:** Military service can be a significant factor in caring for veterans, whether they have served active duty or not. Learning more about the veteran can inform treatment planning and increase the healthcare worker's understanding of the challenges veterans face. Clinicians may access the Community Provider Toolkit: Serving Veterans Through Partnership at the following link: http://www.mentalhealth.va.gov/communityproviders/#sthash. uqPFr2h0.dpbs

- **Self-harm risk:** Self-harm risk is a common problem seen in emergency department settings (Randall et al., 2011). However, to date there is no well-established tool to measure its risk (Quinlivan et al., 2014). The Self Harm Inventory, developed by Sansone and Sansone (2010), is one self-harm inventory that is currently being tested.

The specific types of assessment of forensic nurses vary related to their roles, but all nurses must have basic skills that serve to support the patient in any circumstance. Much of the current literature related to assessment for victimization of violence relates to specific populations (Newton, 2013).

Obtaining Consent to Document

Consent is a major consideration when collecting evidence. Whenever possible, consent from the victim for collection of evidence and photographs taken must be obtained.

Delay with evidence collection can make it more difficult to secure evidence, which ultimately affects the prosecution of the case. In the general healthcare settings, the concerns are the same: where and how to collect the evidence when the victim is unable to consent to evidence collection. Currently there is much debate regarding whether evidence can (may) be collected in instances when consent cannot be obtained. For example, in a case where an unconscious woman who was brutally beaten presents at the emergency department via ambulance and appears to have been raped, it then becomes an important question: Is it okay to collect evidence without her consent? Or should the collection of evidence be delayed until the patient is able to give consent?

The decision as to whether to collect evidence or not in an unconscious patient depends on two considerations (Chasson, 2011):

■ Will the evidence be lost if the clinician waits until the person is conscious?

■ Could the collection of evidence be considered assault and battery once the patient becomes conscious and decides against having the evidence collected?

In some states, the guidelines say that if "a reasonable person would conclude that exigent circumstances justify conducting a forensic examination," then a nurse may collect evidence in an unconscious patient. For instance, in the state of Virginia (SB 205), the law states:

> A judge is allowed to approve the collection of evidence when a sexual assault is suspected, from an adult unable to make an informed decision;
> a minor, 14 years or older, is permitted to consent to a forensic evidence exam for suspected sexual assault; and,
> the collection of forensic evidence from a minor child is allowed without the consent of a parent or guardian.

In some cases, a court order can be obtained. However, each healthcare setting should have protocols in place that address these issues, and hospital legal counsel and ethics committees should be involved with the creation of protocols.

Who can, and should, make the decision, and how do generalist nurses know what their role entails? Of greatest importance is that you know the laws within your state of practice. If not, then know where to seek out that information when needed; preferably, before it is needed.

The nurse clinician may request a forensic nurse, if available, to take over the collection of evidence when a patient presents in any department and it is suspected that that patient is a victim of violence. If a forensic nurse is not available, a nurse should use his or her best judgment in collecting the evidence. Documentation includes written documentation, photo documentation, and the collection of physical evidence.

Identification and documentation of wounds is covered in Chapter 6.

PHOTOGRAPHING EVIDENCE

Forensic photographs can play a pivotal role in the medical documentation of injuries in all forms of interpersonal violence and can be used in a court proceeding. The photograph is a visual representation of observed injury. Written documentation should accompany the photographs. If called to serve as a witness in the case, the nurse can testify that the photographs are true and accurate depictions of the wounds that the nurse observed the day of care.

Digital cameras are now the gold standard for forensic photography, and every hospital should establish policies that provide clear guidelines for how to store and document photographs (Sheridan, Nash, Hawkins, Makely, & Campbell, 2013). These authors created a list of factors that should be taken into consideration when taking forensic photographs:

- **Lighting:** Use as much natural light as possible. Fluorescent lights can cast a green hue on photographs. Show the detail of each photograph as clearly as possible.

- **Scales:** Use a scale in the photographs to show the extent (size) of the injury.

- **Sequence:** Always begin with a full-body photograph followed by a mid-distance photograph and then by a closeup.

- **Labels:** Be sure to place identifying information on the photographs (patient name, hospital number, date of birth, date and time the photo was taken, and the name of the photographer).

- **No deletions:** Keep all photographs, even the ones that do not turn out. It's important to be able to document that no photographs were disposed of.

- **Consent:** A signed consent should be obtained for photography by the victim or by a qualified surrogate. Sometimes the victim is unable to consent, but the clinician recognizes that the injuries are/may be related to a potential forensic issue that may have to be litigated. In those cases, the clinician may take the photographs and obtain consent later (Pasqualone, 1996).

What is most important here is that the nurse understands that she or he can play a positive role in the outcome of a case by being proactive and collecting what photographs can be collected. You don't need to be a professional photographer. Just photograph what you see and what instincts lead the clinician to think that this case may involve forensic issues. Once the photographs are taken, properly label and store them, maintaining the chain of custody so that property security can be testified to in the courtroom.

PACKAGING EVIDENCE

Evidence should be packaged in such a way that there is no question as to whether anyone has tampered with the evidence or affected it in any way. Some important things to remember when packaging evidence:

- **Clothing:** Each item of clothing should be collected and placed in a separate paper bag to avoid cross-contamination. If wet, the clothing should be dried before packaging, or placed in a plastic bag to avoid leakage and cross-contamination until the clothing can be hung and dried and then placed in a paper bag. Bacterial or mold growth can occur if items are not dried. Any patterns of stains or cuts or holes should be noted, and the patterns must be preserved for further analysis. Do not cut through any defects in the fabric. If you must cut clothing off of a patient, cut in a place where patterns are not evident (Cabelus & Spangler, 2013).

- **Weapons:** Safety is always a concern. Whether it be a victim or a perpetrator, the nurse must document and, whenever possible, photograph weapons that are found on an incoming patient. Security measures must be taken to secure the weapon in order to protect staff and others in the facility (Cabelus & Spangler, 2013).

- **Common errors in documentation:** Common errors in documentation may make all the difference in the outcome of the court case. Sloppy jargon, confusing abbreviations (or acronyms) and statements, vague descriptions, and lack of clarity can make the difference in the outcome of a trial (Cabelus & Spangler, 2013). Information as it's reported directly by the patient should be included. Do not edit the patient's statements or omit interventions provided, and record all observations in a timely fashion. Late entries can call the nurse's actions into question.

- **Chain of custody:** Documents record the handling of evidence as it moves from the location where it was collected and ultimately to the laboratory where it will be processed and then presented in court. The documents must provide a paper trail of each change of location of the evidence, dates when it is moved and by whom, and who is responsible for the evidence at each time point. This involves proper packaging and sealing of the evidence. Sexual assault evidence collection kits have a place to record the chain of custody on the box, and most hospitals have a chain of custody document that is used in their facility. The fewer people handling the evidence, the better, because the more people handling the evidence, the more mistakes can be made. This documentation is most likely to be requested at the time of trial in order to establish that no one has tampered with the evidence.

The nurse working in the hospital and community setting is not expected to be an expert in forensic care of patients. However, given the prevalence of violence in society, all clinicians must make themselves aware of warning signs that a patient may actually be a victim of violence. And at the point where they become suspicious of forensic aspects of care, each clinician should perform to the best of his or her abilities in documenting the case and collecting whatever evidence he or she is able to collect.

PREPARING FOR COURT TESTIMONY

Nurses may be called as a witness regarding any forensic case in which they are involved. With all of this said, it must be stressed that the nurse can make a difference in the lives of patients by attending to the important aspects of a case when a patient presents in the healthcare setting with forensic issues. Many nurses are concerned about what might happen if they are subpoenaed to testify in a court case. First, you should remember you're being asked to testify to the facts. You can only testify to what you observed and documented. If documentation was well done, you only have to refer to those original documents before testifying. It's not within your purview as a nurse to determine "what happened," but only to document what is seen and heard once the patient presents in the healthcare system. The evidence will speak for itself.

These tips can help nurses prepare for testifying. And while it's to be expected that testifying is stressful—especially the first time—there are tips on how to ease the process. Remember that it's an important role that nurses can provide. Nurses are often the first to see a victim of an assault and therefore can offer first-hand documentation of what they observe and the evidence they collect.

■ If the lawyer who subpoenaed you doesn't ask to meet with you before the trial, ask him/her to meet with you to discuss what is expected of you.

- Read over all documents to which you will be testifying. This will refresh your memory.

- Dress professionally and comfortably.

- Be on time and prepared.

- When answering questions on the stand, take your time and answer only to what you know.

- Listen carefully to the question and if you do not understand it, ask the lawyer to repeat the question or to clarify the question.

- Make eye contact with the lawyer who is addressing you.

- If you do not know an answer, just state that fact.

- If you can't remember something from the documents, ask to refer to the document. Don't make any guesses.

- Do not become intimidated if the opposing lawyer appears to be "badgering" you. It's not personal. He is just doing his job.

- If an objection is raised, stop speaking and wait for the judge's decision.

- If you feel you cannot answer a question with a simple "yes" or "no," ask the judge if you can clarify your answer.

- You are there to state the facts of what you observed, evidence collected, and what you documented. Nothing else.

- Remain calm and composed throughout your testimony. Do not let the opposing counsel unnerve you. Take a deep breath when questioned and take your time answering.

SUMMARY

This chapter has stressed the importance of the nurse in forensic cases in which s/he is involved. Objective and accurate assessment, documentation, and collection of evidence are of utmost importance when dealing with forensic issues, as the nurse's documentation may be used later in court proceedings. Proper consent procedures, proper collection of various types of evidence, maintenance of the chain of custody of the evidence, and preparing to testify in court are major considerations when caring for the forensic patient. Never forget that your role is an important one and one that can make a difference in the lives of those involved in the case.

REFERENCES

American Medical Association. (1992). Diagnosis and treatment guidelines on domestic violence. Chicago, IL: American Medical Association.

Basile, K. C., Hertz, M. F., & Back, S. E. (2007a). Intimate partner violence and sexual violence vctimization assessment instruments for use in healthcare settings: Version 1. for Injury Prevention and Control; 2007. Atlanta, GA: Centers for Disease Control and Prevention, National Center for Injury Prevention and Control.

Basile, K. C., Hertz, M. F., & Back, S. E. (2007b). Intimate partner violence and sexual violence victimization assessment instruments for use in healthcare settings. Centers for Disease Control and Prevention. National Center for Injury Prevention and Control.

Bond, P., & French, J. (2010). Implementing online tools and resources to help nurses apply evidence based care. *Nurs Times, 106*(1), 20–22.

Cabelus, N. B., & Spangler, K. (2013). Evidence Collection and Documentation. In R. M. Hammer, B. Moynihan, & E. M. Pagliaro (Eds.), *Forensic nursing: A handbook for practice* (2nd ed., pp. 261–284). Burlington, MA: Jones & Bartlett.

Campbell, J. C. (1986). Nursing assessment for risk of homicide with battered women. *Advances in Nursing Science, 8*, 36–51.

Chasson, S. (2011). Legal and ethical issues in forensic nursing roles. In V. A. Lynch & J. B. Duval (Eds.), *Forensic nursing science* (2nd ed., pp. 537–543). St. Louis, MO: Elsevier.

Family Violence Prevention Fund (2003). Interpersonal Violence New Tool for Identification in Health Care Settings, Health Alert, 9, 8–9. Contact Dr. David McCollum at md4peace@earthlink.net.

Feldhaus, K. M., Koziol-McLain, J., Amsbury, H. L., Norton, I. M., Lowenstein, S. R., & Abbot, J. T. (1997). Accuracy of 3 brief screening questions for detecting partner violence in the emergency department. *Journal of the American Medical Association, 277,* 1357–1361.

Ferrell, J. J. (2007). Forensic aspects of emergency nursing. In K. S. Hoyt & J. Selfridge-Thomas (Eds.), *Emergency nursing core curriculum* (6th ed., pp. 1025–1032). St Louis, MO: Saunders.

Hammer, R. M., Moynihan, B., & Pagliaro, E. M. (Eds.). (2013). *Forensic nursing: A handbook for practice* (Vol. 1). Burlington, MA: Jones & Bartlett.

Lee, H. C., & Harris, H. A. (2011). *Physical evidence in forensic science* (3rd ed.). Tucson, AZ: Lawyers and Judges Publishing.

Lynch, V. A. (2011). Evolution of forensic nursing science. In V. A. Lynch & J. B. Duval (Eds.), *Forensic nursing science* (2nd ed., pp. 1–9). St. Louis, MO: Elsevier.

McCracken, L. (1999). Living forensics: A natural evolution in emergency care. *Accident and Emergency Nursing, 7*(4), 211–216.

McFarlane, J., Parker, B., Soeken, K., & Bullock, L. (1992). Assessing for abuse during pregnancy: Severity and frequency of injuries and associated entry into prenatal care. *Journal of the American Medical Association, 267,* 3176–3178.

Morrison, L. J., Allan, R., & Grunfeld, A. (2000). Improving the emergency department detection rate of domestic violence using direct questioning. *The Journal of Emergency Medicine, 19,* 117–124.

Newton, M. (2013). The forensic aspects of sexual violence. *Best practice & research. Clinical obstetrics & gynaecology, 27*(1), 77–90.

Pasqualone, G. (1996). Forensic RNs as photographers: Documentation in the ED. *Journal of Psychosocial Nursing, 34*(10), 47–51.

Queensland Government (1998). Domestic violence initiative screening tool, from http://www.adfvc.unsw.edu.au/PDF%20files/screening_final.pdf

Quinlivan, L., Cooper, J., Steeg, S., Davies, L., Hawton, K., Gunnell, D., & Kapur, N. (2014). Scales for predicting risk following self-harm: An observational study in 32 hospitals in England. *BMJ Open* 2014; 4:e004732. doi: 10.1136/bmjopen-2013-004732

Randall, J. R., Colman, I., & Rowe, B. H. (2011). A systematic review of psychometric assessment of self-harm risk in the emergency department. *Journal of Affective Disorders, 134* (1–3), 348–355. doi: 10.1016/j.jad.2011.05.032

Saferstein, R. (2011). Principles of forensic evidence collection and preservation. In V. A. Lynch & J. B. Duval (Eds.), *Forensic nursing science* (2nd ed., pp. 55–60). St. Louis, MO: Elsevier.

Sansone, R. A., & Sansone, L. A. (2010). Measuring self-harm behavior with the Self-Harm Inventory. *Psychiatry (Edgmont), 7*(4), 16–20.

Sheridan, D. J., Nash, C. R., Hawkins, S. L., Makely, J. L., & Campbell, J. C. (2013). Forensic implications of intimate partner violence. In R. M. Hammer, B. Moynihan, & E. M. Pagliaro (Eds.), *Forensic nursing: A handbook for practice* (pp. 129–144). Burlington, MA: Jones & Bartlett.

Sullivan, M. K. (2011). Forensic investigations in the hospital. In V. A. Lynch & J. B. Duval (Eds.), *Forensic nursing science* (2nd ed., pp. 134–143). St. Louis, MO: Elsevier.

Virginia Senate Bill 205, Forensic evidence; delay in collecting for sexual assault cases. Legis. (2012).

Weiss, S. J., Ernst, A. A., Cham, E., & Nick, T. G. (2003). Development of a screen for ongoing intimate partner violence. *Violence and Victims, 18*, 131–141.

17

TRAUMA-INFORMED CARE

Angela F. Amar, PhD, RN, FAAN; and
Annie Lewis-O'Connor, PhD, NP-BC, MPH, FAAN

"I am not what happened to me; I am what I choose to become."

–C. G. Jung

KEY POINTS IN THIS CHAPTER

- A trauma-informed system has an organizational structure and treatment framework for understanding, recognizing, and responding to the effects of trauma.

- Examining common practices in many healthcare facilities can reveal areas that aren't sensitive to trauma experiences and that can exacerbate mental health responses to trauma.

- Implementation of a trauma-informed care approach requires collaboration and input at all levels of the healthcare system with the goal of meeting health needs and empowering survivors.

Increasingly more individuals, families, and communities experience violence and the devastating aftermath. The experience of violence and trauma alters one's emotional and physical growth, perceptions, responses, and often behavior. Experiencing childhood trauma places one at risk for mental illnesses such as depression, anxiety, post-traumatic stress disorder, alcohol and drug abuse, and personality disorders and for physical health conditions such as cardiovascular disease, lung and liver disease, hypertension, diabetes, asthma, and obesity (Felitti et al., 1998). A report from a United Kingdom correctional facility revealed that 27% of prisoners experienced abuse as a child and 41% observed violence in the home as a child (Williams, Papadopoulou, & Booth, 2012). Additionally, 90% of individuals seeking public mental healthcare and 75% of substance abuse treatment seekers report trauma exposure (Jennings, 2004). The consequences of trauma increase the likelihood that these individuals will seek healthcare in a variety of settings. A recognition and understanding of trauma and its effects is important for optimal patient care. The purpose of this chapter is to define and describe principles of trauma-informed care. It also includes strategies, barriers, and solutions to implementing trauma-informed care.

Individuals who experience trauma develop strategies and resiliency that enable them to continue to function and to manage the trauma. Many of these behaviors appear dysfunctional in other contexts. For example, substance use can provide respite from the trauma, but it can lead to abuse and addiction. Similarly, hypervigilance and hyperawareness help one remain alert to prevent further abuse; these behaviors can also place strains on interpersonal relationships. Sensitivity to touch and not feeling safe can negatively influence healthcare experiences. Although many of the individuals that nurses routinely encounter in their professional practices have experienced trauma, nurses are often unaware of the cumulative effect of trauma. Trauma and undisclosed history of exposure to violence can complicate nursing care and treatment plans.

Trauma-informed care (TIC) is an overarching framework that emphasizes the effects of trauma and guides the entire organization and behavior of individuals in the system (Hopper, Bassuk, & Olivet, 2010). Individuals include patients and staff that experience that organization. Treatment facilities have to consider how trauma could affect parts of their practice, analyze the effect of the environment on trauma survivors, and move to providing trauma-sensitive services.

Understanding Trauma and Trauma-Informed Care

Over the past several years, trauma-informed care (TIC) has emerged as a foundational framework from which to approach all healthcare services.

Trauma and Its Impact

Trauma causes emotional or physical harm to the affected individual and impairs the individual's emotional, social, spiritual, physical, and/or mental wellbeing. Usually a set of circumstances or events, or even one event in particular, can cause an individual to experience trauma. According to the Substance Abuse and Mental Health Services Administration (SAMHSA), trauma can have life-threatening and lasting effects on children and adult survivors (SAMHSA, 2014). A child who is abused may not master the developmental tasks of his or her age and of subsequent stages. The social, emotional, and cognitive effects can be seen in the short and long term.

Trauma exposure is pervasive across the healthcare system and includes both patients and staff. According to the Adverse Childhood Experiences (ACE) Study, over 63% of individuals have experienced at least one form of childhood trauma (Felitti et al., 1998). Trauma has significant physical and mental health effects, and greatly influences how people access and experience healthcare. If providers and healthcare organizations and systems do not consider or understand the impact of trauma, healthcare services can be retraumatizing; treatments may not be effective, and patients may not be able to engage.

Trauma can be individual or collective in nature:

■ *Individual trauma* is the experience of an event or an enduring condition in which an individual's coping capacity is overwhelmed, causing significant distress. Examples of such events or conditions include but are not limited to actual or threatened death, serious injury, and sexual or psychological violation or threat. Individual trauma happens to one person.

■ *Collective trauma* refers to the cultural, historical, insidious, and political/economic trauma that affects individuals and communities across generations. Collective trauma happens to groups or communities.

A Systemic Approach: Trauma-Informed Care Systems

Trauma-informed care (TIC) provides an organizational context for understanding, recognizing, and responding to the effects of all types of trauma. An awareness of the prevalence of trauma necessitates that treatment and care facilities be supportive of healing and not create further harm. Health providers often unintentionally retraumatize trauma survivors. A trauma-informed system designs services that accommodate the vulnerabilities of trauma survivors and promotes service delivery in a manner that avoids inadvertent retraumatization and facilitates patient participation in treatment (Jennings, 2004). By incorporating knowledge about trauma in all aspects of service delivery, treatment minimizes revictimization and facilitates recovery and empowerment. Providers using this systemic approach deliver trauma-specific diagnostic and treatment services within a trauma-informed environment capable of sustaining these services and supporting positive outcomes.

The implementation of trauma-informed care is most successful when it emanates through all areas of the organization, specifically from the highest levels. All staff of an organization, from the receptionist to direct care workers to the board of directors, must understand how violence affects people, so that every interaction is consistent with the recovery process and reduces the possibility of retraumatization (Harris & Fallot, 2001).

Trauma-specific services are designed to treat the actual consequences of physical and sexual abuse (Jennings, 2004). Integrated services include these core areas:

- Outreach and engagement

- Screening and assessment

- Resource coordination and advocacy

- Crisis intervention

- Mental health and substance abuse services

- Trauma-specific services, parenting support, and healthcare

The healthcare system's recognition of the long-term and pervasive impact of trauma validates the survivors' experiences and the difficulties faced in seeking services. The validation increases survivors' sense of hope and safety. Staff working in a trauma-informed system must understand the effects of traumatic life events on individual development, the common coping strategies and adaptations used by survivors, and effective treatment approaches and tools. Staff must self-reflect on how trauma and violence have affected their own lives. Creating a trauma-informed system will require approaches at the individual and system level.

GUIDING PRINCIPLES AND VALUES OF TRAUMA-INFORMED CARE

Implementing a trauma-informed system begins with administrative leadership and requires reconceptualization of the values of the organization. Elliott and colleagues (Elliott, Bjelajac, Fallot, Markoff, & Reed, 2005) provide 10 principles developed by consensus that reflect the values and practices that define a trauma-informed service organization:

- Recognize the impact of violence and victimization on development and coping strategies

- Identify recovery from trauma as a primary goal

- Employ an empowerment model

- Strive to maximize a patient's choice and control over his or her recovery

- Base services in a relational corroboration

- Create an atmosphere that is respectful of survivors' need for safety, respect, and acceptance

- Emphasize patients' strengths, highlighting adaptation over symptoms and resilience over pathology

- Set a goal of minimizing possibilities of retraumatization

- Strive to be culturally competent and to understand each patient in the context of his or her life experiences and cultural background

- Solicit patient input and involve patients in designing and evaluating services

A system that recognizes the effects of violence and victimization validates the experiences of the patients served. This validation and recognition increases the survivor's sense of security and safety. Incorporating trauma questions into the assessment and training staff on best practices for assessment conveys an understanding and recognition of trauma that validates the patients' experiences. The staff recognizes that many behaviors were developed as a means of coping with the trauma. An understanding of the importance of trauma requires provision and integration of services and referrals that promote recovery from trauma.

An empowerment and strength-based model leads to a partnership between the survivor and the provider. This model increases the client's ability to take charge of her life and to have control and choice over her actions. Despite attempts to partner with patients, healthcare systems often exert a patriarchal position with patients. The emphasis on provider as expert can remove choice and agency from patients. An empowerment model attempts to enable patients to make decisions and staff to support this process. A care philosophy of maximizing the survivor's choices and control over the treatment process helps him to regain power and control of his life choices.

Survivors should be involved in designing treatment services and be part of an ongoing evaluation of those services. They can be on an advisory board that reviews program design, serve as paid patient specialists, or participate in focus groups and/or regular forums about how to respond to program evaluations and improve services. Guidelines for creating patient advisory councils can be found at the Institute for Patient- and Family-Centered Care (www.ipfcc.org).

FOSTERING TRUSTING RELATIONSHIPS

Interpersonal trauma occurs in relationships. Interpersonal trauma includes intimate partner violence, child maltreatment, sexual abuse, etc. It differs from the experience of trauma resulting from violence by an unknown assailant. The relationship of the survivor and the perpetrator means that the two were connected and that trust was broken and the relationship betrayed. Therefore, the subsequent healing must also occur within relationships. Many trauma survivors have not had warm and trusting relationships. They have felt betrayed, abused, and used by those that they love. For full healing to occur, survivors must learn that others can be trusted and that relationships can be healthy. The staff creates a safe environment by developing relationships with survivors that are consistent, predictable, nonviolent, and free of shame and blame. The staff and patient/client relationship has an inherent power imbalance. Nurses must recognize that survivors' past relationships have involved an abuse of power and control. When the survivor is in situations that feel like there is a loss of power and control, it becomes untenable. It is important for staff to stress that the client has the right to decline answering questions, decline treatment, or request an alternative treatment.

CREATING A SAFE ENVIRONMENT

Survivors should perceive the physical space as safe, welcoming, and respectful. A welcoming environment includes sufficient space for comfort and privacy, and the absence of exposure to violent or sexual material (magazines in waiting area). Further, given the commonality of violence, healthcare organizations must work to ensure a safe environment for everyone, including staff, patients, and their families. Healthcare systems and services often focus intently on problems, making it easy to miss the survivors' strengths. The medical model highlights pathology and inadvertently gives the impression that there is something wrong with the person rather than an understanding that something wrong was done to the person. Understanding a symptom as an adaptation reduces the client's guilt and shame, increases self-esteem, and provides a guideline for developing new skills and resources. Another commonly missed strength is the person's capacity to serve in valued social roles. Despite problems, a survivor can still serve as parent, employee, neighborhood organizer, and so on. It is important to recognize the strengths that come from these multiple roles and to ensure that patients appreciate their strengths. These varied roles bring skills that survivors can use in the recovery process and that can be highlighted in order to increase the survivors' self-concept.

The goal is to minimize the possibilities of retraumatization. Routine health and dental care have the potential to trigger feelings of an unsafe situation and loss of control over one's body. Invasive procedures can trigger trauma-related symptoms. Once providers recognize this, they can work on strategies to avoid revictimization and promote self-caring activities for the patient. For example, the nurse informs the survivor of what will occur before and during the procedure, and helps the survivor to maintain a sense of safety and control. Other actions by providers can parallel interpersonal dynamics that trigger memories of abuse.

ACCEPTING CULTURAL DIFFERENCES

Cultural competence helps the nurse to fully understand each survivor in the context of life experiences and cultural background. Cultural competency includes having the knowledge and skill to work within the client's culture, and understanding how the nurse's cultural background and the program influence interactions with the client. Healing takes place within the survivor's cultural context and support network. Understanding cultural norms and values for each individual helps us to develop a treatment plan that respects his uniqueness and that uses this to assist the patient. Different cultural groups have unique resources that support healing. For example, some cultures rely on faith more than problem-solving; other cultures promote autonomy rather than community approaches to handling adversity (McGoldrick, Giordano, & Garcia-Preto, 2005). Cultural competence does not require the nurse to know everything about each cultural group; rather, the nurse recognizes the uniqueness of each person and seeks to understand by asking questions relevant to one's culture. Relevant questions include "What kinds of foods do you eat? What are activities your family would do together?" The nurse tries to understand survivors' experiences and responses through the lens of cultural context.

DEVELOPING A TRAUMA-INFORMED CARE SYSTEM

A discussion of organizational implementation must first consider the traditional systems and the barriers to implementing trauma-informed care. Trauma-informed systems are differentiated from other systems of care by philosophy, power and control, authority and responsibility, goals, and language (Harris & Fallot, 2001):

- In traditional systems the staff hold disproportionate power and control.

- Trauma-informed systems use an empowerment and strength-based model that values collaboration and shares power and control with the survivor and promotes autonomy.

A trauma-informed system helps providers shift the focus from what is wrong with a patient to what has happened to this patient. In systems without trauma-informed care, individuals are labeled as pathological with terms such as manipulative, needy, attention-seeking, and non-compliant. Systems without trauma-informed care have higher rates of staff and patient assault and injury; lower treatment adherence; higher rates of adult, child/family complaints; higher rates of staff turnover; lower morale; longer lengths of stay; and increased recidivism (Chandler, 2008; Fallot & Harris, 2002).

Stigma, lack of staff education, lack of trauma sensitivity, lack of common experience, and resistance to change are common barriers (Hodgdon, Kinniburgh, Gabowitz, Blaustein, & Spinazzola, 2013; Latham, Dollard, Robst, & Armstrong, 2010). Trauma-informed systems of care require educating staff at all levels, including the effects of and principal standards of trauma-informed care (Steele, 2009).

Trauma-informed care requires sustained effort. Key areas to consider are discussed in the following sections.

ADMINISTRATIVE COMMITMENT TO CHANGE

Administrative commitment to change ensures that those who control resources are on board (Harris & Fallot, 2001). Key administrators can ensure that all staff are trained and that trauma-informed practices are rewarded and integrated throughout the system (Cook et al., 2005; Fallot & Harris, 2002). Having a dedicated committee or working group ensures that the process of implementation advances within an organization.

UNIVERSAL APPROACH TO SCREENING PATIENTS

Universal screening and awareness for traumatic exposures should be the standard of practice in all clinical settings. Screening should be conducted in both inpatient and outpatient settings. When patients have been admitted to the hospital, it's important to assess soon after admission so that the plan of care can be individualized. Gathering clinically relevant information about violence and trauma in the lives of patients enables providers to determine immediate danger and needs. The provider is careful to elicit only information needed to plan care and not potentially traumatize or trigger the survivor by asking unnecessary questions and details. Staff would use screening measures to determine histories of violence and victimization as well as symptoms of depression and post-traumatic stress disorder (Ursano, Benedek, & Engel, 2012). Trauma screening helps to determine any imminent danger and documents the patient's response and the need for referrals. A positive screen for trauma is followed by an in-depth assessment of trauma and its response. Examples of questions to ask during an in-depth assessment are:

- "I would like to ask you some questions about your childhood and young adult years. Are you okay with that? If at any point you choose to stop, please just let me know."

- "Have you had any events in your life that you feel have had an impact on your health and wellbeing?"

- "Can you share with me two things you wish you could change about your years as a young adult? Your years as a child?"

- "Is there anything else you want to share with me that would help to make you comfortable during your hospitalization [healthcare visit]?"

STAFF REVIEW OF POLICIES AND PROCEDURES

Because all staff interact with consumers in some manner, everyone needs to receive education and training on trauma care (Harris & Fallot, 2001). Perhaps the best course of action is to have all staff receive education during orientation and over time annually or when needed. Organizations may also consider hiring a few individuals who are already sensitive and trained who can serve as champions. These champions can influence treatment teams and guide specific interventions, in part by helping them to consider the connection between behaviors and symptoms and abuse (Harris & Fallot, 2001). Another option is to identify staff that may have an expertise in this area and create a committee and/or working group within the organization. Including Human Resources is critical, because staff may also be trauma survivors—all members of the leadership team require advanced training that facilitates embedding the standards of trauma-informed care into employee services.

An environmental assessment of policies and procedures is needed to determine the opportunities to improve trauma-informed services and for potentially damaging practices that replicate or exacerbate past abuse experiences. Practices such as restraints and seclusion can trigger past abuse memories. Less intrusive measures, such as one-on-one support during times of crisis, or time-outs, can maintain the therapeutic relationship, provide safety, and are less triggering (Fallot & Harris, 2002).

IMPLEMENTING TRAUMA-INFORMED CARE STRATEGIES

A trauma-informed care approach is a strength-based approach grounded in a universal understanding of the impact of trauma. This framework emphasizes:

- The physical, psychological and emotional safety of both providers and survivors

- Creating opportunities at all levels of the healthcare system for survivors to rebuild a sense of control and empowerment

- The need to focus on cultural awareness and patient-centeredness

A patient- and trauma-informed approach ensures that an individual's unique trauma history is an integral component to her healthcare.

A key factor to be assessed are *triggers*, sensory perceptions that remind an individual of the past trauma and set off an action, process, or series of events in response to perceived danger. For the trauma survivor, the present and past are confused. Potential triggers include seeing, hearing, smelling, tasting, or feeling something that reminds one of the trauma. Hospital-based triggers can include bedtime, persons entering the room at night, people getting too close, and constant stimulations in the environment. Each survivor has different triggers. Understanding the survivor's triggers helps the treatment team to prevent the response. The provider wants to identify early signs of escalation so that an eruption is prevented. Survivors can identify coping and calming strategies that the staff can use in times of crisis.

Examples of providing a trauma-informed approach include:

- An environmental scan that assesses for privacy, safety, and access to services

- Ensure that patients have choices and care is individualized

- Establish trust, ensure good listening, balanced relationships, safety, comfort, and time

- Be aware of hierarchal structures that impede fair and equitable access to care

CHILD-SPECIFIC APPROACHES TO TRAUMA-INFORMED CARE

Unfortunately, children experience traumatic events, which result in fear, confusion, distrust, and hurt. How can professionals help children process their exposures to trauma? A trauma-informed and patient-centered strategy can be the first step toward healing. In 2001, SAMHSA funded the National Child Traumatic Stress Initiative (NCTSI) to increase understanding of child trauma and to develop effective interventions for children exposed to different types of traumatic events. The experience of child maltreatment, whether it be physical abuse, sexual abuse, mental abuse, exploitation, or neglect, can be seen as traumatic; trauma that can affect a child throughout his or her life span and into adulthood. The National Child Traumatic Stress Initiative (NCTSI) has a number of resources and fact sheets that provide information on trauma-informed care to many different populations. One relevant resource is found at http://www.nctsn.org/resources/topics/treatments-that-work/promising-practices.

It's important that the healthcare environment feels secure, safe, and welcoming to the child. The care environment should be age-appropriate, comfortable, and calming. The nurse should spend time with pediatric patients and their caregivers to build trust and safety. Often, children lack the cognitive ability to process adverse situations that have occurred in their lives. The nurse should use developmentally appropriate assessment and screening tools. Age-appropriate language should be used in all teaching and explanations. The assessment must include consideration of the parent's or caregiver's history of trauma and how the experiences of the caregiver affect her parenting skills. Psychoeducation is important to ensure that parents/caregivers understand responses to and consequences of trauma.

Lastly but most importantly, healthcare providers must consider self-reflection, recognition of their past traumas, and self-care. Working with traumatized children and their families is distressing to healthcare providers (Craig & Sprang, 2010), and being cognizant of this can help the nurse to be proactive in ensuring his own wellbeing. Healthcare providers should, according to the NCTSI:

- Routinely screen for trauma exposure and related symptoms

- Use culturally appropriate evidence-based assessment and treatment for traumatic stress and associated mental health symptoms

- Make resources available to children, families, and providers on trauma exposure, its impact, and treatment

- Engage in efforts to strengthen the resilience and protective factors of children and families affected by and vulnerable to trauma

- Address parent and caregiver trauma and its impact on the family system

- Emphasize continuity of care and collaboration across child-service systems

- Maintain an environment of care for staff that addresses, minimizes, and treats secondary traumatic stress and that increases staff resilience

FINDING RESOURCES FOR TRAUMA-INFORMED SYSTEMS

Several programs and resources exist that can guide the assessment, development, and implementation of a trauma-informed system.

Women Embracing Life and Living

The Women Embracing Life and Living (WELL) toolkit is geared toward directors of organizations and policy-makers. Members of the Massachusetts State Leadership Council developed this toolkit in the Women, Co-Occurring Disorders and Violence Study to help organizations develop plans to improve the quality of care. It includes principles for trauma-informed treatment of women with co-occurring mental health and substance abuse disorders, self-assessment for provider organizations, organizational assessment, and instructions for using the assessments to move toward providing trauma-informed, integrated care. Several modules were developed that can be used for staff training. Topics include:

- Understanding trauma

- Collaborating with survivors on treatment goals

- Keeping a trauma framework during crises and life-threatening behaviors

- Working with dissociation and staying grounded

- Self-awareness as a tool for clients and helpers

- Vicarious traumatization and integration

- Putting it all together

The toolkit can be found at http://healthrecovery.org/images/products/30_inside.pdf.

Sanctuary Model

The Sanctuary Model is a trauma-informed method for creating and changing organizational culture that effectively provides a cohesive context for healing from traumatic experiences (Jennings, 2004). It can be used in short-term and long-term acute inpatient psychiatric populations of adults traumatized as children, residential settings, domestic violence shelters, group homes, outpatient settings, substance abuse programs, and parenting support programs. The Sanctuary Model has demonstrated effectiveness in reducing post-traumatic stress disorder symptoms (Wright, Woo, Muller, Fernandes, & Kraftcheck, 2003).

TRAUMA RECOVERY AND EMPOWERMENT MODEL

Trauma Recovery and Empowerment Model (TREM) is a group intervention to address the long-term cognitive, emotional, and interpersonal consequences of physical and sexual abuse (Fallot & Harris, 2002). TREM provides a psychoeducational and peer-supportive curriculum organized around the principles of empowerment and skill building. The manualized program occurs over a 24 to 33 session group approach (Jennings, 2004). TREM focuses on survivors' personal and relational experience, with a focus on empowerment and skill building. Members learn strategies for self-comfort and accurate self-monitoring, as well as ways to establish safe physical and emotional boundaries.

TREM provides a supportive (gender-separated) group peer environment in which each survivor can explore current life problems as they relate to past or present experiences of physical, sexual, and emotional abuse. The model helps survivors to overcome fear, grief, and shame. Survivors are helped to reintegrate trauma experiences into a personal life narrative and to reframe the connection between their experiences of abuse and other current difficulties including substance abuse, mental health symptoms, and interpersonal problems. Several sessions focus on skills building, emphasizing self-awareness; self-soothing; communication style; decision-making; problem-solving; regulating overwhelming feelings and emotional modification; and establishing safer, more reciprocal relationships. Throughout, TREM addresses substance abuse problems and relapse prevention. There is a strong evidence base of support for its efficacy (Toussaint, VanDeMark, Bornemann, & Graeber, 2007).

TRAUMA ADAPTIVE RECOVERY GROUP EDUCATION

Trauma Adaptive Recovery Group Education and Therapy (TARGET) uses a strength-based model in a seven-step sequence of skills for processing and managing trauma-related ramifications (Ford & Russo, 2006). Participants receive psychoeducation on the impact of traumatic exposure and post-traumatic stress disorder on the body's stress response system and brain and on a set of practical skills to enable participants to gain control of PTSD symptoms. This 8 to 9 week manualized group treatment uses creative arts throughout the group and individual sessions to facilitate nonverbal learning, self-expression, and social problem-solving.

The mnemonic FREEDOM identifies the key aspects of the treatment (Ford & Russo, 2006, p. 343):

> Participants are helped to self-regulate by focusing, trauma processing via recognizing current triggers, emotions, and cognitive evaluations, strength-based reintegration by defining core goals, identifying currently effective options and affirming core values by making positive contributions.

TARGET has demonstrated effectiveness in the care of trauma survivors (Frisman, Ford, & Lin, 2005).

SUMMARY

Trauma causes emotional or physical harm to the affected individual and is most clearly recognized as an impairment of the individual's emotional, social, spiritual, physical, and/or mental wellbeing. Usually a set of circumstances or events, or even one event in particular, can cause an individual to experience trauma. A trauma-informed care approach is a strength-based approach grounded in a universal understanding of the impact of trauma. This framework emphasizes the physical, psychological, and emotional safety of both providers and survivors; creating opportunities at all levels of the healthcare system for survivors to rebuild a sense of control and empowerment; and the need to focus on cultural awareness and patient centeredness. A patient- and trauma-informed approach ensures that an individual's unique trauma history is an integral component to healthcare.

ADDITIONAL RESOURCES

Adverse Child Experiences Study: http://www.cdc.gov/violenceprevention/acestudy/

National Center on Domestic Violence, Trauma, & Mental Health: http://www.nationalcenterdvtraumamh.org/about/

The National Child Traumatic Stress Network: http://www.nctsn.org/resources/topics/creating-trauma-informed-systems

Substance Abuse and Mental Health Services Administration: http://www.samhsa.gov and http://www.samhsa.gov/nctic

The Trauma Informed Care Project: http://www.traumainformedcareproject.org/

Trauma-Informed Organizational Toolkit: http://www.familyhomelessness.org/media/90.pdf

REFERENCES

Chandler, G. (2008). From traditional inpatient to trauma-informed treatment: Transferring control from staff to patient. *Journal of the American Psychiatric Nurses Association, 14*(5), 363–371.

Cook, A., Spinazzola, J., Ford, J., Lanktree, C., Blaustein, M., Cloitre, M., … van der Kolk, B. (2005). Complex trauma in children and adults. *Psychiatric Annals, 35*(5), 390–398.

Craig, C. D., & Sprang, G. (2010). Compassion satisfaction, compassion fatigue, and burnout in a national sample of trauma treatment therapists. *Anxiety, Stress, & Coping, 23*(3), 319–339.

Elliott, D. E., Bjelajac, P., Fallot, R. D., Markoff, L. S., & Reed, B. G. (2005). Trauma informed or trauma denied: Principles and implementation of trauma informed services for women. *Journal of Community Psychology, 33*(4), 461–477.

Fallot, R. D., & Harris, M. (2002). The Trauma Recovery and Empowerment Model (TREM): Conceptual and practical issues in a group intervention for women. *Community Mental Health Journal, 38*(6), 475–485.

Felitti, V. J., Anda, R. F., Nordenberg, D., Williamson, D. F., Spitz, A. M., Edwards, V., … Marks, J. S. (1998). Relationship of childhood abuse and household dysfunction to many of the leading causes of death in adults: The Adverse Childhood Experiences (ACE) Study. *American Journal of Preventive Medicine, 14*(4), 245–258.

Ford, J. D., & Russo, E. (2006). Trauma-focused, present-centered, emotional self-regulation approach to integrated treatment for posttraumatic stress and addiction: Trauma Adaptive Recovery Group Education and Therapy (TARGET). *American Journal of Psychotherapy, 60*(4), 335–355.

Frisman, L., Ford, J. D., & Lin, H. (2005, October). *Trauma treatment for persons in substance abuse care: Results of a randomized controlled trial.* Paper presented at the annual convention of the American Evaluation Association, Toronto, Canada.

Harris, M., & Fallot, R. D. (2001). Envisioning a trauma informed service system: A vital paradigm shift. *New Directions for Mental Health Services, 89,* 3–22.

Hodgdon, H. B., Kinniburgh, K., Gabowitz, D., Blaustein, M. E., & Spinazzola, J. (2013). Development and implementation of trauma-informed programming in youth residential treatment centers using the ARC framework. *J Fam Violence, 28*(7), 679–692.

Hopper, E. K., Bassuk, E. L., & Olivet, J. (2010). Shelter from the storm: Trauma-informed care in homelessness services settings. *The Open Health Services and Policy Journal, 3*(2), 80–100.

Jennings, A. (2004). *Models for developing trauma-informed behavioral health systems and trauma-specific services.* Alexandria, VA: National Association of State Mental Health Program Directors, National Technical Assistance Center for State Mental Health Planning.

Latham, V. H., Dollard, N., Robst, J., & Armstrong, M. I. (2010). Innovations in implementation of trauma-informed care practices in youth residential treatment: A curriculum for organizational change. *Child Welfare, 89*(2), 79–95.

McGoldrick, M., Giordano, J., & Garcia-Preto, N. (Eds.). (2005). *Ethnicity and family therapy* (3rd ed.). New York, NY: Guilford Press.

Steele, W. (2009). *Trauma informed care: A history of helping, a history of excellence.* Grosse Pointe Woods, MI: The National Institute for Trauma and Loss in Children.

Substance Abuse and Mental Health Services Administration. SAMHSA's Concept of Trauma and Guidance for a Trauma-Informed Approach. HHS Publication No. (SMA) 14-4884. Rockville, MD: Substance Abuse and Mental Health Services Administration, 2014.

Toussaint, D. W., VanDeMark, N. R., Bornemann, A., & Graeber, C. J. (2007). Modifications to the Trauma Recovery and Empowerment Model (TREM) for substance abusing women with histories of violence: Outcomes and lessons learned at a Colorado substance abuse treatment center. *Journal of Community Psychology, 35*(7), 879–894.

Ursano, R. J., Benedek, D. M., & Engel, C. C. (2012). Trauma-informed care for primary care: The lessons of war. *Annals of Internal Medicine, 157*(12), 905–906.

Williams, K., Papadopoulou, V., & Booth, N. (2012). Prisoners' childhood and family backgrounds: Results from the Surveying Prisoner Crime Reduction (SPCR) longitudinal cohort study of prisoners. *Ministry of Justice Research Series, 3,* 12.

Wright, D. C., Woo, W. L., Muller, R. T., Fernandes, C. B., & Kraftcheck, E. R. (2003). An investigation of trauma-centered inpatient treatment for adult survivors of abuse. *Child Abuse and Neglect, 27*(4), 393–406.

18

COMMUNITY VIOLENCE INTERVENTION PROGRAMS

Phyllis W. Sharps, PHD, RN, FAAN; Netanya Frohman, BSN, RN; and Brittany E. Kelly, BSN

"Violence is man-made. It is preventable."

–Teny Gross, Executive Director, The Institute for the Study & Practice of Nonviolence (http://www.nonviolenceinstitute.org/)

KEY POINTS IN THIS CHAPTER

▪ Nursing home visitation programs are promising interventions aimed at reducing child abuse and neglect and maternal intimate partner violence (IVP) and subsequently reducing infants' and young children's exposure to IPV.

▪ Nurses can be involved in community policing strategies by promoting partnerships with local law enforcement, providing feedback from community members to local law enforcement agencies regarding successes and challenges of community policing, and encouraging citizens to support community policing initiatives.

▪ Nurses can support the efforts of communities to establish neighborhood watch programs by providing resources, encouragement, and support when a need or opportunity is recognized.

◼ Social norms campaigns aim to increase equality in male-female roles, reduce the acceptance of violence against women, and empower women toward independence and less acceptance of violence. School nurses can educate students and teachers; however, all nurses can confront misinformation and provide correct information to patients and their families.

Violence is widespread throughout many communities and neighborhoods. The presence of violence in residential neighborhoods and communities affects the health of both the community and the families and children residing in the neighborhoods. In its most severe forms, violence and resultant injuries are the top 15 killers of Americans of all ages (Centers for Disease Control and Prevention [CDC], 2014). Community violence not resulting in death can result in immediate health consequences such as concussions, broken bones, and other injuries, as well as lifelong consequences such as mental health and physical disabilities. Other negative consequences associated with non-fatal violence include disruptions in school, work, and community settings and poor academic performance for many children.

The critical importance of addressing the frequency and severity of violence and the health consequences of violence has also been highlighted by the Healthy People 2020 goals for injury and violence prevention. There are at least 20 Healthy People 2020 goals that address some aspect of violence. These goals focus on the impact of violence on the health and wellbeing of families, children, and communities and reinforce the need and importance of community violence prevention strategies and interventions.

The purpose of this chapter is to describe several community violence intervention strategies such as home visiting, community policing, neighborhood watch, and campaigns to change social norms. The theoretical background supporting these strategies as well as exemplars of each are described.

HOME VISITING PROGRAMS

Nurse home visitation has long been an essential part of public health nursing practice. Home visiting programs for pregnant and parenting women often incorporate pregnancy health promotion strategies and parenting skills to enhance infant and child development. The goal of these home visiting programs is to improve awareness, sensitivity, and understanding of the cues and behaviors of infants and children, thereby reducing parental maltreatment and abuse of their children, reducing subsequent future perpetration of violence by childhood victims upon others, and reducing the perpetuation of adolescent and adult intimate partner violence (IPV) (Sharps, Campbell, Baty, Walker, & Bair-Merritt, 2008). These programs have been viewed as a long-term solution for reducing community violence.

REVIEW OF HOME VISITING PROGRAMS FOR PREVENTING CHILD ABUSE AND NEGLECT

A 2009 review by Howard and Brooks-Gunn of the role of perinatal and early childhood home visiting programs for preventing child abuse and neglect included six of the most widely implemented programs in the United States. Table 18.1 summarizes each program.

TABLE 18.1 EVIDENCE-BASED HOME VISIT PROGRAMS

Program	Program Goals	Population Served	Duration and/or Frequency of Home Visits	Type of Home Visitor
Nurse-Family Partnership (NFP)	Improve maternal health and pregnancy outcomes Improve parenting skills Enhance maternal life course	First-time, low-income mothers	Pregnancy to 24 months after birth	Public health nurses

continues

TABLE 18.1 EVIDENCE-BASED HOME VISIT PROGRAMS   (CONTINUED)

Program	Program Goals	Population Served	Duration and/or Frequency of Home Visits	Type of Home Visitor
Hawaii Healthy Start (HSP)	Identify risks Improve parenting skills Prevent child abuse and neglect	Family assessment questionnaire that identifies as high risk	Birth to 3–5 years	*Lay home visitors
Healthy Families America (HFA)	Identify risks Improve parenting skills Prevent child abuse and neglect	Family assessment questionnaire that identifies as high risk	Prenatal or birth to 5 years or enrollment in Pre-K	*Lay home visitors
Comprehensive Child Development Program (CCDP)	Enhance child development Support parents Help families with economic self-sufficiency	Low-income families with children	1st year to school entry Bi-weekly; 1 hour	*Lay home visitors
Infant Health and Development Program (IHDP)	Enhance development of premature, low birthweight infants	Low birth-weight infants and their families	Birth to 12 months, weekly 13 months to 36 months, biweekly	College graduates with home visiting experience Master's-level supervisor
Early Head Start (EHS)	Enhance child development Support/strengthen families	Low-income families with children	Prenatal or birth to 3 years	Trained lay home visitors

*Paraprofessionals (non-college preparation)

Source: Howard & Brooks-Gunn, 2009.

The review concluded that the quality of the available evidence for the effectiveness of programs for preventing child abuse and neglect is mixed. This conclusion was based on the limitations of existing research on home visiting programs, including the lack of precise measures for assessing child maltreatment, child abuse, and neglect.

The Howard and Brooks-Gunn (2009) review revealed important findings:

- Among the six programs, only the Hawaii Healthy Start program and Healthy Families America had specific goals related to preventing child abuse and neglect; however, Nurse-Family Partnership, Hawaii Healthy Start, and Healthy Families America all evaluated abuse and neglect as outcomes of their home visiting programs.

- The Nurse-Family Partnership (NFP) Home Visitation program (Kitzman et al., 2010; Olds et al., 2007) is the most well-developed home visiting program and is implemented in 26 states, serving more than 20,000 families each year with plans to expand to 100,000 families by 2017.

  The NFP uses baccalaureate-prepared nurses who have received extensive training on the program's comprehensive home visit curriculum, which includes topics such as maternal and pregnancy health, infant and child development, parenting, and family planning. Using the NFP curriculum, nurses provide home visits to first-time pregnant women beginning during pregnancy through 24 months after birth.

  The NFP program has been recognized as the intervention with the best evidence for decreasing child maltreatment (Chalk, 2003; Chalk & King, 1998). The NFP has documented a 48% decline in rates of child abuse and neglect in its 15-year follow-up.

- The Hawaii Healthy Start and all randomized Healthy Families America programs have program goals that include preventing child abuse and neglect among families who have been identified using an assessment questionnaire as high risk for child maltreatment. Both of these programs use lay home visitors, who make home visits beginning during pregnancy or birth and continue until children enter Pre-K. Evaluations from both of these programs have documented significant reductions in substantiated cases of child abuse or neglect as a result of home visiting interventions.

■ Some Healthy Families America programs have evaluated parental self-report of abusive or neglectful behaviors toward their children. Healthy Families America of New York found that families enrolled in their intervention program reported reductions of abusive and neglectful behaviors (Straus, Hamby, Finklehor, Moore, & Runyan, 1998). The Hawaii Healthy Start program concluded that overall, the program did very little to prevent child abuse (Duggan et al., 2004). These limited findings reinforce the need for continued studies that evaluate home visiting programs' effectiveness to prevent child abuse and neglect. The findings of future studies will be strengthened by incorporating more precise measures to collect adequate data about indicators of child abuse and neglect.

REVIEW OF HOME VISITING PROGRAMS FOR VIOLENCE

Other home visiting programs have implemented interventions aimed at reducing violence against women as mothers, including interventions targeting intimate partner violence (Bybee & Sullivan, 2002; Parents as Teachers [PAT], 2013). The goals of these programs are to reduce the negative outcomes related to partner abuse (such as maternal depression, lack of support networks, and isolation) as a long-term strategy for enhancing maternal competence and reducing further victimization of mothers, infants, and children, and reducing the potential for poor parenting.

A review of home visiting programs by Sharps et al. (2008) revealed that few perinatal programs included specific interventions for addressing intimate partner violence (IPV) and that failure to adequately address IPV against pregnant and parenting women limited the ability of the other components of the home visiting program to reduce violence and improve maternal and infant outcomes.

Similarly, a review of the IPV prevention effectiveness of the Olds Nurse-Family Partnership program demonstrated that when the home visitors do not adequately address IPV, the overall program effectiveness was limited for families experiencing IPV (Eckenrode et al., 2000; Jack et al., 2012).

The Domestic Violence Enhanced Home (DOVE) Visiting program is a specific intimate partner violence intervention that has been successfully integrated into perinatal home visiting programs, as well as Parents as Teachers (PAT, 2013). The results found it decreased the severity of violence for pregnant women who participated in the DOVE intervention (Sharps, 2012).

- The DOVE brochure-based intervention, which is delivered by nurses or community health worker home visitors, increases a women's awareness of the impact of IPV on her health and the health of her unborn child and helps the woman to assess the potential dangerousness of her relationship (Campbell, Webster, & Glass, 2009) and make her own personal safety plan.

- The DOVE intervention is delivered during the pregnancy and the early postpartum period.

- Urban and rural health departments that provided perinatal home visiting programs integrated the DOVE IPV prevention intervention into their existing home visit protocols.

- Women enrolled in the health department home visiting programs were randomly assigned to receive the DOVE intervention or the health department's usual IPV prevention intervention.

- Women who received the DOVE intervention reported less IPV as long as 24 months postpartum.

The Nurse-Family Partnership program (NFP) also addressed intimate partner violence in its protocols. Findings from a study by Olds et al. (2013) revealed maternal reports of partner violence by participants in the NFP program. Olds and colleagues have subsequently worked to enhance the NFP program to integrate modifications to specifically address IPV. Their preliminary findings, which have reported extensive training of nurse home visitors and integrating culturally appropriate violence-prevention strategies for pregnant women, suggest that it is feasible to integrate a specific IPV intervention that addresses the needs of pregnant women exposed to IPV (Jack et al., 2012).

The DOVE intervention and modified Nurse-Family Partnership are promising interventions aimed at reducing maternal IPV and subsequently reducing infants' and young children's exposure to IPV. Importantly, adding evidence-based IPV interventions to home visiting programs aimed at reducing child abuse and neglect will also increase their effectiveness.

COMMUNITY POLICING PROGRAMS

According to the U.S. Department of Justice *Office of Community Oriented Policing Services* (COPS) 2014 report, community policing is based on a philosophy that promotes organizational strategies that support the systematic use of partnerships and problem-solving techniques to proactively address the immediate conditions that give rise to public safety issues such as crime, social disorder, and fear of crime (U.S. Department of Justice, 2014). Although community policing strategies vary depending on the specific needs of the communities involved, certain basic principles are common to all community policing approaches. Three key elements have been associated with American policing throughout its history: crime control, order maintenance, and service provision (Trojanowicz & Bucqueroux, 1990). The primary functions of community policing based on its theoretical focus shifts responsibilities for crime prevention to include community partnerships, organizational transformation, and problem-solving (U.S. Bureau of Justice Assistance, 1994).

Effective community policing depends on optimizing positive contact between police officers and community members (Zhao, Lovrich, & Robinson, 2001). According to the 2014 COPS report on community policing, police department implementation of routine patrols of a particular neighborhood or geographic area may be utilized as a preventive strategy to reduce crime in hot-spot neighborhoods or to increase police presence in neighborhoods to reduce fear of crime (U.S. Department of Justice, 2014). Also according to the 2014 COPS report, community policing encourages a rapid response to community calls about crime, which increases the trust level of community members in the willingness and ability of police to respond to crime as it occurs in the community.

Community policing emphasizes proactive problem-solving in a systematic and routine fashion. Rather than responding to crime only while or after it occurs, community policing also encourages communities and law enforcement agencies to proactively develop solutions to the immediate underlying conditions contributing to public safety problems (U.S. Department of Justice, 2014). A strong foundation of trust is the most important value of community policing; it allows the formation of solid community partnerships and problem-solving relationships. Interactive partnerships between community organizations and law enforcement agencies are essential to the success of community policing. In order to successfully accomplish these partnerships, police agencies must look to other government agencies, community members and groups, nonprofits and service providers, private businesses, and the media to develop relationships that promote ways of working collaboratively to improve the impact of policing on the local community (Evans & Owens, 2007).

For community policing to be successful, *organizational transformation* (the alignment of organizational structure, personnel, and information systems) must occur within local law enforcement agencies in order to support established community partnerships and continually initiate proactive problem-solving efforts within the community (Allen, 2002). Proactive problem-solving and the formation of community partnerships must become institutionalized in agency policy to ensure that community policing principles and practices have a positive impact upon policing activities both at the organizational and street level (U.S. Department of Justice, 2014). Examples of organizational transformation to support community policing include a shift to the long-term assignment of officers to specific neighborhoods or geographical areas (Allen, 2002). Furthermore, community policing philosophy emphasizes changes in organizational structure to encourage its adoption across an entire law enforcement agency, not just specialized departments (Novak, Alarid, & Lucas, 2003).

Reports on successful community policing programs and strategies to address and prevent issues of violence and other criminal activity can be found dating back to the early 1980s, when community policing philosophy began to gain popularity in American law enforcement agencies. One early study conducted in Flint, Michigan, revealed that citizens in the community felt safer and believed they were less prone to experiencing violence and other crime when foot patrol officers were "well known and highly visible" in the community (Trojanowicz & Bucqueroux, 1990). Another study of community policing in five small to mid-size American cities showed that awareness of community policing was associated with greater self-protection efforts, lower fear of crime, and stronger feelings of community attachment (Adams, Rohe, & Arcury, 2005). Other studies have shown that although community policing may be successful in the eyes of community members, there are often challenges associated with law enforcement agency adoption of community policing policies and procedures (Allen, 2002). Community policing requires partnerships between officers and communities. Often the perception is that the responsibility lies solely with officers. Departments must work with officers to change from a strictly rule and policy orientation to a new style of problem-solving by working with the community as partners. Disengaged communities present an additional challenge.

Nurses can support the efforts of communities to initiate more community-oriented policing in the communities they serve:

- Public health nurses are in a position, through home visitation and regular interaction with community members, to recognize the need for more community-oriented policing and can proactively suggest a community policing model to local law enforcement agencies and advocacy groups in the area.

- Nurses can provide organizations with evidence of successes in community policing as well as resources supporting the initiation and continuation of a community policing program structure.

- In areas where community policing already occurs, nurses can help keep community policing successful by providing feedback from community members to local law enforcement agencies regarding successes and challenges of community policing, and by encouraging citizens to support community policing initiatives.

NEIGHBORHOOD WATCH PROGRAMS

Similar to community policing philosophy, the purpose of a neighborhood watch is to reduce crime through citizen involvement and police cooperation. The National Crime Prevention Council (NCPC) defines *neighborhood watch* as organized groups of neighborhood residents who watch out for criminal and suspicious behavior and report it to local law enforcement to help prevent crime and promote cooperation among residents and police (NCPC, n.d.). The concept of formulating citizens' watch groups to work with police agencies in protecting local neighborhoods began in the 1960s in response to the rape and murder of Kitty Genovese in Queens, New York, after reports that a dozen witnesses did nothing to save Genovese or apprehend her killer (Rasenberger, 2006). What followed was the establishment of the federally funded National Neighborhood Watch, an organization that remains active to this day. The adoption of community policing by local law enforcement agencies in the 1980s and 1990s contributed to the success of the National Neighborhood Watch and the increased development of neighborhood watch groups.

Most neighborhood watch groups follow standardized guidelines provided by the National Neighborhood Watch organization in selecting their approaches and recommendations, and certain strategies have emerged as successful for encouraging trust in the community as well as for reporting problems in the community such as violence or other suspicious activity:

- The Tucson, Arizona police department encourages its neighborhood watch groups to hold regular block parties and to maintain "block maps" with detailed demographic information about current community residents (City of Tucson, n.d.).

- In Fairfax County, Virginia, a flourishing neighborhood watch program began in 1979 and has developed to include over 900 programs throughout the county (Fairfax County, n.d.). Watch groups in Fairfax offer services such as a free home security inspection for local citizens of the community.

■ The New York State Police agency emphasizes that a watch group can be formed around a block, apartment building, townhouse complex, park, business area, public housing complex, office building, or marina (New York State Police, n.d.).

■ In Stockton, California, neighborhood watch members are invited to regular community advisory board meetings at the local police department to ensure that police officers and community members are regularly in touch regarding neighborhood watch activities and any problems or concerns in the community (City of Stockton, n.d.).

Most neighborhood watch programs commonly encourage regular community meetings and the establishment of effective partnership and communication with local law enforcement agencies. Table 18.2 outlines a few successful neighborhood watch programs.

TABLE 18.2 EXAMPLES OF SUCCESSFUL NEIGHBORHOOD WATCH STRATEGIES

Location	Strategy	Purpose
Tucson, Arizona	Block parties (organized by neighborhood watch group) "Block maps" (detailed demographic information about current community residents)	To encourage trust between members of community To increase awareness of neighborhood watch initiatives To increase accountability of community members to one another by encouraging community members to know each other To facilitate reporting of crime and other emergency situations to police

Fairfax County, Virginia	Free home security inspection (completed by local police officers)	To increase awareness of security presence in community and discourage criminal activity To increase trust between community citizens and local police
Stockton, California	Regular advisory board meetings with local police department	To ensure that police officers and community members are regularly in touch regarding neighborhood watch activities and any problems or concerns in community
New York, New York	Creative neighborhood watch group location structures	To encourage citizens to form neighborhood watch groups to increase security in both traditional and non-traditional community settings, including blocks, apartment buildings, townhouse complexes, parks, business areas, public housing complexes, office buildings, or marinas

THE RISE OF THE NEIGHBORHOOD WATCH

The neighborhood watch movement gained national media attention in February of 2012 when unarmed black teenager Trayvon Martin was fatally shot by Hispanic neighborhood watch volunteer George Zimmerman. Zimmerman's actions of carrying a gun and following Martin were said to have violated typical neighborhood watch protocol (Robinson & Schwartz, 2012). Zimmerman, who was later acquitted of murder charges, was widely accused of targeting Martin because of his race. Immediately following this incident, neighborhood watch remained a popular topic in the media. In June 2012, a *New York Times* article reported that neighborhood watches in the New York City area were growing again after decades of decrease due to lower crime rates (Wilson, 2012). The article also stated that neighborhood watch groups had fallen under scrutiny since the shooting of Trayvon Martin earlier that year.

Some controversy exists around whether or not neighborhood watch programs succeed in strengthening local communities and helping to reduce crime. The Project on Human Development in Chicago Neighborhoods, a research study that assessed the role of neighborhood-level resources in aggressive and delinquent behaviors among youths in urban areas, found that communities with programs such as neighborhood watch were associated with lower levels of aggressive and violent behavior among adolescents (Molnar, Cerda, Roberts, & Buka, 2008). In contrast, however, a 2012 study by Schultz and Tabanico found that community members were more likely to perceive a higher likelihood of being a victim of crime, higher levels of community crime, and lower levels of perceived safety and community quality when neighborhood watch signs were made highly visible in the community (Schultz & Tabanico, 2012).

Nurses can support the efforts of communities to establish neighborhood watch programs by providing resources, encouragement, and support when a need or opportunity is recognized. As discussed, neighborhood watch programs can be adapted to fit a wide variety of community structures, and examples abound of successful neighborhood watch programs throughout the United States. Nurses who recognize a need in a community for increased citizen involvement in safety and security can utilize these resources to suggest and support the formation of neighborhood watch groups and related community efforts.

SOCIAL NORMS CAMPAIGNS

Social norms are defined by societies and their respective social subgroups. These norms are then enacted by members of society and are often reflected in individuals' treatment of one another in relationships (Ellsberg et al., 2014). Social norms regarding masculinity often emphasize men's differences from women, and differences between heterosexual norms and those of gay men (Jewkes, Flood, & Lang, 2014). Social norms involving gender are especially influential on human behavior, particularly with regard to the perpetration of violence by men against women (Jewkes, 2002).

Violence against women and girls has been associated with ideas and behavior influenced by social norms of male and female gender differences and expectations of gender roles in society (Flood, 2011). Likewise, where violence against women and girls is highly prevalent, male experiences of violence as victims are also common, as is interpersonal violence between men (Jewkes, 2002). In addition, studies such as the Campus Sexual Assault (CSA) Study have identified sexual violence as a particularly prevalent problem on college campuses, finding that 1 in 5 women and 1 in 16 men are sexually assaulted while in college (Krebs, Lindquist, Warner, Fisher, & Martin, 2007). Recent updates to Title IX legislation have increased pressure on colleges and universities to proactively prevent and be well-prepared to respond to reports of sexual violence on campus, including new requirements for colleges to publish a policy against sex discrimination, designate a Title IX coordinator, and adopt and publish grievance procedures (U.S. Department of Education, 2014). Title IX is a federal program that prohibits discrimination based on sex in any federally funded education program or activity.

A number of interventions have been developed recently that give consideration to social norms of masculinity and directly involve men and boys in the prevention of violence against women and girls (Flood, 2011; Pease, 2008). These interventions range in tactics that include changing the way men view masculine roles in society to methods that are more woman-focused and aim to strengthen women's awareness of and resilience to violence (Jewkes et al., 2014):

- An evaluation of the Safe Dates program by Foshee et al. showed that the program could be successful without directly addressing social norms of masculine and feminine gender roles in society (Foshee et al., 1998). Other campaigns to change social norms ideas, such as Men Can Stop Rape, have targeted specific concepts associated with masculinity and aimed to change participants' perspectives on such norms (Hawkins, 2006).

- In an effort to utilize male role models to promote non-violence and change social norm ideas on college campuses, the First National Conference for Campus-Based Men's Gender Equality and Anti-Violence Groups highlighted the influence of role models in changing common social perspectives on gender roles (Murphy, 2010). However, this approach was met with controversy, as the typical masculine role model might actually serve to reinforce gender biases instead of the goal of the campaign to change ideas about them.

- A 2009 study suggests that rape prevention programs addressing men in college have less effect on men at a higher risk of committing rape (Stephens & George, 2009).

A number of successful violence intervention and prevention programs have involved pairing non-violent men with men who are perpetrators of violence in a group education setting. Successful programs engage multiple stakeholders with multiple approaches, aim to address underlying risk factors for violence including social norms that condone violence and gender inequality, and support the development of non-violent behaviors (Ellsberg et al., 2014). Interventions that have been successful in reducing violence perpetration have tended to be many hours long, have involved both women and men, and have included critical reflection on social norms and building of relationship skills (Wolfe et al., 2009).

A few examples of programs are:

- *Mentors in Violence Prevention* program in Washington, DC, is considered to be successful in changing social norm ideas about gender equality and male-female roles in society (Jewkes et al., 2014).

- Youth-oriented programs, such as *Coaching Boys Into Men*, address gender norms with positive results, including changed attitudes about gender equality and reduction in self-reported gender-based violence perpetration (Miller et al., 2013).

- Parenting and couples programs such as the international *Men Care* program and *Men's Action for Stopping Violence Against Women* have been evaluated for effectiveness, but more research evidence is needed (Fulu, Kerr-Wilson, & Lang, 2014).

- A study by Potter, Moynihan, Stapleton, and Banyard on the effectiveness of an on-campus poster campaign to encourage bystander participation in the prevention of sexual violence against women showed that students who reported seeing the posters exhibited greater awareness of the problem and greater willingness to participate in reducing sexual violence compared to those who did not report seeing the posters (Potter et al., 2009).

Social norms regarding masculine and feminine roles in society often focus on the differences between men and women as well as those differences between heterosexual and gay men (Jewkes et al., 2014). Acknowledging the similarities that exist between men and women and addressing issues of homophobia is important for transforming ideas and behaviors resulting from social norms and gender-related expectations in society (Jewkes et al., 2014). In addition, women need to be empowered not only economically but also socially and individually, and a need exists to enable critical thought and awareness of the necessity for more equitable social roles and relationships for women in society (Pronyk et al., 2006).

Campaigns to change social norms have been used primarily to change attitudes about male-female roles in society as a means of reducing interpersonal violence. These campaigns advocate for more equality in male-female roles to reduce the acceptance of violence against women and to empower women toward independence and less acceptance of violence. Nurses can play a role in educating the public. School nurses can educate students and teachers. All nurses have the opportunity to confront misinformation and provide correct information to patients and their families.

SUMMARY

Violence in communities and neighborhoods is a significant public health problem as well as a contributing factor in the occurrence of crime and the disorganization of communities. Violence manifests in many ways, including intimate partner violence, child abuse and neglect, dating violence, bullying, crimes such as physical and sexual assaults, destruction of property, and in its most severe forms, homicide. This chapter has described several programs and strategies to address community violence. Home visiting programs have been implemented to prevent child abuse and neglect. The evidence to support these programs is mixed, with the most effective being the Nurse-Family Partnership (NFP) program. Other promising home-based interventions such as DOVE and modifications to NFP address interpersonal violence and aim at reducing IPV against women and reducing infants' and children's exposure to violence. It's believed that reducing IPV against mothers also enhances home visiting programs aimed at reducing child abuse and neglect, and in the long term reduces the potential youth and adult perpetrators.

Other strategies to reduce community violence (generally occurring outside of the home) such as community policing and neighborhood watch were also described. These approaches reduce violence by engaging citizens to become involved in active partnerships with law enforcement agencies to reduce community violence. These programs are most effective if trust is built between the community and law enforcement groups and by adapting a proactive approach to addressing and reducing the occurrence of violence and crime in the community. The evidence to support the effectiveness of these approaches is controversial, on one hand showing an impact on reduction in crimes, but also including stories of aggressive behaviors toward suspected perpetrators resulting in what some have called inappropriate levels of vigilante justice. While the presence of programs such as neighborhood watch have increased even after recent criticisms, they have also come under even closer scrutiny.

These approaches provide evidence for the importance of an integrated approach to prevent and reduce community violence. In addition to the strategies described in this chapter, violence prevention requires the integration of societal values and beliefs as well as the support of faith communities, legislators, business/corporate entities, school systems, and military groups. Nurses are present in many of these communities such as health ministry in churches, school nurses both in school health suites and school-based health centers, college health centers, workplace health programs, and all uniformed services including the military and public health. In each of these communities, nurses can actively provide care and interventions that include assessment and brief counseling for safety planning and referrals to community resources intervention. Nurses can be involved in advocacy for services, policy, funding, and implementation of programs that address all forms of violence such as partner, dating, bullying, and cyber bullying. Nurses can play a role in increasing awareness through implementing educational programs in churches, schools, and higher education, as well as training programs for professionals responding to violence (i.e., law enforcement, schoolteachers, athletic coaches, and other healthcare professionals).

More research is needed that incorporates precise measures of violence and outcomes as well as appropriate proxies for prevention and reduction of violence. Systematic research findings are needed to inform policy-makers and to provide evidence for the most effective community violence intervention and prevention programs. Nurse faculty in research-based settings, as well as hospital- and agency-based nurse researchers, can also design and implement research studies to develop more evidence for the best screening and assessment strategies and interventions for women, families, and perpetrators of violence. Nurses can join other research teams to develop studies and protocols that use interdisciplinary teams to develop evidence-based solutions that address the complex issues related to violent victimization and perpetrations, such as housing stability, job security, chronic physical health problems, mental health problems, and batterer intervention programs for perpetrators of violence. Nurses with specialization in child health and elder health are needed to do more research on the effects of violence on the health and wellbeing of the young and old.

REFERENCES

Adams, R. E., Rohe, W. M., & Arcury, T. A. (2005). Awareness of community-oriented policing and neighborhood perceptions in five small to midsize cities. *Journal of Criminal Justice, 33*(1), 43–54.

Allen, R. (2002). Assessing the impediments to organizational change: A view of community policing. *Journal of Criminal Justice, 30*(6), 511–517.

Bybee, D. I., & Sullivan, C. M. (2002). The process through which a strengths-based intervention resulted in positive change for battered women over time. *American Journal of Community Psychology, 30*(1), 103–132.

Campbell, J., Webster, D., & Glass, N. (2009). The danger assessment: Validation of a lethality risk assessment instrument for intimate partner femicide. *Journal of Interpersonal Violence, 24,* 4653–4674.

Centers for Disease Control and Prevention (CDC). (2014). *Web-based Injury Statistics Query and Reporting System (WISQARS).* Retrieved from http://www.cdc.gov/injury/wisqars/

Chalk, R. (2003). Assessing family violence interventions: Linking programs to research-based strategies. *Journal of Aggression, Maltreatment & Trauma, 4*(1), 29–54.

Chalk, R., & King, P. A. (1998). *Violence in families: Assessing prevention and treatment programs*. Washington, DC: National Academies Press.

City of Stockton. (n.d.). *Neighborhood watch*. Retrieved from http://www.stocktongov.com/government/departments/police/prevNWatch.html

City of Tucson. (n.d.). *Neighborhood watch*. Retrieved from http://www.tucsonaz.gov/police/neighborhood-watch

Duggan, A., Fuddy, L., Burrell, L., Higman, S. M., McFarlane, E., Windham, A., ... Jacobs, F. H. (2004). Randomized trial of a statewide home visiting program to prevent child abuse: Impact in reducing parental risk factors. *Child Abuse & Neglect, 28*(6), 623–643.

Eckenrode, J., Ganzel, B., Henderson Jr, C. R., Smith, E., Olds, D. L., Powers, J., ... Sidora, K. (2000). Preventing child abuse and neglect with a program of nurse home visitation: The limiting effects of domestic violence. *Jama, 284*(11), 1385–1391.

Ellsberg, M., Arango, D. J., Morton, M., Gennari, F., Kiplesund, S., Contreras, M., & Watts, C. (2014). Prevention of violence against women and girls: What does the evidence say? *Lancet, 385*(9977), 1555–1566.

Evans, W. N., & Owens, E. G. (2007). COPS and crime. *Journal of Public Economics, 91*(1–2), 181–201.

Fairfax County. (n.d.). *Neighborhood watch: A community crime prevention program*. Retrieved from http://www.fairfaxcounty.gov/oem/citizencorps/nw.htm

Flood, M. (2011). Involving men in efforts to end violence against women. *Men and Masculinities, 14*, 358–377.

Foshee, V. A., Bauman, K. E., Arriaga, X. B., Helms, R. W., Koch, G. G., & Linder, G. F. (1998). An evaluation of Safe Dates, an adolescent dating violence prevention program. *American Journal of Public Health, 88*, 45–50.

Fulu, E., Kerr-Wilson, A., & Lang, J. (2014). What works to prevent violence against women and girls? Evidence review of interventions to prevent violence against women and girls. *Pretoria: Medical Research Council*.

Hawkins, S. R. (2006). *Evaluation findings: Men can stop rape*. Men of Strength Club. Retrieved from http://www.mencanstoprape.org/images/stories/Images__Logos/Who_We_Are/MOST_Club/Evaluation_Feb-06.pdf

Howard, K. S., & Brooks-Gunn, J. (2009). The role of home visiting programs in preventing child abuse and neglect. *The Future of Children, 19*(2), 119–146.

Jack, S., Ford-Gilboe, M., Walthen, C. N., Davidov, D., McNaughton, D., Coben, J., ... MacMillan, H. (2012). Development of a nurse home visitation intervention for intimate partner violence. *BMC Health Services Research, 12*, 50.

Jewkes, R. (2002). Intimate partner violence: Causes and prevention. *Lancet, 359*, 1423–1429.

Jewkes, R., Flood, M., & Lang, J. (2014). From work with men and boys to changes of social norms and reduction of inequities in gender relations: A conceptual shift in prevention of violence against women and girls. *Lancet, 385*(9977), 1580–1589.

Kitzman, H., Olds, D., Cole, R., Hanks, C., Anson, E., Arcoleo, K., ... Holmberg, J. (2010). Enduring effects of prenatal and infancy home visiting by nurses on children: Age 12 follow-up of a randomized trial. *Archives Pediatric & Adolescent Medicine, 165*(5), 412–418.

Krebs, C. P., Lindquist, C., Warner, T., Fisher, B., & Martin, S. (2007). *The Campus Sexual Assault (CSA) Study: Final report.* Retrieved from http://www.ncjrs.gov/pdffiles1/nij/grants/221153.pdf

Miller, E., Tancredi, D. J., McCauley, H. L., Decker, M. R., Virata, M. C. D., Anderson, H. A., ... Silverman, J. G. (2013). One-year follow-up of a coach-delivered dating violence prevention program: A cluster randomized controlled trial. *American Journal of Preventive Medicine, 45*(1), 108.

Molnar, B. E., Cerda, M., Roberts, A. L., & Buka, S. L. (2008). Effects of neighborhood resources on aggressive and delinquent behaviors among urban youths. *American Journal of Public Health, 98*(6), 1086–1093.

Murphy, M. (2010). An open letter to the organizers, presenters and attendees of the First National Conference for Campus Based Men's Gender Equality and Anti-Violence Groups (St. John's University, Collegeville, MN, November 2009). *Journal of Men's Studies, 18,* 103–108.

National Crime Prevention Council (NCPC). (n.d.). *Strategy: Starting neighborhood watch groups.* Retrieved from http://www.ncpc.org/topics/home-and-neighborhood-safety/strategies/strategy-starting-neighborhood-watch-groups

New York State Police. (n.d.). *A community effort: Neighborhood watch.* Retrieved from http://troopers.ny.gov/crime_prevention/General_Safety/Neighborhood_Watch/

Novak, K. J., Alarid, L. F., & Lucas, W. L. (2003). Exploring officers' acceptance of community policing: Implications for policy implementation. *Journal of Criminal Justice, 31*(1), 57–71.

Olds, D., Donelan, N., O-Brein, R., MacMillan, H., Jack, S., Jenkins, T., ... Beeber, L. (2013). Improving the nurse-family partnership in community practice. *Pediatrics, 132,* S110–S117.

Olds, D. L., Kitzman, H., Hanks, C., Cole, R., Anson, E., Sidora-Arcoleo, K., ... Bondy, J. (2007). Effects of nurse home visiting on maternal and child functioning: Age 9 follow-up of a randomized trial. *Pediatrics, 120*(4), 832–845.

Parents as Teachers (PAT). (2013). *Guidance for identifying and addressing domestic violence with families.* Retrieved from http://www.parentsasteachers.org/images/stories/Guidance_for_DOVE_Screening_11-18-13Rev.pdf

Pease, B. (2008). *Engaging men in men's violence prevention: Exploring the tensions, dilemmas and possibilities.* Sydney, Australia: Australian Domestic & Family Violence Clearinghouse.

Potter, S. J., Moynihan, M. M., Stapleton, J. G., & Banyard, V. L. (2009). Empowering bystanders to prevent campus violence against women. *Violence Against Women, 15,* 106–121.

Pronyk, P. M., Kim, J. C., Morison, L. A., Godfrey, P., Busza, J., Porter, J. D. H., ... Hargreaves, J. (2006). Effect of a structural intervention for the prevention of intimate-partner violence and HIV in rural South Africa: A cluster randomised trial. *Lancet, 368,* 1973–1983.

Rasenberger, J. (2006, October). Nightmare on Austin Street. *American Heritage Magazine, 57*(5).

Robinson, C., & Schwartz, J. (2012, March). Shooting focuses attention on a program that seeks to avoid guns. *The New York Times.* Retrieved from http://www.nytimes.com/2012/03/23/us/trayvon-martin-death-spotlights-neighborhood-watch-groups.html?_r=0

Schultz, P., & Tabanico, J. (2012). *A social norms approach to community-based crime prevention: Implicit and explicit messages on neighborhood watch signs.* San Marcos, CA: National Institute of Justice.

Sharps, P. (2012, March). Domestic violence enhanced home visitation: Evidenced based findings for home visiting protocols. In the 6th Biennial National Conference on Health and Domestic Violence (March 29–31, 2012). nchdv.

Sharps, P., Alhusen, J. L., Bullock, L., Bhandari, S., Ghazarian, S., Udo, I. E., & Campbell, J. (2013). Engaging and retaining abused women in perinatal home visitation programs. *Pediatrics, 132*(Supplement 2), S134–S139.

Sharps, P. W., Campbell, J., Baty, M. L., Walker, K. S., & Bair-Merritt, M. H. (2008). Current evidence on perinatal home visiting and intimate partner violence. *Journal of Obstetric, Gynecologic, and Neonatal Nursing, 37*(4), 480–490.

Stephens, K. A., & George, W. H. (2009). Rape prevention with college men: Evaluating risk status. *Journal of Interpersonal Violence, 24,* 996–1013.

Straus, M. A., Hamby, S. L., Finkelhor, D., Moore, D. W., & Runyan, D. (1998). Identification of child maltreatment with the Parent-Child Conflict Tactics Scales: Development and psychometric data for a national sample of American parents. *Child Abuse and Neglect, 22,* 249–270.

Trojanowicz, R., & Bucqueroux, B. (1990). *Community policing: A contemporary perspective.* Cincinnati, OH: Anderson Publishing.

U.S. Bureau of Justice Assistance. (1994). *Understanding community policing: A framework for action.* Washington, DC: USDOJ.

U.S. Department of Education. (2014). *Questions and answers on Title IX and sexual violence.* Retrieved from http://www2.ed.gov/about/offices/list/ocr/docs/qa-201404-title-ix.pdf

U.S. Department of Justice. (2014). *Office of Community Oriented Policing Services* [2014 Report]. Washington, DC: Author.

Wilson, M. (2012, June 22). Far from a shooting in Florida, an increase in block watchers. *The New York Times.* Retrieved from http://www.nytimes.com/2012/06/23/nyregion/neighborhood-watches-in-new-york-far-from-trayvon-martin-case.html?_r=0

Wolfe, D. A., Crooks, C., Jaffe, P., Chiodo, D., Hughes, R., Stitt, L., … Ellis, W. (2009). A school-based program to prevent adolescent dating violence: A cluster randomized trial. *Archives of Pediatric Adolescent Medicine, 163,* 692–699.

Zhao, J., Lovrich, N. P., & Robinson, T. (2001). Community policing: Is it changing the basic functions of policing?: Findings from a longitudinal study of 200+ municipal police agencies. *Journal of Criminal Justice, 29,* 365–377.

INDEX

C

J – K

jails, 115
Joint Commission for Accreditation of
    Healthcare Organization, 235
Joint Commission Standard, 12, 15
judges, 115
juvenile courts, 115–116
Juvenile Justice and Delinquency Prevention
    Act, 116

L

Labeling Theory, 111
larceny, 133
laws
    death investigations, 248–252
    elder abuse, 219–220
    healthcare of ex-offenders, 276–277
    sexual violence, 178–179
    and statutes for intimate partner violence
        (IPV), 157–158
legal nurse consultants, 11
limbic system, 41–43
Listen, Inquire, Validate, Enhance Safety,
    and Support (LIVES), 154–155
liver mortis (lividity), 255
Locard, Edmond, 22, 23, 287, 288
loose-contact wounds, 98

M

malingering patients, 228–229
management strategies for elder abuse,
    218–221
manner of death, 246
manslaughter, 129
Martin, Trayvon, 335
mass incarceration, 119–120. *See also*
    criminal justice system

material exploitation, elder abuse, 213
McCormack, Mary Ellen, 200
McNaughton rules, 237
Medicaid, 276
medical examiner systems, 245–246
medical histories, 230
medications, psychotropic, 48
medicolegal death investigators (MDIs), 247
memory, 42
men. *See also* women
    male privilege, 90
    male role models, 337
    male specific verification analysis
        techniques, 27
Men Care program, 338
Mendelsohn, Benjamin (types of victims),
    84–85
*Men's Action for Stopping Violence Against
    Women,* 338
mental health
    antisocial personality disorder (APD),
        228
    assessments, 230–231
    case studies, 238–239
    competency/insanity, 236–238
    documentation, 231–232
    forensic mental health nursing, 225–241
    forensic psychiatric issues, 230–238
    malingering patients, 228–229
    responses to violence, 62–65
    safety, 232–235
Mentors in Violence Prevention program,
    338
meteorology, 21
Minnesota Sex Offender Program (MSOP),
    175
mitochondrial DNA (mtDNA), 27–28
mixed death investigation systems, 246
models
    brains, 42
    of care (child maltreatment), 202–204
mortality data, 248
Mullis, Kary, 26

R

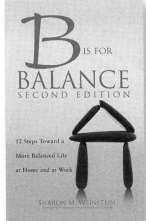
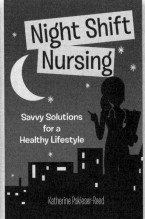
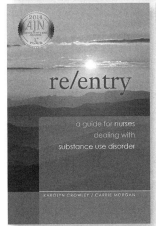
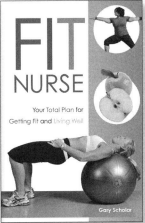

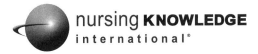

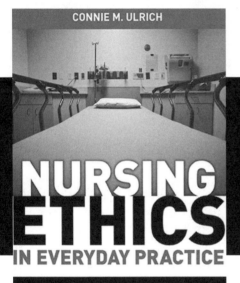
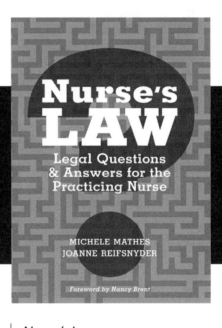

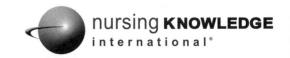